GENE EXPRESSION AND REGULATION IN MAMMALIAN CELLS - TRANSCRIPTION FROM GENERAL ASPECTS

Edited by **Fumiaki Uchiumi**

Gene Expression and Regulation in Mammalian Cells - Transcription From General Aspects
http://dx.doi.org/10.5772/intechopen.70352
Edited by Fumiaki Uchiumi

Contributors

Kevin Gaston, Sheela Jayaraman, Sarah George, Kerry Wadey, Guang-Jer Wu, Youming Zhang, Kumiko Ui-Tei, Tomoko Takahashi, Yuko Nakano, Fumiaki Uchiumi, Masami Nagahama, Toshimichi Yamada, Nobuyoshi Akimitsu, Mari Sogayar, Marina Trombetta-Lima, Carlos DeOcesano-Pereira, Fernando Velloso, Ana Carreira, Carolina Ribeiro, Sheila Winnischofer, Toshinori Nakayama, Atsushi Onodera, Kota Kokubo, Tao Lu, Han Wei, Lakshmi Prabhu, Antja-Voy Hartley, Matthew Martin, Emily Sun, Guanglong Jiang, Yunlong Liu, Irina Vlasova-St. Louis, Calandra Sagarsky, A K M Azad, Alfons Lawen, Jonathan M. Keith, Shen Hu, Li Cui, Xinyuan Zhao, Partha Mitra, Ciriaco Piccirillo, Tomoyuki Honda, Kozue Sofuku

Published by InTech
Janeza Trdine 9, 51000 Rijeka, Croatia

Publishing Process Manager Romina Skomersic
Technical Editor SPi Global
Cover InTech Design team

First published February, 2018
Printed in Croatia
Legal deposit, Croatia: National and University Library in Zagreb

Additional hard copies can be obtained from orders@intechopen.com

Gene Expression and Regulation in Mammalian Cells - Transcription From General Aspects, Edited by Fumiaki Uchiumi
p. cm.
Print ISBN 978-953-51-3855-6
Online ISBN 978-953-51-3856-3

For EU product safety concerns:
IN TECH d.o.o., Prolaz Marije Krucifikse Kozulić 3, 51000 Rijeka, Croatia,
info@intechopen.com or visit our website at intechopen.com.

Meet the editor

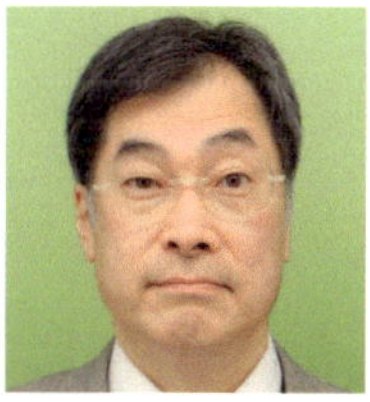

Fumiaki Uchiumi, professor of Pharmaceutical Sciences, Tokyo University of Science, received his bachelor's degree (Chemistry) from Tokyo University of Science in 1987. In 1993, after obtaining his PhD degree (Molecular Biology) from Tokyo University, he joined Professor S. Tanuma's Laboratory at Tokyo University of Science as an assistant professor. He obtained his second PhD degree (Pharmaceutical Science) from Tokyo University of Science in 1999, and in 2000, he was promoted to the position of lecturer at Tokyo University of Science. Professor Uchiumi then went abroad as a postdoctoral researcher for the United States-Japan Cooperative Cancer Research Program in Professor E. Fanning's Laboratory at Vanderbilt University, 2000–2001. Professor Uchiumi was promoted to associate professor and then full professor at Tokyo University of Science in 2010 and 2016, respectively.

Contents

Preface

We have learned that transcription is the most fundamental biological event both in prokaryotic and eukaryotic cells. It plays an essential role in converting information of genomic DNAs into various functions of proteins. Depending on various circumstances, such that in the course of development of mammalian cells, it should be precisely controlled to produce required amounts of ribonucleic acids or RNAs. Recent studies revealed that dysregulation of transcription or gene expression frequently occurs in specific human diseases, including cancer. Therefore, understanding the mechanism of transcription and gene expression in eukaryotic cells from the aspect of basic biochemistry and molecular biology should give us key insights into the development of novel therapies for transcription-dysregulated diseases.

In Section 1, the most primary and essential concept of transcription from recent findings is discussed. In Chapter 1, recent integrative understanding in the mammalian transcription system is reviewed. Chapters 2 and 3 show recent studies in cellular and viral *cis*- and *trans*-elements, respectively, in detail. And we should remember that mathematical analysis of the transcription networking is important, and it is reviewed in Chapter 4.

In Section 2, molecular mechanisms of RNA degradation and functions of ncRNAs are reviewed. We will find Chapter 5 important advising us to pay attention not only to synthesis but also to degradation of RNA molecules. Chapters 6 and 7 make us to realize that ncRNAs are not merely junk but key regulators for cell behaviour. We could expect novel therapies with nucleotide-derivative drugs in the near future.

In Section 3, transcriptional control in differentiation of cells that function in the immune system is reviewed. In Chapter 8, regarding the development of B cells, transcriptional control on class switch recombination is reviewed with recent findings. Regulation of T-cell development and differentiation by epigenetic control system are thoroughly explained in Chapters 9 and 10.

In Section 4, focusing on the molecular mechanisms that control cell behaviour, including proliferation and migration, the relationships between transcription and cancer generation are discussed. Chapter 11 describes that phosphorylation of homeobox protein regulates proliferation and migration of cells. Cell adhesion will send signals to control transcription, and the details are discussed in Chapter 12. The functions of well-known NF-kB and SOX proteins in the regulation of cancer generation are thoroughly commented with recent findings in Chapters 13 and 14, respectively.

The "central dogma" can be metaphorically said here as a kind of ancient war. Then, this book volume (1) could be a voyage. Visiting various islands (subjects and topics), we meet a lot of scientists who are the experts studying mechanisms of transcription and gene expression in mammalian cells. The authors show us current progresses in the field of basic biological studies by excellent articles. But how could we reach the goal? Is it safe? Is goddess still patiently waiting for us to arrive? We would be just anticipating that these questions are answered in Volume 2.

Fumiaki Uchiumi, PhD
Professor, Department of Gene Regulation
Tokyo University of Science
Japan

Section 1

Introduction

Chapter 1

Introductory Chapter: Current Studies in Transcriptional Control System; Toward the Establishment of Therapies against Human Diseases

Fumiaki Uchiumi

Additional information is available at the end of the chapter

http://dx.doi.org/10.5772/intechopen.71701

1. Introduction: the RNA world

We have already learned how the genetic codes or biological information are transcribed into mRNAs, and then how they are translated into amino acid sequences of various polypeptides. This is widely known as "Central Dogma", the most fundamental and important concept in molecular biology. In the translation process, polypeptides are synthesized by ribosomes with a template mRNA. Thus, in this context, we tend to take it for granted that the main function of RNAs is just transporting genomic information from nuclei to cytoplasm. However, if we regard a ribosome as a polypeptide-synthesizing protein-RNA complex, which contains all major RNAs, mRNA, rRNA, and tRNA, we will realize that the RNAs have biologically important roles as enzymatic machinery to synthesize proteins. RNAs are not only required for the translation system, but also for splicing/processing of RNAs and telomere elongation, contained in the protein-RNA complexes, snRNPs, and *TERC* subunit of the telomerase, respectively. Moreover, recent studies revealed that non-coding RNAs (ncRNAs, siRNAs, or miRNAs) regulate transcription and translation.

Because, as described, RNAs have both information and function, it is suggested that they might have been the most fundamental and primary molecules from the beginning of chemical evolution before living organisms emerged on earth. Even in the DNA replication process, RNAs are required as primers for the leading strand synthesis. Recent study in initiation site sequencing (ini-seq) revealed that the human DNA replication origins very frequently overlap with transcription start sites (TSSs) and G-quadruplex (G4) motifs [1]. In other words, a number of biologically essential events or reactions are dependent on the synthesis of the RNA molecules. Thus, it has been proposed that an origin of life has come from an "RNA

World" [2], which might have given a chance to develop the most biologically essential reactions for life, including replication, transcription, and translation.

Based on the concept that RNAs are the most essential molecules for living things, in this book project, it is worth to focus on topics discussing on how transcription is regulated and how it becomes if it is dysregulated.

2. Transcriptional controlling system in eukaryotic cells

It is already known that three types of RNA polymerases participate in the synthesis of different types of RNAs. The RNA polymerase (RNA pol) I and III catalyzes production of rRNAs, tRNAs, and snRNAs. Although they are essentially important enzymes to generate functional RNAs, much of the interest have been directed to RNA pol II, which catalyzes both protein-encoding and non-coding gene transcription. Up to present, molecular mechanisms of how each protein-encoding gene is expressed have been well studied. Most of the textbooks in molecular biology describe in detail how general transcription factors, including TBP, TFIIB, TFIID, TFIIE, TFIIF, and TFIIH, co-operatively work to recruit RNA pol II appropriately onto the TSSs [3]. Recently, structure of the eukaryotic RNA pol II complex, containing elongation factors, Spt4/5, Elf1, and TFIIS, has been revealed [4]. The entire transcription reaction system from initiation to termination on DNA template will be elucidated in the near future.

In eukaryotic cells, epigenetic regulation or chromatin modification affect gene expression. After unwinding the chromosomes, each gene will be correctly transcribed from TSS in the core promoter region. The promoter activity is regulated by enhancer or proximal promoter regions, where various transcription factors (TFs) access to bind. These TFs usually recognize specific DNA sequences or *cis*-elements, and the enhancement of transcriptional activity is dependent on the combinations of TFs, their binding sites, or distances from TSS. Thanks to the completion of human genome project, and with a development of Next Generation Sequencing (NGS) and especially Chromatin Immune Precipitation sequencing (ChIP-seq) technique [5], we can now refer TF-binding sequences and TSSs of most of the genes by a number of online programs, including NCBI, JASPAR, and DBTSS databases [6–8]. Promoters and enhancers, which might be digital landmarks on genomes for TFs, can determine transcription-initiation frequency. After transcription is completed, RNAs should be appropriately processed and modified. These processes are regulated by RNA binding helicases and ncRNAs [9]. It should not be ignored that RNAs are degraded in RNA exome complexes [10]. The degradation is required for the quality control of RNAs and gene expression. Then, mRNAs are incorporated in mRNPs that are to be exported from nuclei to cytoplasm with a help of export-component proteins, including TREX [11]. Thus, matured mRNA molecules are made through a complicated multistep process, though it would be advantageous for cells to fine tune gene expression system overall. If unpredictable and undesired expression of some specific genes happened, it may lead to dysfunctions in mitochondria, immune response, and DNA-repair/epigenetic controlling systems. If it were deleterious for organisms, it may cause diseases, including cancer.

3. Non-coding RNAs (ncRNAs)

Not all of the information on the genomes encodes protein. It is estimated that most (about 95%) of the genomes consist of non-coding regions. Recent transcriptome analyses, including Cap-Analysis Gene Expression (CAGE), revealed that large amount of ncRNAs are contained in total transcripts [12]. Because ncRNAs do not encode proteins, they have long been thought as "junks" in the genome. However, recent studies discovered that some of them are not junks, rather "jewels" in nuclei having essential roles in controlling cell growth, development, and function. The ncRNAs are classified into two groups as short ncRNAs (miRNAs, piwiRNAs, and snRNAs) and long ncRNAs (lncRNAs), consisting of over 200 ribonucleotides in the molecule. The more analytical methods in sequencing RNA molecules developed, the more lncRNAs were identified with increasing in number, which are estimated over 35,000 at present. The lncRNAs are transcribed by RNA pol II, and their TSSs are frequently (65%) found at bidirectional promoter regions [13]. In mouse embryonic cells, transcribed lncRNAs recruit TFs and splicing factors to activate neighboring or bi-directional partner gene expression [14]. Therefore, lncRNAs may give accurate platforms or TSSs for bi-directional partner genes. Recent study with genome editing system identified lncRNA loci regulate genes neighborhood [15]. In addition, it was revealed that specific lncRNAs are contained in nuclear bodies, including nuclear speckle (*MALAT1*), paraspeckle (*NEAT1*), and polycomb body (*TUG1*) [16], suggesting that lncRNAs affect chromosomal integrity. More importantly, the lncRNAs have certain effects on epigenetic gene regulation systems [17]. The famous example is that X inactive specific transcript (*Xist*) silences X chromosome genes, interacting with transcriptional suppressor proteins [18]. Not only *Xist*, but also other lncRNAs, such as *HOTAIR*, *LUNAR1*, and *MALAT1* are required as scaffolds for DNA methylation/demethylation factors, chromosome looping factors, and splicing factors, respectively [17]. Additionally, enhancer RNA (eRNA), which is transcribed at active enhancer, can function as a scaffold for histone acethyltransferase CBP to modulate gene expression [19].

4. Epigenetic control of gene expression

Gene expression pattern could be altered by epigenetic regulation [20]. The epigenetic control, which mainly regulates expression of sets of genes, is driven by DNA methylation, histone modifications, chromatin remodeling, and ncRNAs [20, 21]. A lot of factors that are involved in the epigenetic controlling system have been identified and characterized. Methyl groups could be transferred to both DNAs and histone proteins by enzymatic reactions. DNA methylation plays pivotal roles in the regulation of nuclear events, including gene expression [22]. Especially, when silencing of DNA repair genes occurred, it may boost mutation rate, and it will be resulted in the genome instability. Therefore, DNA methylation is regarded as one of the essential biomarkers in cancer [23]. The reaction is catalyzed by at least three independent DNA methyltransferases (DNMTs): DNMT1, DNMT3A, and DNMT3B [24], using S-adenosyl-L-methyonine (AdoMet) as a methyl group donor [25]. The ten-eleven translocation (TET) family proteins, including TET1, TET2, and TET3, are the 5-methylcytosine hydroxylases that remove methyl group from an oxidized form of the cytosine (5mC), 5-hydroxymethylcytosine (5hmC), and other forms [20, 22]. Recent study revealed that intragenic DNA methylation assists fidelity in genome transcription initiation [26]. NRF protein preferentially accesses to unmethylated genomic regions, indicating that DNA methylation status restricts binding of methylation sensitive TFs onto their recognition sequences [27]. A methylation sensitive SELEX analysis indicated that transcription factor ETS protein binding was inhibited by mCpG, but homeobox proteins, such as POU and NFAT, preferentially bind to the methylation introduced site [28]. The results suggest that DNA recognition mechanism of several TFs that mainly act in the development of organisms is dependent on the methylation of DNA.

Histone proteins could be modified by attachment of various molecules, including methyl-, acetyl-, hydroxyl-, SUMOyl-, and poly ADP(ribosyl)-groups [20, 29]. In addition, they are acylated on the Lys residues to regulate transcription of genes that encode metabolic-response factors [30]. These modifications are recognized by different proteins, such as bromodomain-containing proteins [31], double PHD finger domain proteins [30, 32], YEATS domain proteins [30], WD40 proteins [33], and Ankyrin-repeat proteins [34].

As described above, epigenetic regulation is tightly linked with genome stability, and it is affected by modifying group molecules or metabolites, including acetyl-CoA, AdoMet, and NAD^+ [35]. These observations suggest that aging is not only determined by genetic information, but also by environmental stresses, including nutrient conditions [36]. Interestingly, recent study indicated that lactate dehydrogenase LDHA promotes IFN-γ expression through an epigenetic mechanism [37]. The results suggest that LDHA-mediated aerobic glycolysis could enforce mitochondria to generate more acetyl-CoA that is to be utilized for histone modification. Poly(ADP-ribosyl)ation is a protein modification reaction that is catalyzed by PARP enzymes using NAD^+ as a substrate. The poly(ADP-ribosyl)ation occurs on histones, non-histone proteins, DNA-repair factors [38], and TFs to regulate gene expression [39, 40]. In summary, nutrients or food intake may have some roles in regulating transcription because they can induce epigenetic changes [41].

5. Transcription disorders and human diseases

The great progresses in the whole genome sequencing (WGS) techniques enabled us to study subtle differences in genomic sequences between cancer and normal cells [42]. Somatic mutations on driver genes in various cancers have been identified [43] and the statistical data will be applied on diagnosis or even on the prediction of cancer risks and incidences [44]. Very recently, it was proposed that analysis of WGS data from circulating tumor cells could be applied for personalized therapy for malignant cancer [45]. Importantly, mutations in 5′-upstream region of the human *TERT* gene are frequently identified in melanoma [46, 47]. It should be noted that in certain cancers, especially in melanomas, the rate of somatic mutations is highly increased at active TF-binding sites, where they interfere accession of nucleotide excision repair (NER) machinery [48, 49]. Thus, cancer-related mutations are not only present in the protein-coding regions, but also in the gene expression regulatory regions, including promoters and enhancers in the genomes.

Various diseases may be caused by dysregulations in transcription. For example, Yes-associated protein (YAP) and TAZ proteins, which activate inflammatory gene expression, are involved in the atherosclerosis [50]. In several neurological and neuromuscular disorders, including Huntington disease, muscular dystrophy, and amyotrophic lateral sclerosis (ALS), accumulation of repeat containing RNAs in aberrant foci in nucleus have been observed [51]. Moreover, shRNA screening system *in vitro* showed that transcription elongation factors, including JMJD6, help cells to survive in the microenvironment of glioblastoma [52]. The result suggests that the transcription elongation machinery could be an effective therapeutic target. It was recently reported that ENL protein, which possesses acetyl lysine recognizing YEATS domain [30], acts as an activator of leukemia-diving factor encoding gene expression [53, 54]. Therefore, targeting the ENL protein could be an effective therapeutic strategy against aggressive leukemia. Currently, candidate drugs that target HDAC [55–57] and DNMTs [56, 57] are under clinical tests and expected to contribute to the development of novel cancer therapeutics. Epigenetic alterations on genomic DNAs is not only associated with cancer generation, but also with neurologic diseases [58], autoinflammatory diseases [59], and metabolic diseases, including type II diabetes [60]. Toward establishment of new therapies for these diseases, epigenetic modulators will be the right targets for effective treatment with lowered side effects [61]. We should remember drug resistance of cancer could be caused by compounds that induce epigenetic reprogramming, and thereby alter transcriptional state, which is regulated by SOX proteins, Jun/AP1, and GGAA-recognizing factors [62]. Therefore, secondly effects of drugs on transcription system should be examined. In summary, next generation therapeutics may have to put gene expression systems under control.

6. Future prospects

Overall, most of the cellular responses to signals and stresses from the environment, including DNA damage, nutrient condition, viral infections, and some specific drugs, could affect transcription or gene expression profile. Presently, it has been shown that introduction of several TFs (OKSM factors or Yamanaka factors) into somatic cells can reprogram and convert them with pluripotency [63, 64]. Very recently, it was experimentally shown that iPS cell-derived dopaminergic neurons could be applied for the treatment of Parkinson's disease [65]. These experimentally supported evidences suggest that introduction of certain combination of TFs into cancer cells might enforce them to reprogram transcription profile so that they could stop proliferation but acquire DNA repair with more accuracy.

Clinical application of gene therapy [66] with appropriate set of expression vectors to induce DNA repair or mitochondrial function associated genes will soon be established. Not only vectors, which deliver TF-encoding genes into cell nuclei, but also nucleic acids, including siRNAs, lncRNAs, or RNA aptamers, should be also improved for the strategy. In addition, genome editing on the promoter or enhancer regions of some target genes of patient derived cells will be an effective approach to treat specific diseases. For example, it was recently reported that genome editing to delete α-globin enhancer reduces its excessed expression in primary human hematopoietic stem cells, strongly suggesting the clinical use of the technique could be applied as a potential therapy for β-thalassemia [67]. Therefore, genome editing on transcription regulatory elements will be an alternative novel gene therapy for leukemia and cancer, in accordance with a progress in gene delivery system. In the near future, the continuing studies in the transcription controlling systems will successfully contribute to establish novel therapeutics for various human intractable diseases, including cancer, immunological diseases, and neuro-degenerating diseases.

Author details

Fumiaki Uchiumi

Address all correspondence to: uchiumi@rs.noda.tus.ac.jp

Department of Gene Regulation, Faculty of Pharmaceutical Sciences, Tokyo University of Science, Noda, Chiba-ken, Japan

References

[1] Langley AR, Gräf S, Smith JC, Krude T. Genome-wide identification and characterization of human DNA replication origins by initiation site sequencing (ini-seq). Nucleic Acids Research. 2016;**44**(21):10230-10247

[2] Cech TR. The RNA world in context. In: Atkins JF, Gesteland RF, Cech TR, editors. RNA Worlds: From Life's Origins to Diversity in Gene Regulation. Cold Spring Harbor, NY: Cold Spring Harbor Laboratory Press; 2011. pp. 1-5

[3] Carey MF, Peterson CL, Smale ST. A primer on transcriptional regulation in mammalian cells. In: Carey MF, Peterson CL, Smale ST, editors. Transcriptional Regulation in Eukaryotes: Concepts, Strategies, and Techniques. 2nd ed. Cold Spring Harbor, NY: Cold Spring Harbor Laboratory Press; 2009. pp. 1-45

[4] Ehara H, Yokoyama T, Shigematsu H, Yokoyama S, Shirouzu M, Sekine S. Structure of the complete elongation complex of RNA polymerase II with basal factors. Science. 2017;**357**(6354):921-924

[5] Mundade R, Ozer HG, Wei H, Prabhu L, Lu T. Role of ChIP-seq in the discovery of transcription factor binding sites, differential gene regulation mechanism, epigenetic marks and beyond. Cell Cycle. 2014;**13**(18):2847-2852

[6] NCBI. Gene [Internet]. Available from: https://www.ncbi.nlm.nih.gov/gene/

[7] The JASPAR database [Internet]. Available from: http://jaspar.genereg.net/

[8] DBTSS [Internet]. Available from: http://dbtss.hgc.jp/

[9] Bourgeois CF, Mortreux F, Auboeuf D. The multiple functions of RNA helicases as drivers and regulators of gene expression. Nature Reviews. Molecular Cell Biology. 2016;**17**(7):426-438

[10] Wickramasinghe VO, Laskey RA. Control of mammalian gene expression be selective mRNA export. Nature Reviews. Molecular Cell Biology. 2015;**16**(7):431-442

[11] Kilchert C, Wittmann S, Vasiljeva L. The regulation and functions of the nuclear RNA exosome complex. Nature Reviews. Molecular Cell Biology. 2016;**17**(4):227-239

[12] Schein A, Carninci P. Complexity of mammalian transcriptone analyzed by RNA deep sequencing. In: Kurokawa R, editor. Long Noncoding RNAs. Tokyo, Japan: Springer Japan KK; 2015. pp. 3-22

[13] Kurokawa R. Initiation of transcription generates divergence of long noncoding RNAs. In: Kurokawa R, editor. Long Noncoding RNAs. Tokyo, Japan: Springer Japan KK; 2015. pp. 69-91

[14] Engreitz JM, Haines JE, Perez EM, Munson G, Chen J, Kane M, McDonel PE, Guttman M, Lander ES. Local regulation of gene expression by lncRNA promoters, transcription and splicing. Nature. 2016;**539**(7629):452-455

[15] Joung J, Engreitz JM, Konermann S, Abudayyeh O, Verdine VK, Aguet F, Gootenberg JS, Sanjana NE, Wright JB, Fulco CP, Tseng YY, Yoon CH, Boehm JS, Lander ES, Zhang F. Genome-scale activation screen identifies a lncRNA locus regulating a gene neighbourhood. Nature. 2017;**548**(7667):343-351

[16] Mannen T, Chujo T, Hirose T. Long noncoding RNAs as structural and functional components of nuclear bodies. In: Kurokawa R, editor. Long Noncoding RNAs. Tokyo, Japan: Springer Japan KK; 2015. pp. 111-129

[17] Kondo Y, Shinjo K, Katsushima K. Long non-coding RNAs as an epigenetic regulator in human cancers. Cancer Science. DOI: 10.1111/cas.13342

[18] Engreitz JM, Ollikainen N, Guttman M. Long non-coding RNAs: Spatial amplifiers that control nuclear structure and gene expression. Nature Reviews. Molecular Cell Biology. 2016;**17**(12):756-770

[19] Bose DA, Donahue G, Reinberg D, Shiekhattar R, Bonasio R, Berger SL. RNA binding to CBP stimulates histone acetylation and transcription. Cell. 2017;**168**(1-2):135-149

[20] Ann Blakey CA, Litt MD. Epigenetic gene expression—An introduction. In: Huang S, Litt MD, Ann Blakey C, editors. Epigenetic Gene Expression and Regulation. London, UK: Academic Press; 2016. pp. 1-19

[21] Ann Blakey CA, Litt MD. Histone modifications—Models and mechanisms. In: Huang S, Litt MD, Ann Blakey C, editors. Epigenetic Gene Expression and Regulation. London, UK: Academic Press; 2016. pp. 21-42

[22] Neidhart M. DNA methylation—Introduction. In: Neidhart M, editor. DNA Methylation and Complex Human Disease. London, UK: Academic Press; 2016. pp. 1-8

[23] Neidhart M. DNA methylation and epigenetic biomarkers in cancer. In: Neidhart M, editor. DNA Methylation and Complex Human Disease. London, UK: Academic Press; 2016. pp. 9-27

[24] Jeltsh A. Molecular enzymology of mammalian DNA methyltransferases. Current Topics in Microbiology and Immunology. 2006;**301**:203-225

[25] Pradhan S, Esteve PO. Mammalian DNA (cytosine-5) methyltransferases and their expression. Clinical Immunology. 2003;**109**(1):6-16

[26] Neri F, Rapelli S, Krepelova A, Incarnato D, Parlato C, Basile G, Maldotti M, Anselmi F, Oliviero S. Intragenic DNA methylation prevents spurious transcription initiation. Nature. 2017;**543**(7643):72-77

[27] Domcke S, Bardet AF, Ginno PA, Hartl D, Burger L, Schübeler D. Competition between DNA methylation and transcription factors determines binding of NRF1. Nature. 2015;**528**(7583):575-579

[28] Yin Y, Morgunova E, Jolma A, Kaasinen E, Sahu B, Khund-Sayeed S, et al. Impact of cytosine methylation on DNA binding specificities of human transcription factors. Science. 2017;**356**(6337):aaj2239

[29] Choudhary C, Weinert BT, Nishida Y, Verdin E, Mann M. The growing landscape of lysin acetylation links metabolism and cell signaling. Nature Reviews. Molecular Cell Biology. 2014;**15**(8):536-550

[30] Sabari BR, Zhang D, David Allis C, Zhao Y. Metabolic regulation of gene expression through histone acylations. Nature Reviews. Molecular Cell Biology. 2017;**18**(2):90-101

[31] Smith SG, Zhou MM. The bromodomain as the acetyl-lysine binding domain in gene transcription. In: Zhou MM, editor. Histone Recognition. Switzerland: Springer International Publishing AG; 2016. pp. 1-26

[32] Gatchalian J, Kutateladze TG. PHD Fingers as histone readers. In: Zhou MM, editor. Histone Recognition. Switzerland: Springer International Publishing AG; 2016. pp. 27-47

[33] Wilson JR, Justin N. Histone recognition by WD40 proteins. In: Zhou MM, editor. Histone Recognition. Switzerland: Springer International Publishing AG; 2016. pp. 83-100

[34] Collins RE, Chang X. Histone recognition by WD40 proteinMethyl-lysine recognition by Ankyrin-repeat proteins. In: Zhou MM, editor. Histone Recognition. Switzerland: Springer International Publishing AG; 2016. pp. 101-124

[35] Gut P, Verdin E. The nexus of chromatin regulation and intermediary metabolism. Nature. 2013;**502**(7472):489-498

[36] Benayoun BA, Pollina EA, Brunet A. Epigenetic regulation of aging: Linking environmental inputs to genome stability. Nature Reviews. Molecular Cell Biology. 2015;**16**(10):593-610

[37] Peng M, Yin N, Chhangawala S, Xu K, Leslie CS, Li MO. Aerobic glycolysis promotes T helper 1 cell differentiation through an epigenetic mechanism. Science. 2016;**354**(6311): 481-484

[38] Tanuma S, Sato A, Oyama T, Yoshimori A, Abe H, Uchiumi F. New insights into the roles of NAD+-poly(ADP-ribose) metabolism and poly(ADP-ribose) glycohydrolase. Current Protein & Peptide Science. 2016;**17**(7):668-682

[39] Verdone L, La Fortezza M, Ciccarone F, Caiafa P, Zampieri M, Caserta M. Poly(ADP-ribosyl)ation affects histone acetylation and transcription. PLoS One. 2015;**10**(12):e0144287

[40] Martin KA, Cesaroni M, Denny MF, Lupey LN, Tempera I. Global transcriptome analysis reveals that poly(ADP-ribose) polymerase 1 regulates gene expression through EZH2. Molecular and Cellular Biology. 2015;**35**(23):3934-3944

[41] Brant JO, Yang TP. Epigenetic effects of environment and diet. In: Huang S, Litt MD, Ann Blakey C, editors. Epigenetic Gene Expression and Regulation. London, UK: Academic Press; 2016. pp. 339-365

[42] Chang F, Liu GL, Liu CJ, Li MM. Somatic diseases (cancer): Ampligication-based next-generation sequencing. In: Kulkarni S, Pfeifer J, editors. Clinical Genomics: A Guide to Clinical Next Generation Sequencing. London, UK: Academic Press; 2015. pp. 297-319

[43] Ku CS, Cooper DN, Ziogas DE, Halkia E, Tzaphlidou M, Roukos DH. Research and clinical applications of cancer genome sequencing. Current Opinion in Obstetrics & Gynecology. 2013;**25**(1):3-10

[44] Vogelstein B, Papadopoulos N, Velculescu VE, Zhou S, Diaz LA Jr, Kinzler KW. Cancer genome landscapes. Science. 2013;**339**(6127):1546-1558

[45] Gulbahce N, Magbanua MJM, Chin R, Agarwal MR, Luo X, Liu J, Hayden DM, Mao Q, Ciotlos S, Li Z, Chen Y, Chen X, Li Y, Zhang RY, Lee K, Tearle R, Park E, Drmanac S, Rugo HS, Park JW, Drmanac R, Peters BA. Quantitative whole genome sequencing of circulating tumor cells enables personalized combination therapy of metastatic cancer. Cancer Research. 2017;**77**(16):4530-4541

[46] Huang FW, Hodis E, Xu MJ, Kryukov GV, Chin L, Garraway LA. Highly recurrent TERT promoter mutations in human melanoma. Science. 2013;**339**(6122):957-959

[47] Horn S, Figl A, Sivaramakrishna Rachakonda P, Fischer C, Sucker A, Gast A, Kadel S, Moll I, Narore E, Hemminki K, Schadendorf D, Kumar R. TERT promoter mutations in familial and sporadic melanoma. Science. 2013;**339**(6122):959-961

[48] Perera D, Poulos RC, Shah A, Beck D, Pimanda JE, Wong JW. Differential DNA repair underlies mutation hotspots at active promoters in cancer genomes. Nature. 2016;**532**(7598):259-263

[49] Sabarinathan R, Mularoni L, Deu-Pons J, Gonzalez-Perez A, López-Bigas N. Nucleotide excision repair is impaired by binding of transcription factors to DNA. Nature. 2016;**532**(7598):264-267

[50] Wang L, Luo JY, Li B, Tian XY, Chen LJ, Huang Y, Liu J, Deng D, Lau CW, Wan S, Ai D, Mak KK, Tong KK, Kwan KM, Wang N, Chiu JJ, Zhu Y, Huang Y. Integrin-YAP/TAZ-JNK cascade mediates atheroprotective effect of shear flow. Nature. 2016;**540**(7634):579-582

[51] Jain A, Vale RD. RNA phase transitions in repeat expansion disorders. Nature. 2017;**546**(7657):243-247

[52] Miller TE, Liau BB, Wallace LC, Morton AR, Xie Q, Dixit D, Factor DC, Kim LJY, Morrow JJ, Wu Q, Mack SC, Hubert CG, Gillespie SM, Flavahan WA, Hoffmann T, Thummalapalli R, Hemann MT, Paddison PJ, Horbinski CM, Zuber J, Scacheri PC, Bernstein BE, Tesar P, Rich JN. Transcription elongation factors represent *in vivo* cancer dependencies in glioblastoma. Nature. 2017;**547**(7663):355-359

[53] Wan L, Wen H, Li Y, Lyu J, Xi Y, Hoshii T, Joseph JK, Wang X, Loh YE, Erb MA, Souza AL, Bradner JE, Shen L, Li W, Li H, Allis CD, Armstrong SA, Shi X. ENL links histone acetylation to oncogenic expression in acute myeloid leukemia. Nature. 2017;**543**(7644): 265-269

[54] Erb MA, Scott TG, Li BE, Xie H, Paulk J, Seo HS, Souza A, Roberts JM, Dastjerdi S, Buckley DL, Sanjana NE, Shalem O, Nabet B, Zeid R, Offei-Addo NK, Dhe-Paganon S, Zhang F, Orkin SH, Winter GE, Bradner JE. Transcription control by the ENL YEATS domain in acute leukemia. Nature. 2017;**543**(7644):270-274

[55] Eckschlager T, Plch J, Stiborova M, Hrabeta J. Histone deacetylase inhibitors as anticancer drugs. International Journal of Molecular Sciences. 2017;**18**(7):1414

[56] Faleiro I, Leão R, Binnie A, de Mello RA, Maia AT, Castelo-Branco P. Epigenetic therapy in urologic cancers: An update on clinical trials. Oncotarget. 2017;**8**(7):12484-12500

[57] Yin B, Li X, Johnson A, Yang Y, Jian W, Qin Y. Epigenetic drugs for cancer therapy. In: Huang S, Litt MD, Ann Blakey C, editors. Epigenetic Gene Expression and Regulation. London, UK: Academic Press; 2016. pp. 397-423

[58] Woodhoo A. Genome-wide epigenetic studies in neurologic diseases. In: Fraga M, Fernández AF, editors. Epigenomics in Health and Disease. London, UK: Academic Press; 2016. pp. 209-234

[59] Álvarez-Errico D, Vento-Tormo R, Ballestar E. Genetic and epigenetic determinants in autoinflammatory diseases. Frontiers in Immunology. 2017;**8**:318

[60] Rönn T, Ling C. DNA methylation as a diagnostic and therapeutic target in the battle against type 2 diabetes. Epigenomics. 2015;**7**(3):451-460

[61] Dawson MA. The cancer epigenome: Concepts, challenges, and therapeutic opportunities. Science. 2017;**355**(6330):1147-1152

[62] Shaffer SM, Dunagin MC, Torborg SR, Torre EA, Emert B, Krepler C, Beqiri M, Sproesser K, Brafford PA, Xiao M, Eggan E, Anastopoulos IN, Vargas-Garcia CA, Singh A, Nuthanson KL, Herlyn M, Raj A. Rare cell variability and drug-induced reprogramming as a mode of cancer drug resistance. Nature. 2017;**546**(7658):431-435

[63] Takahashi K, Yamanaka S. Induction of pluripotent stem cells from mouse embryonic and adult fibroblast cultures by defined factors. Cell. 2006;**126**(4):663-676

[64] Apostolou E, Hochedlinger K. Chromatin dynamics during cellular reprogramming. Nature. 2013;**502**(7472):462-471

[65] Kikuchi T, Morizane A, Doi D, Magotani H, Onoe H, Hayashi T, Mizuma H, Takara S, Takahashi R, Inoue H, Morita S, Yamamoto M, Okita K, Nakagawa M, Parmar M, Takahashi J. Human iPS cell-derived dopaminergic neurons function in a primate Parkinson's disease model. Nature. 2017;**548**(7669):592-596

[66] Naldini L. Gene therapy returns to centre stage. Nature. 2017;**526**(7573):351-360

[67] Mettananda S, Fisher CA, Hay D, Badat M, Quek L, Clark K, Hublitz P, Downes D, Kerry J, Gosden M, Telenius J, Sloane-Stanley JA, Faustino P, Coelho A, Doondeea J, Usukhbayar B, Sopp P, Sharpe JA, Hughes JR, Vyas P, Gibbons RJ, Higgs DR. Editting an α-globin enhancer in primary human hematopoietic stem cells as a treatment for β-thalassemia. Nature Communications. 2017;**8**(1):424

Section 2

Transcription Factors, Regulatory Elements, and Cross Talk Networking System

Chapter 2

Regulation of Mammalian Gene Expression

Partha P. Mitra

Additional information is available at the end of the chapter

http://dx.doi.org/10.5772/intechopen.72848

Abstract

Regulation of mammalian gene expression has been an ever growing subject in the field of Biology and the biomedical science research. In the last several decades, extensive amount of research together with the implementation of the latest technologies revealed that the whole process is regulated at the multiple stages with a series of interconnected complex biochemical and molecular pathways. Unearthing this complexity in one hand helps us in understanding the concerted effort put by the respective cellular machinery to regulate the whole process, and on the other hand, it provides a new insight about the development of several diseases where gene expressions play a pivotal role. Discussions here focus on the involvement of transcription factors or cofactors and the linkage of the transcription network with the signal transduction pathways. Besides proteins as a regulator, the role of the nucleic acids such as miRNA, chromosomal conformation and the modification of DNA bases or core histone proteins, in gene expression has also been explored. The purpose of this chapter is to provide the big picture of the diverse regulatory network and the phenomenal complexity of the regulation of gene expression.

Keywords: transcription factor, gene expression, structure-function relation

1. Introduction

Over the past few decades, extensive amounts of research have been carried out to understand the regulation of mammalian gene expression. Studies were originally started with bacteriophage, yeast and other lower order eukaryotes, and the acquired knowledge was later implicated to understand the mammalian systems, including the human cells. Several milestone discoveries in early days helped scientists to draw the very basic picture of gene expression, which includes lysogenic to lytic phase transition of the bacteriophage lambda (λ), inducible gene regulation in bacteria (lac operon system) and the sequential gene expression during early development of Drosophila embryo. All those studies clearly demonstrated that gene expression is an outcome of a concerted participation, triggered by intracellular or extracellular stimuli, of several intracellular protein factors and cofactors. At the same time, it was assumed that the scenario will be more complicated for the higher order eukaryotes simply due to presence of multistep regulatory processes with the involvement of more factors and cofactors. Until recently, a substantial amount of studies clearly depicted that the regulation of mammalian gene expression is more complicated than we thought ever before. This complex regulatory process comprises of a sequential or simultaneous involvement of at least four major steps and those are as follows:

A. transcriptional

B. posttranscriptional

C. epigenetic

D. translational

Due to the lack of space, rather than going in to the intricate details, a broad overview of each step would be provided taking the example of a few very well-studied systems.

Transcriptional control: Studies on transcriptional regulation are perhaps the most investigated segment in understanding the complexity of mammalian gene expression. Before going into the detail, discussion about the regulatory mechanisms, we should have a very clear idea about the process of transcription. Broadly, it is a process where the enzyme RNA polymerase (RNA Pol) decodes the genetic information, in the form of RNA that stored in the chromosomal DNA. The transcription machinery produces five types of RNAs, which includes messenger RNA (mRNA) contributes between 1 and 2% of the total transcripts, ribosomal RNA (rRNA) that covers more than 80% of the total transcripts, transfer RNA (tRNA, required for translation), the recently discovered micro RNA (miRNA) and small interfering RNA (siRNA). Among the several subtypes of RNA produced at any time, only mRNA translates into proteins. All different types of RNA molecules, synthesized by 5′ to 3′ movement of polymerases, are not produced by a single type of enzyme. For example, mRNA is transcribed by RNA PolII, whereas rRNA is produced by RNA PolI, and obviously, the regulation of transcription to synthesize each subtypes of RNA is significantly diverse and complicated. Our discussion here is mostly focused on the regulation of RNA PolII driven transcription, which has been investigated most rigorously.

Almost 24% of the human genes contain an evolutionary conserve DNA sequence element (5′TATAAA3′) in the core promoter or a variant of it called as TATA box or also known as Goldberg-Hogness box located 25–35 bp upstream of the transcription start site. The advantage of this AT rich sequence is that it facilitates the unwinding of the promoter DNA upon binding of the specific protein TBP (TATA binding protein) which is part of the TFIID complex. This huge multiprotein TFIID complex is specifically playing a very important role because it is associated with CDK7, −8, or −9 which are required for the phosphorylation of the C-terminal domain (CTD) of RNA PolII. TFIIA, which is another core factor, stabilizes the TFIID-DNA complex. Once the binding is stabilized, then RNA-PolII recognized the protein complex and recruited to make the PIC (pre-initiation complex). Among the other core factors, TFIIH plays a very important role in the transcription initiation because this multifunctional protein comprises of DNA-dependent ATPase, helicase and protein kinase activities [1].

Recent bioinformatics studies on human genome indicated that about 80% of the genes are transcribed from the promoter where TATA box does not exist. Such TATA-less genes are characterized by the presence of multiple promoters and transcription start sites and generate several transcripts. However, the question that remains unanswered here was how the transcription starts in this class of promoter? Or, is there any other role of TBP here? Earlier studies [2] indicated that the transcription factor TFIID and TBP were also involved in the initiation of transcription. The involvement of TFIID is conceivable because the associated CDK's are required for the CTD phosphorylation of RNA PolII but the function of TBP was not clear. Recent studies [3] on unicellular eukaryote showed that the DNA binding domain of TBP was not required for the transcription, which implied that TBP does other essential functions which could be a subject of further studies.

Transcriptions in mammalian cells are regulated at multiple stages and several protein factors and cofactors are involved at each stage. In general, a transcriptionally active gene is controlled by a stretch of DNA sequence mostly situated at the upstream of the transcription start site (−500 bp to −1000 bp) defined as promoters which is a docking site of several proteins termed as transcription factors (TF). Mammalian cells synthesize around 3000 transcription factors [4], and each one harbors a specific DNA sequence binding motif.

Transcription factors (TF) are the fundamental regulators of eukaryotic transcription. Therefore, to understand the complexity of transcription, we should have a very clear idea about correlation between the structural diversities and the functional activities of these proteins. TFs can be subdivided into two major categories based on the mechanisms by which they control the gene expression. TFIIA, TFIIB, TFIID, TFIIE, TFIIF and TFIIH are known as basal transcription factors because they are required to form a complex with RNA PolII, known as the PIC, for the transcription of the majority of the mammalian genes irrespective of the nature of cells or tissue types [5].The PIC is a huge multiprotein complex with multiple functions that include binding of the DNA sequence at the transcription start site, recruitment of RNA PolII, creating the bubble by changing the helical structure of the DNA so the polymerase can move after phosphorylation of the CTD.

Ubiquitous TFs are a class of DNA proteins bind to the promoter proximal region of a vast range of mammalian genes after recognizing a unique and conserved DNA sequence. Transcription factors such as Sp1 binds to the 5′-GGGCGG-3′ and AP1 binds to the 5′-TGA(G/C)TCA-3′ across the species. In general, ubiquitous transcription factors such as AP1 and SP1 are engaged in two major functions. One is the DNA binding and other is the recruitment of associated factors to initiate the transcription and in this context, structure-function relation plays a very important role. In case of TF, DNA binding introduces an inevitable change in the three-dimensional structure of the protein, which makes it interactive to the other cofactor proteins. This altered structure promotes to make a functionally active multiprotein complex that is essential in establishing the link with the extra and intracellular signal transduction pathways and at the same time, passing this signal effectively to the transactivation domain for transcription initiation.

Structurally, TFs can be subdivided into four major categories such as (1) helix-turn-helix proteins, (2) zinc finger proteins, (3) leucine zipper proteins and (4) helix-loop-helix proteins. Significant amount of studies were conducted to understand the impact of the three-dimensional structure with the functional activity of the protein. Each structural motif contributes to the (A) binding of the protein to the DNA, (B) homo- or heterodimer formation and (C) subsequent transactivation. To understand the structure-function relationship, we could further discuss citing examples of zinc finger proteins.

Mammalian cells produce about 1000 different types of zinc finger proteins and a significant part of them work as a transcription factor. The very well-studied Sp1 protein contains three zinc finger domains at the C-terminal end of the protein, which are responsible for the DNA binding activity of this protein. To make a higher order multiprotein complex, SP1 interacts with a variety of proteins which is often mediated by the zinc finger domains. For example, SP1 interacts with the CyclinD1 and the retinoblastoma protein pRB to regulate the transcription of the human keratin4 gene in squamous epithelium cells [6]. Our studies with zinc finger transcription factor HiNF-P very clearly demonstrated that the zinc finger domains are responsible for the DNA binding as a well as for the interaction with negative cell cycle regulator protein p57/kip2 (the zinc finger domains third and fourth domain from the N-terminal end of HiNF-P are required, (**Figure 1**). Our studies demonstrated that the HiNF-P-p57/Kip2 interaction is required for the downregulation of H4 gene transcription and the HiNF-P-NPAT/220 association, which is discussed further, not mediated through Zn finger domain, is required for the transcription activation [7].

Transcription factors that belong to the class of helix-turn-helix proteins, leucine zipper proteins and helix-loop-helix proteins are evolutionary conserve group of proteins and are responsible for the expression of the genes associated with cellular differentiation, lineage commitments and

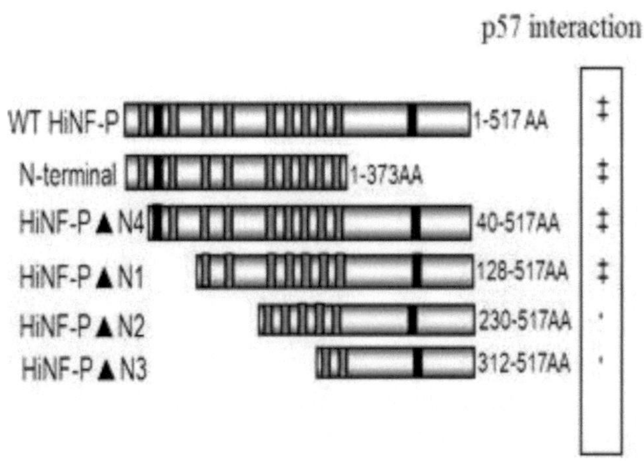

Figure 1. Zn-finger domain of HiNF-P is responsible for the interaction with p57. Zn fingers are marked as vertical gray rectangles. N-terminal deletion mutants of HiNF-P were co-expressed with p57 to perform co-immunoprecipitation experiments. Numbers of amino acids present in each deletion mutant are mentioned at the end of the c-terminal domain. Interaction with p57 of each deletion mutants is mentioned in a separate table at the right-hand side of the figure with +ve (interacting) or –ve (noninteracting).

http://dx.doi.org/10.5772/intechopen.72848

organogenesis. The conserve helical structure contributes to the binding of the major groove of the DNA and the dimerization. In addition to form homodimer, they also form heterodimer and often found that this heterodimer is the functionally active transcription promoting complex. For example, the leucine zipper transcription factor c-Fos cannot bind the DNA unless it forms a heterodimer with another leucine zipper protein c-Jun and interestingly, this heterodimer formation enhances the binding efficiency around 30-fold.

Therefore, it can be concluded that the mammalian gene expression is primarily regulated by the general and a set of ubiquitous transcription factors. However, the next level of regulation begins with the binding of a set of gene selective transcription factor to the promoter proximal region. Most of the cases, these gene-selective transcription factors are connected to the extra- or intracellular signal transduction pathways, which act as master regulator to switch ON or OFF the gene expression. This fact can be illustrated further by taking a very well-studied cell cycle regulated transcription of human histone H4 gene.

Transcription of H4 gene upregulates several fold at the onset of S-phase of the mammalian cell cycle in order to package the newly synthesized DNA. The one part of the proximal promoter, close to the transcription start site (Site-II) of the H4 gene contains the binding site of three major gene specific transcription factor HiNF-M/IFR-2, HiNF-D/CDPcut and HiNF-P (**Figure 2**). HiNF-M/IRF2 is a downstream target of master transcription factor E2F, which also regulates the expression of cell cycle check point controlling cyclins and CDKs. On the other hand, HiNF-P binds with its cofactor NPAT/p220, which is a direct subject of CyclinE/CDK2 that controls the G1/S transition, whereas HiFND/CDPcut is a multimeric protein with homeodomain protein CDPcut participates in DNA binding. Ectopic expression of HiNF-P and HiNF-M activates the H4 gene transcription but HiNF-D/CDPcut downregulates the transcriptional activity, which is an indication that transcription can be positively or negatively regulated depending upon the relative abundance of these factors at this region of the promoter.

The other part of the proximal promoter located further from the transcription start site (site-I) is the binding location for the ubiquitous transcription factors such as AP1 and SP1. Further studies

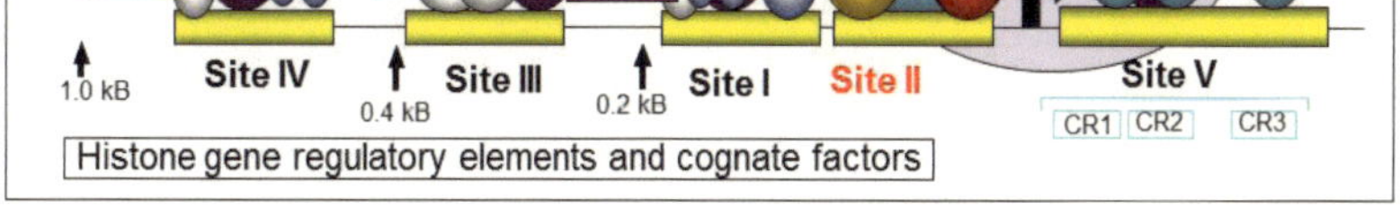

Figure 2. Human H4 gene promoter and the transcription factor binding sites. H4 gene is regulated at the G1/S cell cycle check point by a series of basic and the gene elective transcription factors binding over span of 1.0 kb DNA sequence. The Site-II DNA sequence is considered as the cell cycle element because it is the binding site of the cell cycle regulatory transcription factors as mentioned in the text.

provided clear evidence that the binding of the gene-specific transcription factors at site-II was conditional. A complete loss of HiNF-M/IFR-2, HiNF-D/CDPcut and HiNF-P binding was noticed when cells switch over to differentiation where the H4 gene transcription is shut down completely, but the bindings of AP1, SP1 were observed to be unaffected under this condition. Now the question is how histone H4 gene transcription is connected to the cell cycle check point? Growth factor-dependent signal activated CyclinE/CDK2 complex phosphorylates many essential proteins including NPAT/p220. Upon phosphorylation, NPAT/p220 binds to HiNF-P and makes the functionally active complex, which binds to the HiNF-P binding element at site-II and activates the transcription. At the late S phase, the CyclinE/CDK2 complex becomes inactivated, which in turn fails to phosphorylate the NPAT/p220-HiNF-P complex (**Figure 3**). Therefore, the H4 gene transcription model reveals, in a very simple way, how growth factor-dependent signal transduction pathway controls the gene expression. In order to keep our discussion very focused,

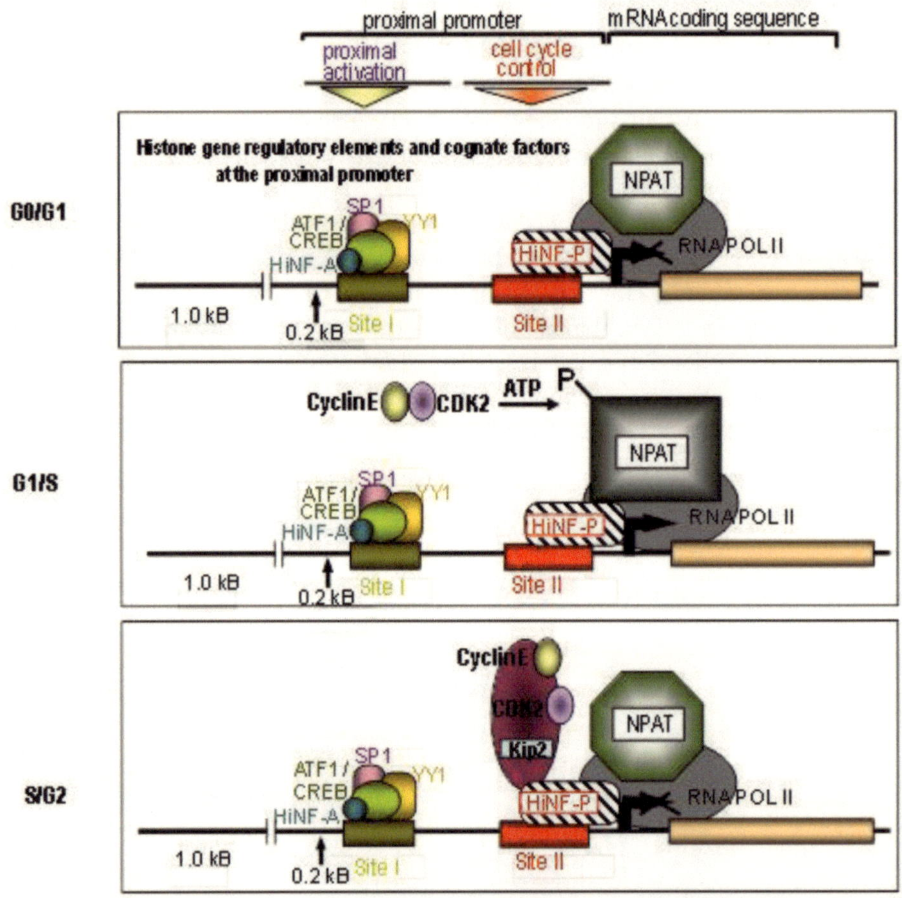

Figure 3. Regulation of human h4 gene transcription at the G1/S transition occurs through transcription complex formation. At the onset of G1/S transition, in association with other cognate Site-II specific binding factor, CyclinE/CDK2 mediated activation of NPAT-HiNF-P complex by phosphorylation is a prime driver of the transcription. At the end of S phase, the complex is functionally inhibited due to the inactivation of the CyclinE/CDK2 complex by the cellular kinase inhibitor p57/kip2.

the involvement of other cognate factors in other sites of this promoter is excluded. However, several important questions are yet to be answered regarding this H4 gene transcription regulation and perhaps one of them is how all three site-II specific factors act in a coordinate fashion to regulate the transcription [8–12].

So far our discussion focused on the effect of promoter and the associated factors or cofactors in the regulation of transcription. Recent studies revealed that besides the promoter, DNA sequence element located several megabases up or downstream of the transcription start site, termed as enhancers, also play a very important role in the regulation. The effect of enhancer on gene expression was revealed long time ago when researchers were trying to understand the massive transcription upregulation of the β-globin gene. However, the mechanism through which the enhancer controls the gene expression was very elusive. The most obvious question was how these cis-acting elements, located so far form the coding region, could control the transcription of a specific gene? The hypothesis that was put forward to explain the regulatory role of enhancers pointed towards the three-dimensional chromatin looping. Mammalian genome has been considered as a series topologically associated domain (TAD) comprises several megabases of DNA connected through intergenic sequence. Genome-wide Chromosomal Conformation Capture (3C) experiments, a recently developed method to estimate the looping in chromosome, indicated that proteins such as CTCF and cohesion are responsible for the TAD formation. Within a TAD, though promoter and enhancer are separated by megabases but due to the loop formation mediated by CTCF and cohesion, the enhancer comes closer to the promoter [13, 14].

The contribution of chromosome folding, which brings the enhancer in the close proximity to the promoter were very well demonstrated in one of the recent studies on transcriptional regulation of mouse c-MYB gene. This gene encodes a transcription factor that activates several downstream genes to support cell proliferation. However, at the onset of differentiation, the transcription of this gene is turned OFF completely. Interestingly, transcription of c-MYB is attenuated at the first intron where a CTCF binding exist, and the enhancer elements are located 36 kilobase (kb), 68, 81 and 108 kb upstream of the transcription start site. When cells are actively proliferating, the three-dimensional conformation of chromosome is changed to make an active transcriptional hub where all those enhancer elements are brought in close proximity of the conserved CTCF binding site located within the intron. On the other hand, during differentiation, the 3D structure of the chromosome is perturbed which in turn destabilizes the formation of active transcriptional hub and downregulates the transcription up to several folds (**Figure 4**).

Posttranscriptional regulation: In order to understand the posttranscriptional regulation, we should have a much updated vision about the movement of RNA Pol through the gene bodies, which is an integral part of the transcription and was a subject discussion for a long period of time. Crystallographic studies of RNA PolII provide very important information about the structural aspects of transcription. Several recent high resolution crystallographic studies in this field indicated that two major transcription bubble fork forms at the upstream and the downstream of the DNA associated with the polymerase. The transcription bubble is a small amount of unwound double stranded DNA (11 bp), which is exposed to polymerase to synthesize the

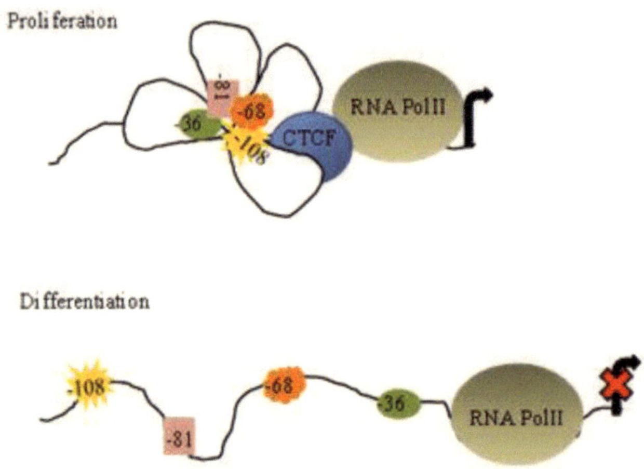

Figure 4. Enhancer-dependent regulation of mouse c-MYB gene. Transcription is upregulated several folds during proliferation when enhancer elements, located several kilobases away, fold to make an active transcription hub mediated through CTCF binding at the intronic region. During differentiation, loss of CTCF binding unfolds the structure and downregulates the transcription.

nascent RNA. The upstream fork forms a more open conformation and participates in DNA annealing and the synthesis of RNA transcripts; on the other hand, the downstream fork forms a rigid or closed domain with the non-template strand. This synchronized shift of open to close conformation allows the polymerase to translocate through the gene bodies [15].

Mammalian RNA Pol is a multi-subunit protein and the C-terminal domain (CTD), which is the biggest subunit of this protein, has several heptapeptide repeats (YSPTSPS). Phosphorylation of amino acid at the Serine-2 (Ser-2), Ser-5 and Ser-7 is very crucial for polymerase to start the transcription and several cofactors such as TFIIH (responsible for ser-5 phosphorylation) and cyclin-dependent kinase-7 (CDK7) or CDK9 (responsible for Ser-2 phosphorylation) mediate those phosphorylations.

Genome-wide chromatin immunoprecipitation (ChIP) experiments using antibodies against phospho-RNA PolII, followed by massive parallel sequencing, opened a new window about our understanding in transcriptional regulation particularly focusing on the movement and the distribution of RNA polymerase throughout the gene bodies. Several such studies indicated about 70% of the actively transcribing mammalian gene, the peak of the RNA PolII binding is located at the transcription start site and the availability of the polymerase along the gene body tapers off as we move along to the 3′ direction. Transcription starts after Ser-5 residues are phosphorylated predominantly by the cofactor TFIIH, whereas Ser-2 phosphorylation is insignificant [16]. For the remaining 30% of the gene, the major peak is located several bases downstream of the putative transcription start site indicating the polymerase stalls, though it initiated the transcription at the start site. In the presence of appropriate signal, the transcription complex recruits the P-TEFb complex, which is a heterodimer of CyclinT1 and CDK9. When RNA polII is stalled, it is associated with two major protein complexes those are DRB sensitivity inducing factor (DSIF) and negative elongation factor (NELF). Upon recruitment of P-TEFb complex, the CDK9 phosphorylates the CTD of RNA PolII and the NELF and DSIF. The phospho-NELF is dissociated and DSIF continues with the polymerase and the process continues until the signal dies away. The function of P-TEFb complex is also regulated by 7SK snRNP-a small nuclear ribonucleoprotein associated with a core noncoding RNA bound with RNA binding protein HXIM (HXIM1 and 2). P-TEFb complexed with 7SK snRNP and HXIM1 are considered to functionally inactive and mammalian bromodomain protein Brd4 and human immunodeficiency virus Tat protein can replace the 7SK snRNP and make the functionally active P-TEFb complex [17, 18].

Discoveries of this pausing mediated regulation raised a few fundamental questions about the regulatory process. (A) Why nature devised this kind of additional regulatory system and (B) what are those genes that belong to this category?

Depending upon the nature of expression, mammalian genes can be classified into two categories. The genes that belong to the constitutive active class are expressing themselves in a continuous fashion. Most of the genes, that encode proteins to carry out biochemical and the metabolic pathways, transcribe almost continuously. However, cells possess another class of genes which are expressed under certain conditions. Expressions of those genes are restricted because abandoned expression may cause abnormalities in the biochemical or molecular pathways that control the natural activities of mammalian cells. This phenomenon was first noticed in the expression of the Drosophila heat-shock gene expression where the proteins are expressed under the exposure of a particular stress condition such as low or high temperature, UV exposure and starvation or under hypoxia (less oxygen tension). Detailed study underpinned that the polymerase synthesizes 25–30 nucleotide (nt) short RNA before it pauses and stays there at least 10 min before it moves. However, during heat shock condition, the RNA polII stays only less than ~4 s. In mammalian cells, most of the developmentally and immediate response genes are regulated following this mechanism. Now, how these immediate response genes in the mammalian system are regulated by this complex mechanism can be discussed further by taking an example of a well-studied system [19].

The human oncogenic transcription factor c-MYB (a counter part of the mouse gene described earlier) is responsible for the development of certain types of breast cancer and leukemia. Overexpression of this protein promotes uncontrolled cell proliferation by activating a bunch of genes that drive the proliferation. In human breast epithelial cells, the transcription of this gene is absolutely regulated by the hormone estrogen. In the absence of estrogen, the transcription is paused at the 1.7 kb downstream of the transcription start site and generates a short transcript with a stretch of poly adenylated (poly A) tail and in the presence of estrogen the polymerase resumes the transcription beyond the pausing site (**Figure 5**). The analysis of DNA sequence indicated that the nascent RNA generated under this condition has the potential to form a secondary hair pin structure, which is considered as a docking site of the P-TEFb complex. Estrogen receptors (ESR1) are a group of nuclear proteins that have ligand (estrogen)-binding domain as well as DNA binding and transactivation domain. Genome-wide ESR1 binding studies and our independent investigations identified a solo ESR1-binding domain close to the upstream of the transcription pausing site. Our in depth studies to understand the underlying mechanism of ESR1-mediated overcoming of the pausing revealed

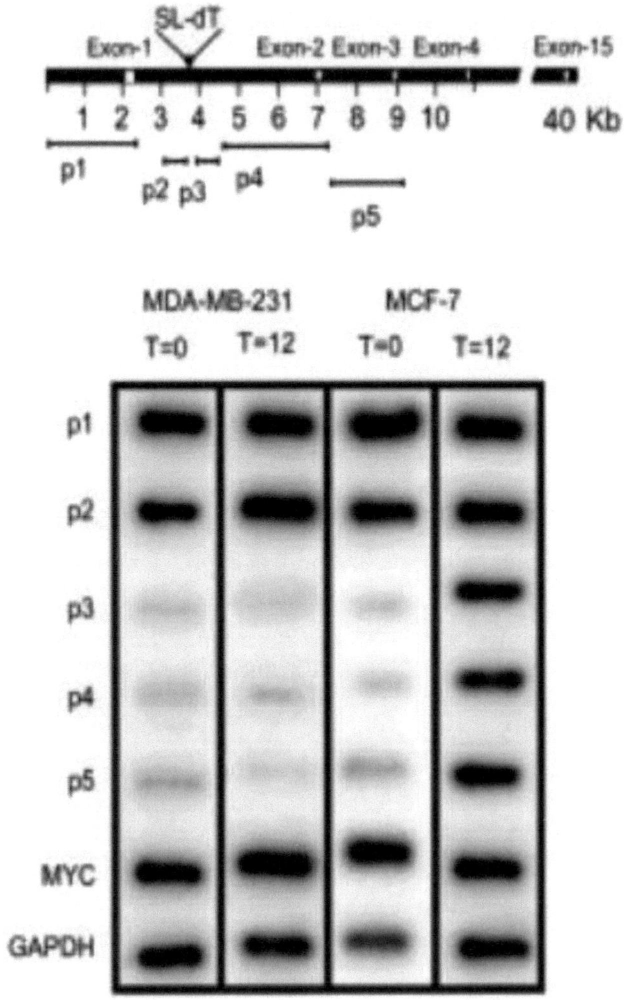

Figure 5. Estrogen-dependent transcription of c-MYB in breast cancer cells. A schematic diagram of human c-MYB gene showing exons and introns and the pausing site (SL-dT, Upper Panel). Nuclear run-on experiment showed that the transcription continues beyond the pausing site in the presence of estrogen in MCF7 cells but not in MDA-MB-231 cells, which do not express MYB (lower panel). Probes used in this hybridization were marked as P1, P2, P3, P4 and P5, and time of estrogen treatment was mentioned as T0 (control) and T12 (12 h).

that the ESR1 makes a tripartite complex with CyclinT1 and CDK9 and thus recruited the P-TEFb complex at the docking site. This recruited CDK9 phosphorylates the Ser-2 residue of the CTD of PolII and drives the transcription (**Figure 6**). Understanding the transcription regulation of oncogenic proteins also has significance in the field of cancer drug discovery. For example, the CDK9, which is playing such a pivotal role in the transcription of *c-MYB,* is a targetable molecule to develop a novel anticancer drug, and several such CDK9 inhibitors are currently under clinical trials to test their efficacies [20–22].

Epigenetic regulation: By definition, epigenetic modification is an inheritable process of regulation of gene expression without changing the DNA base pairs. The modifications take place

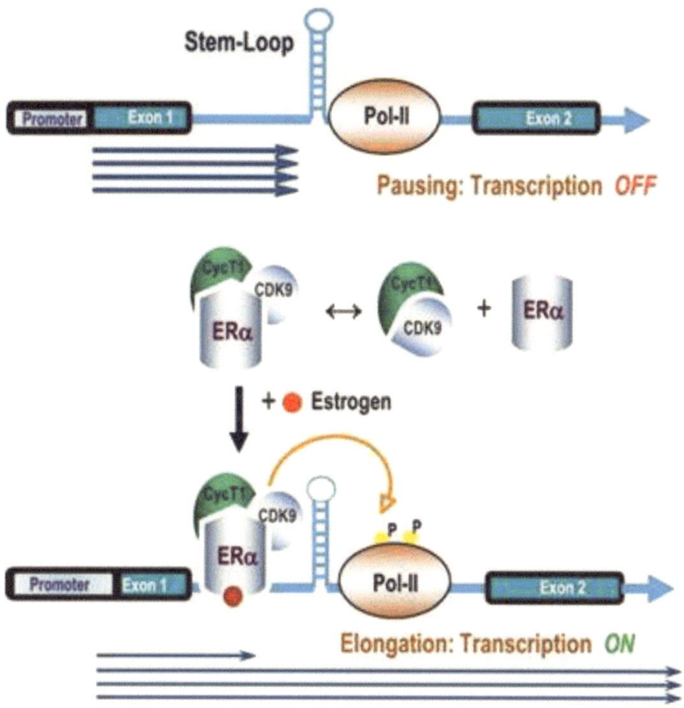

Figure 6. Estrogen-dependent transcription of *c-MYB* in breast cancer cells. In the absence of estrogen, the transcription is attenuated at the pausing site (upper panel). ERα forms a complex with CyclinT1 and CDK9 and in the presence of ligand; it binds DNA close to the pausing site, and the transcription resumes with subsequent phosphorylation of the CTD of the RNA PolII.

by enzyme-mediated inclusion or removal of the methyl groups in the nucleotides of the double stranded DNA or modifications of histone proteins by, for example, acetylation or deacetylation. Changes in the DNA bases or modification of the core histone proteins allow a particular portion of the chromatin accessible for the transcription complex or the repressor proteins to control the gene expression. Enzymes, those are responsible for the modification of DNA or histone proteins have been considered recently in a subject of in depth research in the context of their function and drug development in several diseases. Attempts are underway to develop novel therapeutics against diseases like cancer where the abnormal gene expression, caused by epigenetic modifications, contributes to the uncontrolled cell proliferation.

As discussed earlier, the epigenetic modifications can be subdivided into two different categories such as DNA modification and histone proteins modification. Traditionally, DNA modifications such as methylation happens when the enzyme DNA methyltransferases transfers the methyl group of a donor such as S-adenosylmethionine to a cytosine base and in most of the cases, it happens at the CpG (where the cytosine is connected to the guanosine by phosphate bonding) dinucleotide residues. Most of the CpG methylation in mammalian genome occurs at the outside of a stretch of elevated C- and G-rich region of the DNA called as CpG island and in case of human genome, this stretch is around 1 kb long and overlaps with the promoter region of the 60–70% of the gene. Therefore, CpG methylation in the genome acts as a landmark for the transcription complex to locate site of the chromosomes ready for transcription. DNA methylation at the promoter site contributes significantly in the gene expression as it can be understood that this modification acts like a 'mask', which attenuates the access of the transcription factors. However, it was also very well demonstrated that this methylation is a dynamic and a completely reversible process, which further emphasizes the fact that gene expression can be controlled by manipulating the methylation of the promoter sequence. It was also observed that DNA methylation is abandoned in lots of genes which are permanently silent; on the other hand, significant DNA methylations were observed in several actively transcribing genes [23, 24]. Therefore, further research is needed to understand the significance of DNA methylation in mammalian gene expression.

DNA methylation and its relation to the gene expression have been found to be strongly correlated with the development of diseases such as cancer. A large scale meta-analysis of the methylation profiles of target genes, which includes oncogenes and tumor suppressor proteins in several cancer tissues such as breast, colon and lung indicated that the promoter methylation patterns are significantly different in those tissues in comparison to their normal counter parts. The above statement can be illustrated further by using the very well-studied WNT-β-catenin pathway which is one of the most frequently dysregulated in renal cancer. The proto-oncogene β-catenin, which is the downstream target of WNT pathway, activates the expression of several proteins that promotes tumorigenesis such as proto-oncogene c-MYC and CyclinD1. Expressions of several key regulators that negatively regulate the WNT-β-catenin pathway are controlled by the promoter methylation, which eventually drives to the uncontrolled synthesis of β-catenin and the activation of the downstream target genes. For example, in case of renal carcinoma, expression of several WNT-inhibitor factors (WIF1, at least four, Dickkopf (DKK1 or 2) and IGFBP1 (insulin-like growth factor binding protein 1) are downregulated by promoter methylation [25]. In their studies, Moarii et al. [26] showed a significant amount of modification of the promoter methylation in the cancer tissues targeting to the transcription factor. Expression of several genes that are reported to be associated with the cell cycle (p16INK4a, p15INK4b, p14ARF), DNA repair (hMLH1, MGMT), apoptosis (DAPK), tumor suppression (p53) are downregulated or modified due to promoter methylation. For example, in case of p53, in vitro promoter methylation studies indicated that the DNA methylations can downregulate more than 90% of the mRNA expression. A further support of these data came along when the analysis of p53 expression in correlation to the promoter methylation was studied in vivo in patient samples. Several such studies indicated that the aberrant DNA hypermethylation of the p53promoter strongly correlates with the attenuated expression of this gene in a significant portion of the primary hepatocellular carcinoma, breast cancer, acute lymphoblastic leukemia (ALL) and chronic lymphocytic leukemia (CLL) patients. An increased expression of DNA methyltransferase (DNMT) activities have been noticed in several cancer cells which encouraged scientist to proposed the hypothesis that this enhanced activities hypermethylate the promoter of the tumor suppressor genes such as p53, which eventually promotes tumor development [27]; and therefore, a promising approach would be to develop an inhibitor against DNMTs to upregulate the expression of the tumor suppressor genes. Two of such inhibitors, azacytidine and decitabine, have been considered as the most successful drugs though their applications are restricted due to the toxic side effect. However, this outcome encouraged researchers to develop new drugs with less toxic side effects, and currently few of them are under clinical trials with promising results [28].

Posttranslational modification of histone proteins is one of the very well-studied epigenetic modifications. The mammalian chromosomes are compacted into the nucleus by forming the primary and several higher order structures by the building block nucleosomes. Each nucleosome comprises a histone octamer (four core histones H2A, H2B, H3, and H4 in duplicates) surrounded by 146 base pair of DNA where the amino terminal (N-terminal) part of histone protein protrudes out of the histone-DNA assembly. The N-terminal modification of the core histone proteins is very common and those modifications are acetylation, phosphorylation, methylation, sumoylation and ubiquitination. All those modifications are unique in a sense because each one of them introduces a specific change in the secondary and higher order structure of the chromatins which in turn contributes to the gene expression. For example, histone acetylation occurs at the lysine residue by the enzyme histone acetyl transferases (HATs) and it is associated with the transcription activation. However, the histone deacetylases (HDACs) remove the acetyl group and thereby suppresses the transcription. Dynamic regulation of acetylation and deacetylations of chromosomes have shown to play a very important role in the regulation of gene expression and propagation of disease. Acetylation of histone by HATs has been shown to open the chromatin structure, which allows the transcription factor to access that region. Research in last more than one decade established a strong connection between HATs and HDACs with diseases such as cancer. Extensive research in this field revealed that the malfunction of enzymes related to these activities can cause aberrant cell proliferation and differentiation. Recent studies established a very strong correlation between histone acetylation and deacetylation with the development of several types of cancer such as in hematopoietic malignancies and observed that HAT or HDACs are the common target of mutagenesis. Due to their significant role in disease development, HAT and HDACs are considered as important targets of drug development. One of the HDAC inhibitors suberoylanilide hydroxamic acid (SAHA, marketed by Merck as Zolinza) has been shown to be remarkably effective in the treatment of cutaneous T-cell lymphoma (CTCL). Another HDAC inhibitor, Panobinostat (marketed by Novartis) has been approved to treat multiple myeloma and currently under clinical trials to develop as a drug to treat ovarian and certain types of blood cancer. Similarly, modification of histones by methylation also contributes to the transcription. The methylation marks on chromosomes are recognized by the transcription factor or cofactors to locate the region of the chromosome ready for transcription. The amount of methylation also contributes to the activation and the repression of genes. For example, monomethylation of histone H3 lysine-4 form the N-terminal end (H3K4) is associated with both activation and repression, whereas trimethylated H3K4 is only associated with the repression (**Figure 7**).

Translational regulation: So far, we have discussed the regulation of mammalian gene expression where proteins such as enzymes or transcription factors play the key role in turning/ switching ON or OFF the gene expression. In the beginning of early 1990s, researchers discovered a short stretch of non-coding RNA, known as miRNA, highly conserved across the species, regulates gene expression at the level of translation. Since then, list of miRNAs has been piling up each year and currently more than 2000 miRNAs were reported with their functional association in gene expression, cell proliferation and differentiation. The analysis of human genome

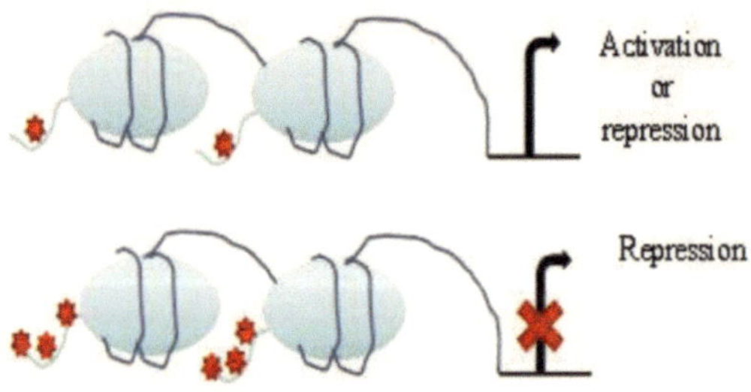

Figure 7. Methylation of histone is a mark of transcriptional activity. Transcription can still be active under monomethylated condition (black stars) of core histone protein but completely or permanently shuts down when histones are trimethylated.

sequence indicated that genes encode miRNA are located either in the intergenic (between two genes) or in the intragenic (located within the gene) region. The intergenic miRNA are transcribed by the independent promoter, whereas intragenic one is transcribed by the same gene-specific promoter. Both miRNAs are synthesized in the form of pre-miRNA that are several kilobases long and later are processed in the nucleus and in cytoplasm to generate a short hair pin, functionally active form.

Extensive studies in the last decade or more have generated a significant amount of evidence describing the mechanism of action of those miRNAs. Nevertheless, it is a subject of ongoing

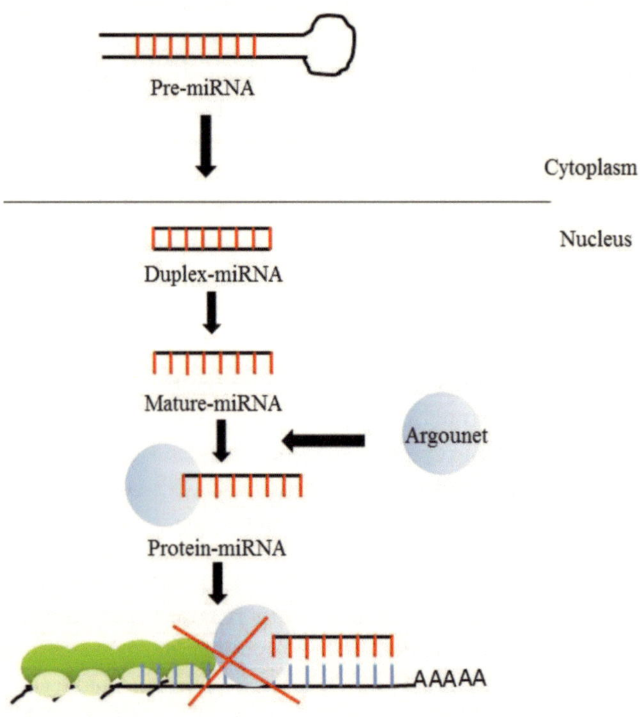

Figure 8. A model of miRNA-mediated regulation of gene expression. Several base pair long pre-miRNA is processed to short duplex miRNA. The sense strand forms a complex with RNA binding protein Argonaut. The RNA strand hybridizes with the 3′UTR of the target gene and the complex blocks the movement of the ribosomes.

study to understand how miRNAs are controlling gene expression. The posttranscriptional regulation is perhaps one of the most established mechanisms for the miRNA mediated control of gene expression. Several observations suggest that miRNA form a complex with the protein Argonaut, which is a highly conserved RNA binding protein. The specificity of the base pairing between miRNA-mRNA follows the Watson-Crick law where the 5′ proximal end of the miRNA forms a 2–8 bp of double-stranded RNA with the 3′ untranslated region (3′UTR) of the target mRNA. This miRNA-mRNA hybridization initiates several processes simultaneously to inhibit the gene expression. For example, the secondary structure form due to the hybridization causes premature termination and slowed elongation of translation, and at the same time, it stimulates the ribosomal drop off. The miRNA-protein complex recruits several factors and co-factors including the endonucleases to degrade the template RNA. On the other hand, Argonaut competes with the 5′mRNA CAP binding protein and elongation factor to prevent transcription initiation. Besides downregulating the gene expression, miRNA mediated upregulation has also been reported (**Figure 8**). However, the mechanism by which the activation occurs is not clear, but it has been proposed that the miRNA-protein complex perhaps inactivates the other miRNA that downregulates the gene expression. Understanding of the function of miRNAs and the complexity of their function was further revealed by the fact that a single miRNA has been shown to be acting like an activator or a repressor. The miR-145 upregulates the expression of the gene myocardin, which encodes a transcription factor that requires muscle cell differentiation. However, the expression of the Rho-associated coiled-coil contain ing protein kinase 1(ROCK1) is downregulated by the same miRNA-145 during osteosarcoma [29].

2. Conclusion

The complexity of the mammalian gene expression is more than what has ever been previously conceived due to the continuous accumulation of information over the period of last several decades. Researchers are trying to understand the molecular basis of every step associated with this process by utilizing cutting edge technologies and thus generating an enormous amount of data, which will take perhaps several decades to validate. The author's effort here is to provide a broad overview of the regulation of gene expression in the mammalian cells. It is hoped that this content will motivate readers to put their efforts to explore further the phenomenal complexity underlying the entire process and translate that knowledge in developing new therapeutics.

Acknowledgements

The data and the models presented here were generated based on the published data from the laboratory of Prof. Gary Stein, Chairman, Department of Biochemistry, University of Vermont and Prof. Thomas J. Gonda, University of South Australia. The generous support of Prof. Erik Thompson, Queensland University of Technology, was also appreciated for providing necessary resources to write the manuscript.

Author details

Partha P. Mitra

Address all correspondence to: p.mitra@uq.edu.au

School—Biomedical Sciences, Queensland University of Technology, Australia

References

[1] Dvir A, Conaway RC, Conaway JWA. Role for TFIIH in controlling the activity of early RNA polymerase II elongation complexes. Proceedings of the National Academy of Sciences of the United States of America. 1997;**94**(17):9006-9010

[2] Pugh BF, Tjian R. Transcription from a TATA-less promoter requires a multisubunit TFIID complex. Genes & Development. 1991;**5**(11):1935-1945

[3] Kamenova I, Warfield L, Hahn S. Mutations on the DNA binding surface of TBP discriminate between yeast TATA and TATA-less gene transcription. Molecular and Cellular Biology. 2014;**34**(15):2929-2943

[4] Baatar D, Jones MK, Pai R, Kawanaka H, Szabo IL, Moon WS, et al. Selective cyclooxygenase-2 blocker delays healing of esophageal ulcers in rats and inhibits ulceration-triggered c-Met/hepatocyte growth factor receptor induction and extracellular signal-regulated kinase 2 activation. The American Journal of Pathology. 2002;**160**(3):963-972

[5] Allen BL, Taatjes DJ. The mediator complex: A central integrator of transcription. Nature Reviews Molecular Cell Biology. 2015;**16**(3):155-166

[6] Opitz OG, Rustgi AK. Interaction between Sp1 and cell cycle regulatory proteins is important in transactivation of a differentiation-related gene. Cancer Research. 2000;**60**(11):2825-2830

[7] Mitra P, Ghule PN, van der Deen M, Medina R, Xie RL, Holmes WF, et al. CDK inhibitors selectively diminish cell cycle controlled activation of the histone H4 gene promoter by p220NPAT and HiNF-P. Journal of Cellular Physiology. 2009;**219**(2):438-448

[8] van Wijnen AJ, van den Ent FM, Lian JB, Stein JL, Stein GS. Overlapping and CpG methylation-sensitive protein-DNA interactions at the histone H4 transcriptional cell cycle domain: Distinctions between two human H4 gene promoters. Molecular and Cellular Biology. 1992;**12**(7):3273-3287

[9] Aziz F, van Wijnen AJ, Vaughan PS, Wu S, Shakoori AR, Lian JB, et al. The integrated activities of IRF-2 (HiNF-M), CDP/cut (HiNF-D) and H4TF-2 (HiNF-P) regulate transcription of a cell cycle controlled human histone H4 gene: Mechanistic differences between distinct H4 genes. Molecular Biology Reports. 1998;**25**(1):1-12

[10] Vaughan PS, Aziz F, van Wijnen AJ, Wu S, Harada H, Taniguchi T, et al. Activation of a cell-cycle-regulated histone gene by the oncogenic transcription factor IRF-2. Nature. 1995;**377**(6547):362-365

[11] Mitra P, Xie RL, Medina R, Hovhannisyan H, Zaidi SK, Wei Y, et al. Identification of HiNF-P, a key activator of cell cycle-controlled histone H4 genes at the onset of S phase. Molecular and Cellular Biology. 2003;**23**(22):8110-8123

[12] Miele A, Braastad CD, Holmes WF, Mitra P, Medina R, Xie R, et al. HiNF-P directly links the cyclin E/CDK2/p220NPAT pathway to histone H4 gene regulation at the G1/S phase cell cycle transition. Molecular and Cellular Biology. 2005;**25**(14):6140-6153

[13] Ghirlando R, Felsenfeld G. CTCF: Making the right connections. Genes & Development. 2016;**30**(8):881-891

[14] Ong CT, Corces VG. CTCF: An architectural protein bridging genome topology and function. Nature Reviews Genetics. 2014;**15**(4):234-246

[15] Barnes CO, Calero M, Malik I, Graham BW, Spahr H, Lin G, et al. Crystal structure of a transcribing RNA polymerase II complex reveals a complete transcription bubble. Molecular Cell. 2015;**59**(2):258-269

[16] Ghamari A, van de Corput MP, Thongjuea S, van Cappellen WA, van Ijcken W, van Haren J, et al. In vivo live imaging of RNA polymerase II transcription factories in primary cells. Genes & Development. 2013;**27**(7):767-777

[17] Zaborowska J, Egloff S, Murphy S. The pol II CTD: New twists in the tail. Nature Structural & Molecular Biology. 2016;**23**(9):771-777

[18] Chen R, Yik JH, Lew QJ, Chao SH. Brd4 and HEXIM1: Multiple roles in P-TEFb regulation and cancer. BioMed Research International. 2014;**2014**:232870

[19] Lis JT, Mason P, Peng J, Price DH, Werner J. P-TEFb kinase recruitment and function at heat shock loci. Genes & Development. 2000;**14**(7):792-803

[20] Drabsch Y, Hugo H, Zhang R, Dowhan DH, Miao YR, Gewirtz AM, et al. Mechanism of and requirement for estrogen-regulated MYB expression in estrogen-receptor-positive breast cancer cells. Proceedings of the National Academy of Sciences of the United States of America. 2007;**104**(34):13762-13767

[21] Mitra P, Pereira LA, Drabsch Y, Ramsay RG, Gonda TJ. Estrogen receptor-alpha recruits P-TEFb to overcome transcriptional pausing in intron 1 of the MYB gene. Nucleic Acids Research. 2012;**40**(13):5988-6000

[22] Mitra P, Yang RM, Sutton J, Ramsay RG, Gonda TJ. CDK9 inhibitors selectively target estrogen receptor-positive breast cancer cells through combined inhibition of MYB and MCL-1 expression. Oncotarget. 2016;**7**(8):9069-9083

[23] Graff J, Kim D, Dobbin MM, Tsai LH. Epigenetic regulation of gene expression in physiological and pathological brain processes. Physiological Reviews. 2011;**91**(2):603-649

[24] Illingworth RS, Bird AP. CpG islands—'a rough guide'. FEBS Letters. 2009;**583**(11):1713-1720

[25] Bennett LB, Taylor KH, Arthur GL, Rahmatpanah FB, Hooshmand SI, Caldwell CW. Epigenetic regulation of WNT signaling in chronic lymphocytic leukemia. Epigenomics. 2010;**2**(1):53-70

[26] Moarii M, Boeva V, Vert JP, Reyal F. Changes in correlation between promoter methylation and gene expression in cancer. BMC Genomics. 2015;**16**:873

[27] Saldana-Meyer R, Recillas-Targa F. Transcriptional and epigenetic regulation of the p53 tumor suppressor gene. Epigenetics. 2011;**6**(9):1068-1077

[28] Gnyszka A, Jastrzebski Z, Flis S. DNA methyltransferase inhibitors and their emerging role in epigenetic therapy of cancer. Anticancer Research. 2013;**33**(8):2989-2996

[29] Valinezhad Orang A, Safaralizadeh R, Kazemzadeh-Bavili M. Mechanisms of miRNA-mediated gene regulation from common downregulation to mRNA-specific upregulation. International Journal of Genomics. 2014;**2014**:970607

Chapter 3

Mammalian Cis-Acting RNA Sequence Elements

Irina Vlasova-St. Louis and Calandra Sagarsky

Additional information is available at the end of the chapter

http://dx.doi.org/10.5772/intechopen.72124

Abstract

Cis-acting regulatory sequence elements are sequences contained in the 3′ and 5′ untranslated region, introns, or coding regions of precursor RNAs and mature mRNAs that are selectively recognized by a complementary set of one or more trans-acting factors to regulate posttranscriptional gene expression. This chapter focuses on mammalian cis-acting regulatory elements that had been recently discovered in different regions: pre-processed and mature. The chapter begins with an overview of two large networks of mRNAs that contain conserved AU-rich elements (AREs) or GU-rich elements (GREs), and their role in mammalian cell physiology. Other, less conserved, cis-acting elements and their functional role in different steps of RNA maturation and metabolism will be discussed. The molecular characteristics of pathological cis-acting sequences that rose from gene mutations or transcriptional aberrations are briefly outlined, with the proposed approach to restore normal gene expression. Concise models of the function of posttranscriptional regulatory networks within different cellular compartments conclude this chapter.

Keywords: cis-elements, posttranscriptional gene regulation, mRNA splicing, translation, mRNA stability, decay, AU-rich elements (AREs) or GU-rich elements (GREs)

1. Introduction

The control of gene expression is fundamental to mammalian cell life. Although much of this control occurs at the level of transcription, posttranscriptional control is both prevalent and momentous [1]. Work over the past quarter century has resulted in the identification of unifying concepts in posttranscriptional regulation. One unifying concept states that posttranscriptional regulation is mediated by two major molecular components: cis-acting regulatory sequence elements and trans-acting factors. Cis-acting regulatory sequence elements are subsequences contained in the 5′ untranslated region (UTR), 3′ UTR, introns, and coding regions of precursor RNA and mature mRNA that are selectively recognized by a complementary set of one or more trans-acting factors to regulate posttranscriptional gene expression. The lists of conserved cis-elements have been expanding over the past decade, but the mechanisms of the precise assembly of RNA-binding complexes in an orchestrated temporal and spatial manner have not been comprehensively described. Conserved sequences within pre-mRNAs play a major role in determining the mRNA's configuration, stability, and ultimately the posttranslational fate of protein products. Mammalian pre-mRNAs contain almost as much conserved sequence as that ascribed to transcriptional regulatory elements, and many of these cis-elements can be attributed to known molecular functions, as described in the following paragraphs.

Trans-acting factors include RNA-binding proteins (RNA-BPs) and microRNAs (miRNAs), which are able to influence the fate of mRNA by controlling processes such as translation and mRNA degradation (reviewed in Refs. [2–5]). The combinatorial interplay between RNA-BPs, various miRNAs, and a given mRNA allows for the transcript-specific regulation critical to many cellular decisions during cell division, cell quiescence, or cell senescence [6]. RNA-BP classification is growing and becoming more defined as more structural data become available. Significant progress has been made in defining RNA-binding domains, such as an RNA recognition motif (RRM), zinc fingers, double-stranded RNA-binding domains, K homology domains, pumilio homology domains, and others, that were recently reviewed in [7, 8].

In the pre-genomic era, very few cis-acting RNA sequences had been discovered, for example, AU-rich elements (AREs) in the 3′ UTR of cytokine mRNAs [9]. Advances in genomic methodologies escalated the discoveries and functional identifications of cis-acting sequences. Microarray-based studies that evaluated mRNA stability and translation on a genome-wide basis have provided valuable information about the role of posttranscriptional regulation of a wide variety of transcripts that have an important physiological function [10–12]. Genome-wide measurements of mRNA decay and bioinformatic sequence motif discovery methods were used to identify the GU-rich element (GRE) as a highly conserved sequence that was enriched in the 3′ UTR and other regions of mRNA transcripts [13]. Various experimental approaches have been developed to understand the functional importance of cis-acting sequence interactions and the network of transcripts that they regulate. One of the most widely used techniques involves immunopurification of specific RNA-binding proteins from cellular extracts followed by a high-throughput analysis of the co-purified RNA species [14]. The coupling of this technique to powerful bioinformatic analysis has led researchers to understand the binding specificity of cis-acting elements [15]. The advent of new technology such as next generation sequencing (NGS) and chemical cross-linking procedures has allowed for fine-scale mapping of cis-binding motifs as well as for the refinement of RNA-binding protein-binding sites. A variety of methods have been developed to identify the *in vivo* target RNAs of a given RNA-BP, including microarray (Chip) or high-throughput sequencing (Seq) of RNA isolated by RNA-BP immunoprecipitation (RIP-Chip, RIP-Seq, and RIPiT-Seq), photo-activatable ribonucleoside-enhanced cross-linking and immunoprecipitation (RIP-CLIP), individual-nucleotide resolution cross-linking and immunoprecipitation (iCLIP), or UV cross-linking and immunoprecipitation (HiTS-CLIP) [16–20]. These methodologies involve RNA immunoprecipitation techniques with RNA-BP, followed by the NGS analysis of associated mRNA or microRNA transcripts and genome-wide identification of cis-elements within RNA target transcripts. More novel techniques such as sequence-specificity landscapes (SEQRS), HiTS-Kin/HiTS-EQ, and digestion optimized (DO)RIP-Seq focus on the identification of multiple trans-acting factors [7, 21, 22]. These techniques allow for the evaluation of the specificity of cellular RNA-BP/RNA-binding patterns from cell lysates under different conditions and might aid in the interpretation of a multiprotein complex formation and RNA-BP competition for RNA substrate. Identified RNA-binding complexes can then be isolated and interrogated *in vitro* using structural and cell-based reporter assays.

This chapter focuses on mammalian cis-acting regulatory elements that have been recently discovered in different regions of mRNA: preprocessed and mature. First, we summarize recent observations of two large networks of mRNAs that contain conserved AREs or GREs in their pre-mRNA splicing sites, polyadenylation sites, and 3′/5′ UTRs. We outline the known roles for ARE and GRE in regulation of mRNA stability or translation and their role in mammalian cell physiology, with a particular emphasis on their role in the dynamic response toward environmental and developmental signals. Second, we describe advances in the identification of other conserved cis-acting elements and their functional role in different steps of RNA maturation and metabolism. We briefly outline the molecular characteristics of pathological cis-acting sequences raised from gene mutation or transcriptional aberration and overview novel approaches to restore normal gene expression. We conclude with an overview of a concise predictive model of the function of posttranscriptional regulatory networks within different cellular compartments.

2. AU-rich element (ARE)

It was noted over a quarter of a century ago that mRNAs exhibit substantial variations in turnover rate upon exposure to different cell stimuli [23–25]. Of the prominent discoveries in the mammalian cis-acting elements field, the AU-rich element was the most notable as it was the most robust determinant of mRNA instability in cytokines and early response genes [26]. Insight into the biological significance and physiological function of ARE as a coordinate regulator of posttranscriptional network was revealed through the experimental identification of ELAVL1 (HuR) and ZNF36 (TTP) proteins [27–29]. The structure of AREs is defined as a repeating pentamer (AUUUA) with 1 or 2 A to U substitutions [9]. Bioinformatic searches throughout the human transcriptome have provided computational estimation of sequence characteristics and nucleotide lengths of ARE sequences required for mRNA to be unstable [30, 31]. The number of pentamers has an additive effect on mRNA decay and deadenylation processes. AREs are classified into five clusters depending on their sequence content and position of A or U. Cluster I AREs contain up to five copies of AUUUA motifs with a nearby U-rich region and cause synchronous RNA deadenylation [32]. Cluster II AREs are composed of at least two overlapping copies of the AUUUA with an adjacent (U/A) nonamer region and cause asynchronous deadenylation. Clusters III through V AREs were identified to contain more U-rich regions and were rather 'poorly structured' (**Table 1**), with an inconsistent deadenylation pattern. This classification system has proved to be helpful in understanding the observed behavior and function of ARE-containing transcripts [25].

Trans-acting factors	Functional categories	ARE sequences	Cluster	GRE sequences	Functional categories	Trans-acting factors
ELAVL1 ELAVL2 ZFP36 KSRP TIA1, TIAL1 HNRNPC1 HNRNPD GAPDH	Cytokines, Chemokines Growth factors; Cell signaling; Apoptosis	**AUUUAUUUAUUUAUUUAUUUA**	**I**	**GUUUGUUUGUUUGUUUGUUUG**	Transcription factors; Cell cycle; Cell metabolism; Cell–cell communication regulators	CELF1 CELF2 ELAVL4 RBM38 TARDBP FUS
		AUUUAUUUAUUUAUUUA	**II**	**GUUUGUUUGUUUGUUUG**		
		WAUUUAUUUAUUUAW	**III**	**GUKUGUUUGUKUG**		
		WWAUUUAUUUAWW	**IV**	**KKGUUUGUUUGKK**		
		WWWWAUUUAWWWW	**V**	**KKKU/GUKUG/UKKK**		

ARE and GRE mRNAs were clustered (with allowance for one mismatch) into five subclasses based on the number of pentameric repeats (AUUUA or GUUUG) and surrounding sequences. W indicates A or U. K indicates G or U. This table was made based on previous publications [33, 47, 74, 75, 77]. ARE- or GRE-containing transcripts in clusters I and II contain four or more overlapping AUUUA or GUUUG pentamers and are each represented by only a few hundred transcripts. Most of the transcripts in these clusters are cytokines, transcription factors, and early response genes. Clusters III through V contain shorter sequences with less sequence repetition and contain up to several thousand members.

Trans-acting factors that bind to ARE (far left column) or GRE (far right column) are: ELAVL1,2,4 (embryonic lethal, abnormal vision)-like 1,2,4; ZFP36, zinc finger protein 36; TIA1, T-cell intracellular antigen 1; TIAL1, TIA1-cytotoxic granule associated RNA-binding protein like 1; KSRP, KH-type splicing regulatory protein; HNRNP C1,D, heterogeneous nuclear ribonucleoprotein C1, D; GAPDH, Glyceraldehyde 3-phosphate dehydrogenase; CELF1,2, CUGBP-ELAV-like family member 1,2; RBM38, RNA-binding protein 38; TARDBP, Tat RNA regulatory element (TAR) DNA-binding protein; FUS, fused in sarcoma.

Table 1. Structural and functional comparison of AU-rich and GU-rich elements.

Genome-wide analyses of mRNA transcript half-lives showed that many labile transcripts contain conserved ARE sequence elements in their 3′ UTRs [21]. Overall, 3′ UTR-ARE-containing transcripts represent approximately 5% of the transcriptome [33]. Human mRNAs encoding cytokines and members of the NFkB cascade are particularly enriched for AREs (**Table 1**). AREs play decisive roles in regulating the effects of cytokines on inflammatory responses since mutation of the ARE in cytokines such as TNF-alpha, IFNG, or IRF5 [34] resulted in profound autoimmune-like inflammatory syndrome [35, 36]. In general, transcripts containing functional AREs have short half-lives, although they can be rapidly stabilized in different cell types or stimulation conditions through complex posttranscriptional mechanisms involving trans-acting factors [10, 37]. Numerous trans-binding factors interact with AREs (e.g., ELAVLs, ZFP36, KSRP, TIA1, TIAL1, HRNPC1, and others, which are described in other chapters of this book) and determine the outcomes for harboring ARE transcripts. The majority of these proteins shuttle between the cytoplasm and the nucleus, where they can affect RNA splicing and 3′-end processing, in addition to altering the rate of decay in the cytoplasm [38]. In this respect, it is interesting to note that AREs are also found in intronic regions of pre-mRNAs [39–42]. This observation leads to the speculation that trans-acting factors could bind ARE in the nucleus and fulfill a function that is different from their cytoplasmic one. Furthermore, a considerable overlap in the binding sites for ARE-BP with other cis-elements, such as GU-rich and poly-U sequences, warrants further investigation since the formation of secondary RNA structure might involve all of the above and subsequently rule the coordinate behavior of RNA-BPs in different cellular compartments or under different cellular stimuli [43–45].

3. GU-rich element (GRE)

GU-rich elements (GREs) are recognized as essential regulators of mRNA splicing, stability, and translation in mammalian cells [11, 46]. GU-rich containing RNAs represent approximately 8% of transcripts of the human transcriptome [47]. Genome-wide analyses of mRNA decay rates allowed for discovery of non-ARE-containing cohorts of mRNAs that exhibited rapid turnover. Computational *de novo* motif search identified conserved sequence elements in their 3′ UTRs in a form of a consensus U(GUUUG)n sequences [13] or GU repeats [48]. These elements were first tested *in vivo* in reporter systems and conferred instability onto reporter mRNAs. A well-utilized rabbit beta-globin reporter system identified GREs as sequences that regulate the decay of exogenously expressed GRE-containing reporter transcripts within cells [13]. Further verification of GRE-mediated mRNA decay came from the observation that siRNA-mediated knockdown of protein CELF1 led to the stabilization of GRE-containing beta-globin reporter transcripts as well as endogenous GRE-containing transcripts [49–51]. These studies also showed that both GU-rich sequences and GU repeats are also enriched in unstable mRNAs, though a number of GUUUG pentamers in the GRE do not seem to correlate with the mRNA decay rate. GREs were subsequently tested for RNA-binding specificities to CELF1 and CELF2 proteins in systemic evolution of ligands exponential enrichment, yeast three-hybrid system selection methods, and surface plasmon resonance quantitative binding assays, revealing that the CELF family preferentially bind to 15–22 nucleotide GU-rich RNA sequences [52–54]. Several studies reported that other proteins bind to very short UG repeats with higher affinity, but dropped once the repeats became longer than 15 nucleotides (e.g., TARDBP, FUS) [55, 56]. Binding to dispersed GRE pentanucleotides (mostly by RRM-containing proteins) have also been reported, although unified functional consequences of it are just beginning to emerge (refer to a comprehensive review in Ref. [57]).

Using whole genome microarrays and high-throughput NGS methodologies, GRE targets have been identified in a number of mammalian cells, for example, resting and activated human T cells, mouse brain cells, and myoblasts or human malignant cell lines [48, 58–61]. The majority of studies extensively characterized GREs as binding sites located predominantly in 3′ UTRs and caused mRNA decay (or stabilization) depending upon the cellular and environmental context [62]. These UG-rich sequences serve as binding sites for the family of CELF and ELAVL proteins. Interestingly, these two families of RNA-binding proteins share over 80% of sequence conservation within RNA recognition motifs but cause opposite outcomes: the CELF family binding to GRE leads to mRNA degradation, but the ELAVL family function as mRNA stabilizers [63]. In addition, several studies reported that UGU repeat sequences were enriched in introns, with the same frequency as AREs [64, 65]. The authors found significant enrichment of short UG-rich motifs in intronic regions flanking exons, supporting a role for GRE in alternative splicing [66, 67], which activate or repress the splicing of pre-mRNA targets through a competitive binding by MBNL and CELF proteins. This is not surprising, as an estimated 90% of human genes produce alternatively spliced mRNA transcripts [68, 69]. Alignment of the genomic regions adjacent to canonical and alternative polyadenylation sites identified UUCUG and UGUU as conserved cis-elements, which are essential for mRNA maturation and polyadenylation site utilization [70–73].

Thus, ARE and GRE can regulate pre-mRNA splicing, translation, and/or mRNA deadenylation or decay depending on the repertoire of proteins they interact with in different intracellular settings. The classification of AREs and GREs has been described in multiple manuscripts [74–77], and an overview is shown in **Table 1**. Single nucleotide polymorphism studies in humans demonstrated that SNPs in ARE and GRE sites are associated with higher risk of human diseases that involve adaptive immune response; mutations in these conserved cis-acting elements resulted in changes in RNA stability and binding preferences for RNA-BPs (reviewed in ref. [44, 63, 78, 79]). The opposing effects of RNA-BP on mRNA turnover may have important implications for the role of posttranscriptional regulation in proliferative diseases such as cancer. Most existing data suggest that the unbalanced expression and function of ARE-BPs appears to drive neoplastic growth and proliferation and contribute to cancer pathogenesis [44, 80]. A definitive causal connection, that is clinically relevant to human pathology, has not yet been demonstrated.

4. Poly(A) tail and polyadenylation sequences

The addition and removal of the poly(A) tail are the rate-limiting steps of maturation and degradation processes that the majority of mammalian mRNAs undergo [81–83]. Two tightly coupled reactions – cleavage and polyadenylation – involve a large number of protein components. Alternative polyadenylation of RNA is a posttranscriptional modification that plays an important role in gene expression, as it produces mRNAs that share the same coding region, but differ in their 3′ UTRs. This process is highly tissue specific and results in the generation of alternative mRNA isoforms with different stability rates and translational efficiency and even subcellular localization [84–86]. In mammals, the poly(A) cleavage/polyadenylation site is composed of three sets of consensus cis-elements: the highly conserved AAUAAA hexamer and less conserved U/GU-rich and UGUA elements. A bioinformatics analysis showed that an overwhelming majority of mammalian mRNAs harbor a conserved AAUAAA or a close canonical variant, AUUAAA, sequences [87, 88]. Flanking sequences are very important for the poly(A) site to function [89]. For example, two downstream U/GU-rich regions are both necessary for binding of the specific cleavage polyadenylation complex [90, 91]. A number of trans-binding factors regulate poly(A) site utilization and the efficiency of pre-mRNA processing in the nucleus, including five large families of CPSF, HNRNP, CF, MBNL, and CSTF proteins as well as snoRNAs [92–95]. These families have opposing effects on polyadenylation site utilization in nascent RNAs, determining the final pool of mature mRNA isoforms and subsequent choreography and activity of trans-binding factors in the cytoplasm (reviewed in [96, 97]). Immediately after cleavage, poly(A) polymerases (PAPs) promote lengthening of the poly(A) tail, completing the mRNA maturation process [98, 99]. Genome-wide polyadenylation site (PAS) analysis in mammalian cells identified a great diversity of PAS utilization in different tissues and organs [73, 100]. Mutations can cause the loss of the canonical adenylation signal and subsequent switch to alternative PAS utilization [101].

Another conserved regulatory cis-element is the cytoplasmic polyadenylation element (CPE). Many mammalian RNAs contain a CPE, a UUUUA/U sequence, located in the 3′ UTR. The CPE serves as a binding site for cytoplasmic polyadenylation element-binding (CPEBs) proteins 1–4 [102]. The most obtrusive differences in the CPE usage have been described under conditions of stress [103].

The nuclear poly(A)-binding proteins (PABPs) act as poly(A) keepers during the mRNA processing through first binding to newly added $(A)_{12}$ nucleotides and allowing the poly(A) tail to grow up to 250 nucleotides before the mRNA is exported into the cytoplasm [104, 105]. In the cytoplasm, the poly(A) tail acts as a cis-regulatory element and mediates mRNA translation. Recently developed methodologies make it affordable to count differentially polyadenylated mRNAs and assess the length of the poly(A) tail [106–108]. In somatic cells, mRNA deadenylation can lead to the degradation or stabilization of translationally silent transcripts; however, the importance of the poly(A) tail length in these processes is currently under scrutiny as there is an evidence that the translation is regulated independently of their poly(A) tail length in the somatic cell cycle [109]. As for embryonic developmental processes, translationally repressed mRNAs can be reactivated by cytoplasmic poly(A) tail elongation at the precise time when their encoded proteins are needed to be translated [108, 110].

5. Other intermediate cis-elements

A number of ARE-like transcripts have been identified in several mammalian systems to regulate important posttranscriptional networks of gene expression.

Poly (U) sequences are the third most conserved cis-element after ARE and GRE, which have been recently found within sequence composition at cross-link nucleotides site using the CLIP assay [111]. Frequencies of poly(U) are most highly enriched for UUUUU pentanucleotides. The HNRNPC and HNRNPD (AUF1) can recognize and bind to U sequences in pre-mRNAs, mature mRNAs, and non-coding RNAs and influence target transcript diversity in the nucleus through pre-mRNA splicing and the stability in the cytoplasm [41]. It is interesting to note that clusters V of ARE and GRE elements (see **Table 1**) include hundreds of mRNAs harboring U-pentanucleotides in the 3′ UTR, suggesting that CELF and ELAVL families can also bind to poly(U) tracts under certain conditions, perhaps with lower affinity [112].

Uridylation is an independent biochemical process that is facilitated by uridylation enzymes such as ZCCHC11 and ZCCHC6. In mammalian cells, uridylation readily occurs on deadenylated mRNAs through the recognition of short poly(A) tails (<25 nt). Protein PABPC1 antagonizes uridylation of polyadenylated mRNAs, contributing to changes in mRNA half-lives [113]. MicroRNA can also induce uridylation of its targets; however, selectivity of mRNA uridylation has not been decisively demonstrated. The development of novel methods, such as TAIL-Seq, allows for genome-wide discovery of alternative mRNA tailing processes such as uridylation and guanylation at downstream sites of shortened poly(A) tails [114]. Dynamic control of mRNA tailing is implicated in turnover and translational control and is fundamental for early embryonic development [115].

GC-rich sequences were also found to be conserved in coding and non-coding regions of mammalian mRNAs. Classified as GC-rich elements (GCREs), these were identified in NCL (nucleolin), PCBP1 and UPF protein-binding complexes [116]. GCREs regulate mRNA stability, decay, and translational efficiency [117]. Several lines of evidence establish primary function for GCRE as regulators of mRNA transcription [118].

The CU-rich element (CURE) is a target for several RNA- or DNA-binding proteins, for example, PCBP1 [119] and PTBP1 [120, 121] and regulates gene expression via a broad, but poorly defined spectrum of posttranslational mechanisms.

Oligonucleotides (T/C)nGGG/G from four separate strands can be folded into stacked tertiary structures known as G-quadruplexes, forming polymorphic loops of three G-quartet layers with four G-tracts [122–124]. Folded G-structures $(Gs)_{2–7}$ are found in 3′ and 5′ UTRs, but are very rare in coding and intergenic regions, and could influence all aspects of RNA metabolism [125, 126]. Studies have shown that 3′ UTR G-quadruplexes can bind more than two dozen proteins that interact with the Gs structure and serve as regulators of transcription, splicing, processing, localization, and stability and have been recently discussed in excellent reviews [127, 128]. Moreover, bioinformatics and computational scans have shown the prevalence of intermolecular DNA–RNA G-quadruplexes and $(Gs)_4$ pairing with miRNA in mammalian cells [129, 130]. These observations imply almost endless possibilities of intermolecular interactions, which undoubtedly would have significant impact on our understanding of transcriptional and posttranscriptional gene expression and regulation in mammalian cells.

Internal ribosome entry sites (IRESs) are heterogeneous cis-acting regulatory elements located primarily in 5′ untranslated regions of mammalian mRNAs. IRESs facilitate alternative mRNA translation, skipping the need for the m7GpppN cap structure and many translation initiation trans-acting factors in the recognition process of the translation initiation codon (e.g., AUG) by ribosomal subunits [131]. Since the length of IRES can be several hundred nucleotides long, it was difficult to identify IRES′ structural elements that are important for the common secondary structures or functions [132, 133]. In depth sequence scans through the human transcriptome identified a variety of poly-U, poly-A, and CU-rich *k*-mers that seem to be important determinants of the IRES activity [134]. These k-mers represent binding sites for IRES trans-acting factors and are located at positions less than 150 nt upstream of the AUG start-codon [135]. Translation initiation mediated by IRES is commonly presented as a cell survival mechanism in response to stress; however, the significance of this process and implications to human diseases are unknown due to lack of solid *in vitro* experimental results that would unambiguously demonstrate the effect *in vivo* [136].

Pumilio response element (PRE) is another cis-element that is well defined in nonmammalian systems. A consensus 5′- UGUANAUA was derived from gel shift, RIP, PAR-CLIP, and crystal structure approaches [137]. It is present in almost 3000 mammalian mRNAs and serves as a cis-element for the PUM family of proteins [138, 139]. PUMs exert two modes of mRNA translational repression: deadenylation-mediated repression and a deadenylation-independent mechanism [140].

Another novel 3′ UTR motif (UAAC/GUUAU) is also prevalent (7% of mammalian 3′ UTRs contain one or more copies) and has strong species conservation [141]. This motif is a binding target for HNRNP A2/B1 and A1 and is involved in mRNA deadenylation. A fundamental role of UAAC/GUUAU and similar elements as regulators of the mammalian mRNA translational activation or repression is yet to be demonstrated [142].

6. Short multivalent regulatory motifs

Mapping mammalian pre-mRNA positional enrichment of short intronic splicing regulatory elements (ISREs) is another example of the identification of cis-acting elements that are most important for pre-mRNA splicing. *De novo* searches for multivalent RNA motifs identified a number of conserved tetra- to hexamers that mediate the position-specific combinatorial binding by RNA-binding proteins [143, 144]. The position of short motifs can predict the tissue-specific RNA isoform abundance and can serve as an intronic splicing enhancer or silencer during embryonic development and in adult organisms [145]. Since the consensus sequence elements of splice sites are very short (e.g., 5′-UUAGGU, AAGGAC, AAGAAC, CCUCUG, GCUGCG, CUGCUG-3′), the mechanism by which the spliceosome distinguishes them as authentic splice sites remains a long-standing question. One of the explanations provided in [146, 147] suggests that these sequences form specific secondary structures that increase binding affinities to RNA-binding motifs across many RNA-BPs. The strong association of ISREs with differences in splicing patterns, but poor evolutionary conservation, suggests the role for these motifs to act as cis-acting splice codes that allow for the progressive divergence of alternative splicing in vertebrates [148].

7. MicroRNAs (miRNAs)

MicroRNAs are conserved regulatory sequences that pervasively act, in trans, toward mRNA. miRNA-binding sites are important regulators of mRNA half-life and activity. The majority of miRNAs influence mRNA life span through biochemical interactions with mRNA and/or RNA-BPs [149]. This could be achieved through direct competition for a shared binding site or through remodeling of the mRNA structure to favor (or impede) miRNA association nearby [150]. In support of this, a recent bioinformatics analysis determined that UUUGUUU motifs, which bear an uncanny resemblance to GRE-binding sites, are enriched in the adjacent to many miRNA-binding sites, and their presence tends to augment miRNA activity [151]. On the other hand, any miRNA that contains a UGUKUGU or UAUKUAU seed sequences (K represents G or U) could in theory bind and occlude GRE-BP- or ARE-BP-binding motifs, which prevent any interaction with cis-elements within mRNA. For example, the mir-122 interaction with CELF1 has been demonstrated, proposing that CELF1 can play a role in the degradation of GRE-containing miRNAs [152]. It has been computed that the proximity of RNA-BP-binding sites and residues pairing to miRNA can quantitatively predict mRNA cis-element performance for several intensely studied RNA-BPs and miRNAs [153–155]. Although mechanistic details of interplay between cis-acting elements, RNA-BPs, and miRNAs are understudied, they perhaps should be a high priority, given recent observations that miRNA expression and/or processing are affected in many human diseases and disorders [156–158]. Significant progress has been made by bioinformaticians and biologists to better understand system biology of the RNA life cycle; several useful metadata hubs were created, which incorporate existing experimental data and computational approaches [159, 160]. The comprehensive list of available software and websites has been recently reviewed in Ref. [161]. However, we are still far from having a comprehensive understanding of mechanisms of RNA biogenesis and its relevance in physiological and pathological conditions.

8. Pathological cis-elements

The human genome contains a large number of short repetitive sequences that are prone to higher than average mutation rates and transcriptional errors [162], which can engender a tandem repeat expansion in cis-acting elements of 3′ or 5′ UTR, introns, or coding regions, and cause a large variety of inherited human diseases. For example, endogenous nucleotide repeat expansions are implicated in many human autosomal dominant diseases and have emerged as new groups of repeat expansion disorder associated with tri- or pentanucleotide repeat expansion pathogenesis. Pathological repeats can elicit toxicity that is triggered by toxic RNA or abnormally translated protein dipeptide or homopolymeric peptides [163]. Disorders as such include, but are not limited to the following conditions:

- Spinocerebellar ataxia (SCAs types 1–37) is the largest and the most diverse group of inherited neurological diseases in which neurological dysfunction is driven by defects known as ataxias. Several mutations in tandem repeat expansions were discovered, including coding (CAG)n mutations in SCA1, 2, 3, 6, 7, and 17 genes; non-coding (CTG)n in *SCA8* [164]; non-coding (CAG)n in SCA12; (ATTCT)n – in SCA10; (TGGAA)n – in SCA31; and (GGCCTG) – in SCA36 (please see OMIM.org for details).

- Myotonic dystrophies (DM), where (DM1) is associated with >300 CUG, repeats in the DMPK mRNA; and (DM2) – with >CCUG repeats in ZF9 mRNA [165].
- Amyotrophic lateral sclerosis (ALS) and frontotemporal dementia are associated with GGGGCC/CCCCGG repeat expansion in the non-coding region of the C9orf72 (C9ALS/FTD) gene [166].
- Huntington's disease is caused by CAG expansion repeats in the HTT gene [167];
- Fragile X syndrome (FXS) arises when the FMR1 gene reach <230 CGG repeats.
- Fragile X-associated tremor/ataxia syndrome (FXTAS) is associated with CGG/CCG repeat expansion in the fragile X gene, FMR1 [168].

Molecular pathogenesis of endogenous nucleotide repeat expansion diseases is complicated and pertained to the presence of repeat-associated non-AUG translation (RAN), where translation of mutant polypeptides is initiated without an AUG-initiation codon or it is driven by the open reading frame shifts due to expanded three-base-pair repeats during skipped mispairing in the course of DNA synthesis (reviewed in [169, 170]). Although the posttranscriptional modification state of these transcripts (e.g., mRNA capping and polyadenylation) is unknown, two translational pathways are described: (1) ATG-initiated translation produces multiple polypeptides if there are multiple ORFs within the transcript. (2) RAN translation of the expanded repeat can produce up to six distinct RAN polypeptides: poly-Gln, poly-Ala, and poly-Ser RAN proteins (from CTG/CAG repeats); and poly-Leu, poly-Ala and poly-Cys polypeptides from the CAG/CUG repeat mRNA. Repeats located in antisense transcripts of above listed genes are also substrates for RAN translation, further expanding the number of pathological dipeptides or homopolymeric RAN proteins produced during disease pathogenesis.

An interesting common aspect of these pathologies is that they are caused by mutated cis-elements and are often produced through bidirectional transcription. Resultant toxic RNA causes intracellular stress and sequestration of RNA-BPs toward expanded sequence repeats [171], which changes the biochemistry of posttranscriptional regulatory networks in affected tissues. The abovementioned diseases represent an incomplete list of a growing number of disorders that can potentially have similar therapeutic opportunities. The recently developed 'base editor' CRISPR-Cas9 methodology has demonstrated a high power of nucleotide-level precision editing, making this approach suitable for repeat excision as genetic therapies for the above listed conditions [172] and may also correct many other RNA pathologies, for example, those driven by nonsense-mediated mRNA decay [173].

9. Models for the effects of cis-acting elements

mRNA molecules move through different cellular compartments within messenger ribonucleoprotein (mRNP) complexes in dynamic association with RNA-binding proteins that bind to conserved cis-elements shared by subsets of transcripts [174]. The association of specific trans-binding factors with conserved regulatory cis-elements shared by subsets of mRNAs coordinates the fate of these bound transcripts through posttranscriptional processes such as splicing, intracellular localization, translation, storage, or mRNA decay [175, 176]. Not surprisingly, very few transcripts have only one type of regulatory element. Focusing on individual scenarios, we built a concise predictive model of higher-order complexes that can be formed simultaneously within different cellular compartments, starting in from the nucleus and moving into the cytoplasm.

A. Regulation of splicing by cis-elements (**Figure 1A**):

The cis-elements within precursor RNA are catalyzed by different components of the spliceosome during constitutive splicing events [177]. Binding by RNA-BP to short intronic splicing regulatory elements (ISREs) regulates exon inclusion or exon skipping during stage-specific constitutive splicing transitions, in a position-dependent manner [67]. These processes are orchestrated by biochemical recognition and binding on a competitive basis by a family of U proteins that compose the spliceosome.

RNA-BPs also bind to multivalent intronic sequences in precursor mRNA and regulate the alternative splicing (e.g., exon skipping, alternative splice site retention, or intron retention). Alternatively-spliced transcripts may contain different 3′ or 5′ UTRs that can be subject to differential translational regulation of mature transcripts. An important regulators of alternative splicing efficiency are PTBP, SR, RBM, and HNRNP families of proteins and snRNAs. The use of alternative exons leads to the production of transcripts with different open reading frames (ORFs) and diversifies the repertoire of encoded proteins, giving rise to protein isoforms with alternative N- and C- termini.

B. Regulation of adenylation by cis-acting elements (**Figure 1B**):

Alternative polyadenylation (APA) occurs in a tandem manner with splicing. Many splicing factors are also 3′-end processing factors within the mRNA 3′-end cleavage and polyadenylation (CPA) complexes. The recognition of cis-elements upstream of canonical or alternative PAS serves as a docking site for specific RNA-binding proteins (e.g., CPSF, CF, CSTFs, HNRNPs, MBNL, and CPEB), which in turn recruit canonical poly(A) polymerases (PAPOL). The CPA complex requires stabilization by a downstream GU/GC-rich sequence element (DSE) and its interaction with the CPSF-processing factors. The upstream sequence element (USE) is U-rich and serves an auxiliary role, binding to CF and PAPOL, and also stabilizes the cleavage complex.

The cleavage and polyadenylation specific factor (CPSF) binds weaker noncanonical polyadenylation (AUUAAA) signals and cuts at the proximal polyadenylation site (PAS). The utilization of distal canonical PAS results in the processing of the full mature transcript. Cleavage at the proximal PAS leads to shortening of the 3′ untranslated region and loss of regulatory sequences within the 3′ UTR (e.g., ARE or GRE or miRNA-binding sites). MBNL can mask the region upstream of weak noncanonical PA signals, blocking the binding of cleavage factor I (CF).

The CPEB1 protein binds the cytoplasmic polyadenylation element (CPE, consensus sequence 5′-UUUUUAU -3′) located upstream of non-canonical PA signals within the

http://dx.doi.org/10.5772/intechopen.72124

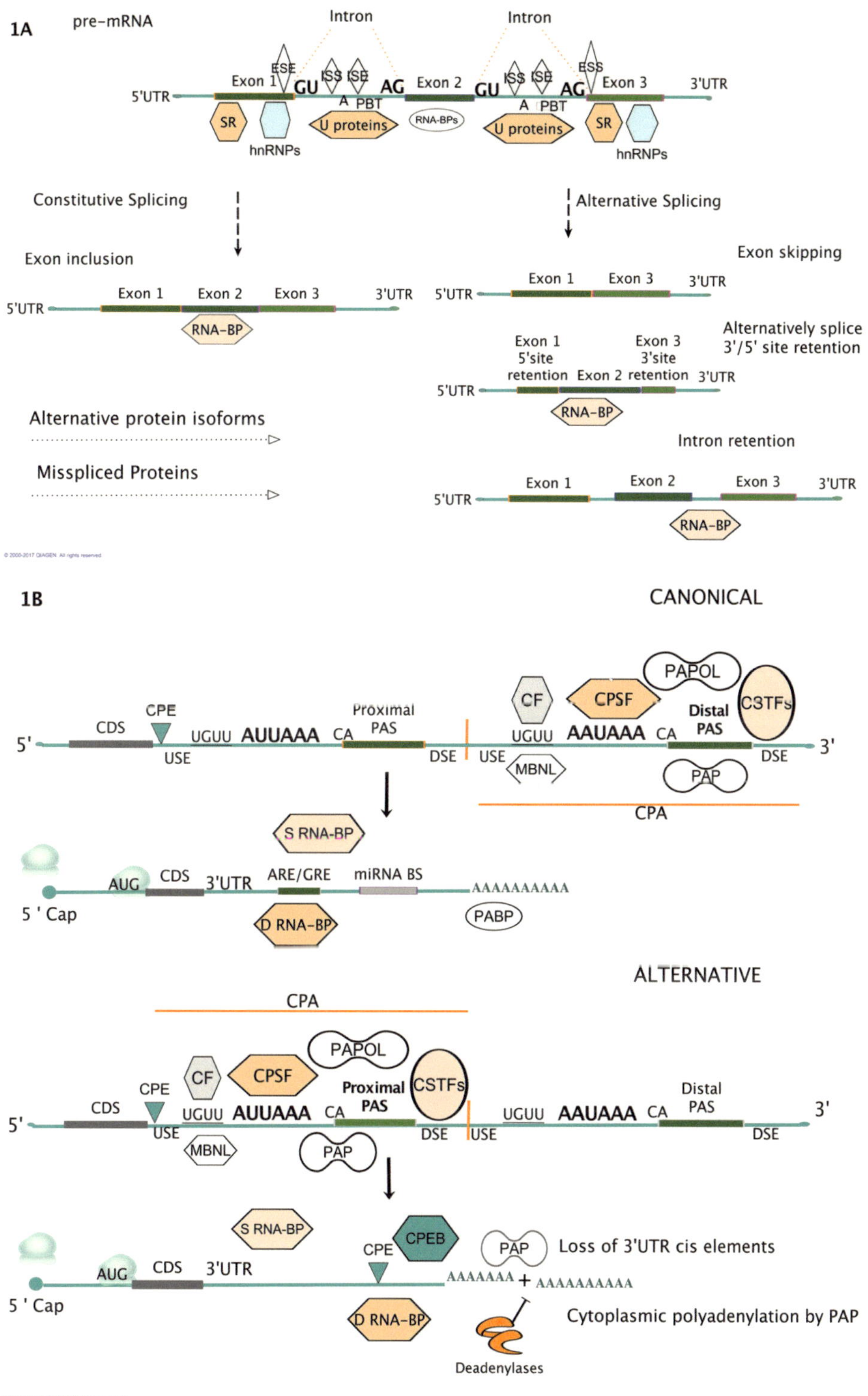

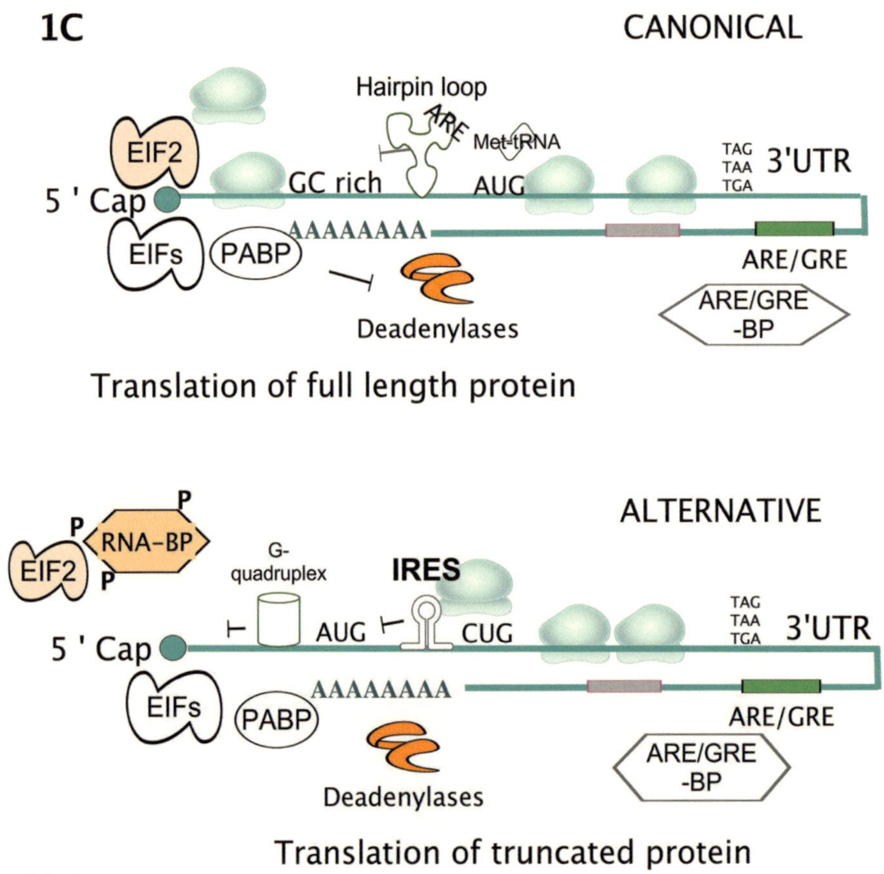
1C
CANONICAL
Hairpin loop
ARE
Met-tRNA
EIF2
GC rich
AUG
TAG
TAA
TGA
3'UTR
5 ' Cap
AAAAAAAA
EIFs
PABP
ARE/GRE
ARE/GRE
-BP
Deadenylases
Translation of full length protein
ALTERNATIVE
P
RNA-BP
P
EIF2
P
G-
quadruplex
IRES
AUG
CUG
TAG
TAA
TGA
3'UTR
5 ' Cap
AAAAAAAA
EIFs
PABP
ARE/GRE
ARE/GRE
-BP
Deadenylases
Translation of truncated protein

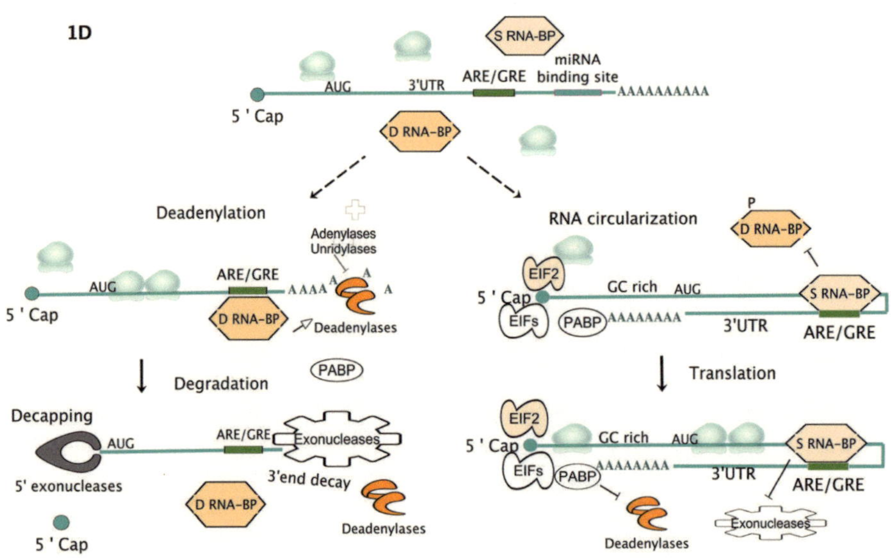
1D
S RNA-BP
miRNA
binding site
AUG
3'UTR
ARE/GRE
AAAAAAAAAA
5 ' Cap
D RNA-BP
Deadenylation
Adenylases
Unridylases
RNA circularization
P
D RNA-BP
AUG
ARE/GRE
AAAA
5 ' Cap
D RNA-BP
Deadenylases
EIF2
5 ' Cap
GC rich
AUG
S RNA-BP
EIFs
PABP
AAAAAAAA
3'UTR
ARE/GRE
Degradation
PABP
Translation
Decapping
AUG
ARE/GRE
Exonucleases
3'end decay
5' exonucleases
D RNA-BP
Deadenylases
5 ' Cap
EIF2
5 ' Cap
GC rich
AUG
S RNA-BP
EIFs
PABP
AAAAAAAA
3'UTR
ARE/GRE
Exonucleases
Deadenylases

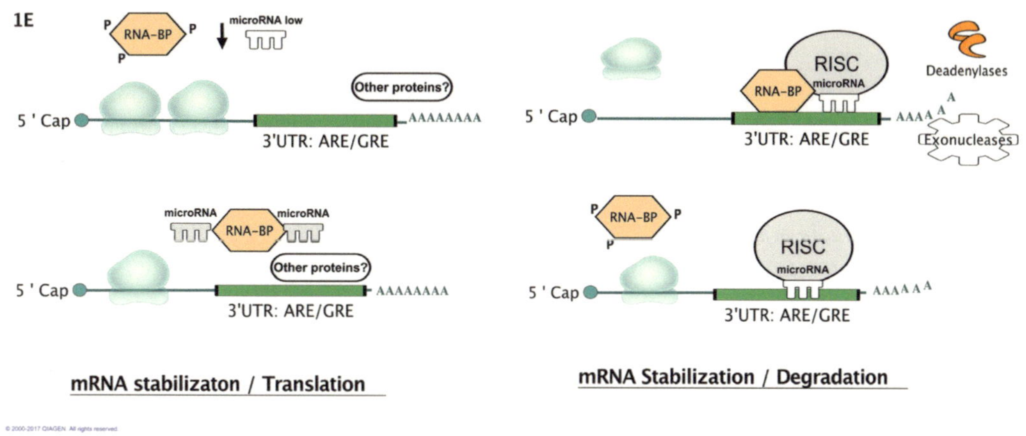

Figure 1. Predictive scenarios of cis-element effects and trans-binding factors behavior on mRNA splicing, adenylation, translation, and decay. Blunt arrows indicate direct suppression; arrows represent activation. These figures are made by using the ingenuity pathway analysis software based upon the observations from previous studies or suggested regulatory mechanisms. A. Consensus multivalent sequences represent the intronic splice sites that are recognized by a family of small nuclear ribonucleoproteins (U snRNPs). These regulatory cis-elements can be divided into two types: (1) intronic regions which almost always begin with the dinucleotide GU and end with AG; and (2) intronic regions which have either AU and AC termini or GU and AG termini. Introns are also rich with pyrimidine nucleotides that cumulatively compose a pyrimidine binding tract, which also have a unique poly(A) branch point sequence upstream. Of the other four types of cis-acting elements: two are located within exons (exonic splicing enhancers, ESEs, and exonic splicing silencers, ESSs), and two are located within introns (intronic splicing enhancers, ISEs, and intronic splicing silencers, ISSs). The key trans-acting splicing factors are shown: SR, serine/arginine-rich (SR) proteins; U1 small nuclear ribonucleoproteins (U1 snRNPs); HNRNPs, heterogeneous nuclear ribonucleoproteins, PTB, polypyrimidine tract binding protein. B. Adenylation of pre-mRNA is triggered by cis-regulatory sequences named poly(A) signals: AAUAAA or/and AUUAAA; the U/GU-rich and UGUA elements. By direct analogy to splicing, canonical adenylation is regulated by RNA-BPs or snRNAs. CF, cleavage factor; CSTF, cleavage stimulation factor; CPSF, cleavage polyadenylation specificity factor; MBNL, muscle blind like protein; PAP, poly(A) polymerase; PABP, poly(A) binding protein; CPEB, cytoplasmic polyadenylation element binding protein; miRNA BS, miRNA binding sites; S RNA-BP, stabilizing RNA-binding protein; D RNA-BP, destabilizing RNA-binding protein; CPA, cleavage polyadenylation assembly; CPE, cytoplasmic polyadenylation element. C. Cis-mediated regulation of canonical and alternative translation includes sequences in all parts of mRNA. In canonical translation, the initiation factors (RNA-BPs) bind the 5′ m7GpppN cap, and then linearly scan through the 5′ UTR until reaching an AUG start codon. For simplicity, the components of the translation machinery are shown as eIF2 and eIFs (eukaryotic early translation initiation factors). PABP, poly(A) binding protein; IRES, internal ribosomal entry site; P, phosphorylation of RNA-BP. D. Schematic illustration of the cytoplasmic mRNA decay complex formation. The details for this scenario are provided in the text. S RNA-BP, stabilizing RNA-binding proteins; D RNA-BP, destabilizing RNA-binding proteins; PABP, poly(A)-binding protein; eIF2 and eIFs, eukaryotic early translation initiation factors. E. Scenarios for miRNA mediated mRNA translational repression or decay pathways. The details for this scenario are provided in the text. RISC, RNA-induced silencing complex; P, phosphorylation of RNA-BP.

mRNA and shuttles it into the cytoplasm. The cytoplasmic CPEB1-CPE complex recruits poly(A) polymerase (PAP), which promotes the lengthening of the poly(A) tail and increases translation efficiency. The greater the distance between CPE and poly(A) tails of transcripts, the weaker the rate of adenylation.

C. Regulation of **translation** by cis-acting elements (**Figure 1C**):

Most eukaryotic mRNAs are translated by the cap-dependent mechanism, which requires recognition of the cap structure (m7GpppN) at the 5′ end by early initiation factor complexes (eIFs). EIFs recruit ribosomal subunits and initiator Met-tRNA and scan along the

5′ UTR of the mRNA to reach the start codon (an AUG triplet). During the scanning, the secondary RNA structure unwinds in an ATP-dependent manner. The 5′ UTR is rich in GC-content and is prone to folding into secondary structures, which may hinder ribosomal assembly [178]. Hairpin loops as secondary structure regulatory elements were described only for a handful of mRNAs, and their role in genome-wide translation is not known. A combination of new ribo-sequencing with fluorescent visualization might shed light on the role of hairpin loops in translation in the near future [179–182]. Other internal 5′ UTR cis-element structures are AREs and GREs. Their effects on translation are mediated by a combination of RNA-BPs. They are often found to be part of hairpin loops. Visualizing a folded hairpin structure *in vivo* is not possible at current resolution limits.

The translation initiation via internal ribosomal entry site (IRES) occurs in a cap-independent manner. Mammalian IRES facilitates bypassing of the eIF4E-m7GpppN cap interaction and recruitment of the small and large ribosomal subunits and tRNA to the transcript, initiating translation at the canonical AUG start codon.

G-quadruplexes within/near IRES may potentiate alternative translation. However, G4 structures in 3′ or 5′ UTRs and an open reading frame mainly repress cap-dependent translation (reviewed in Ref. [183]).

The poly(A) tail also plays a role in translation as an mRNA stabilizer and a facilitator of mRNA circularization, which promotes translation. De-adenylation processes tend to slowdown the translation rate and eventually lead to mRNA degradation.

D. Regulation of mRNA stabilization or decay by cis-acting elements (**Figure 1D**):

In mammalian cells, mRNA stabilization or decay is regulated by cis-elements in the 3′ UTR. Numerous known RNA-BPs serve as trans-binding factors for ARE/GRE and other elements to facilitate transcript deadenylation and subsequent decay by exonucleases. There are also a number of RNA-BPs with the opposite function, which stabilize and promote mRNA translation. Posttranslational alteration of RNA-BPs (particularly within RNA-binding domains) can lead them to dissociate from RNA-binding complexes, and be replaced by other competitors, thereby contributing to mRNA de/stabilization [76]. A fine-tuned balance must be reached in cells for proper function at the organismal level.

E. Interplay between mRNA, miRNA and RNA-BPs (**Figure 1E**):

The estimates on how different miRNA and mRNA are loaded into the RNA-BP-bound RISC (RNA-induced silencing complex) were derived from CLIP assays results [184–186]. Several scenarios are possible to extract from these: If both miRNA and RNA-BP are bound to the 3′ UTR of mRNA, they will be sufficiently close to each other and the complex can be identified by CLIP. They would work cooperatively to promote the assembly of decay machinery. Independent binding by a competitor RNA-BP might disrupt this complex. The strength of miRNA-mRNA canonical and noncanonical bond formation can be computed to project possible biochemical outcomes [187–189].

The mRNA 3′ UTR length and secondary structure formation can greatly influence both miRNA and RNA-BP-binding efficiency; it can also disrupt or assuage the assembly of

RNA-BP complexes by providing high affinity or multioccupancy binding sites. The outcomes of this scenario could be anywhere from marginal translational repression to accelerated mRNA degradation.

Cis-acting sequences within miRNAs that resemble cis-elements (ARE or GRE) have perfect complementarity to RNA-BP's RNA-recognition motifs (RRMs). They can, in theory, occlude RRM-binding sites, acting as alternative inhibitors of RNA-BP activity. This could potentiate (or hinder) translational repression and mRNA degradation of target mRNA, depending on which RNA-BP was affected.

10. Conclusions and perspectives

Examples given in this chapter suggest that mRNA regulation is important in multiple aspects of mammalian biology; however, it is largely unknown how the combinatorial regulation is achieved at the biological complexity of the organisms. Transcriptome-wide mapping of cis-elements and trans-binding sites demonstrates huge regulatory potentials for non-coding parts of mRNA. The more details we learn about cross-talk, molecular assembly, and compartmentalization of RNA-protein complexes, the more unifying principles we may find. Understanding of the factors and elements involved in the regulation of a particular gene expression in a single cell [190] is of paramount importance when designing molecular therapies or when attempting to modulate the expression of a target gene. Thus, scientists and geneticists have exciting opportunities ahead in the field of therapeutic genome editing.

Acknowledgements

This work is supported by University of Minnesota department of Medicine start-up fund to I. V-S. We acknowledge the University of Minnesota Supercomputing Institute for providing the access to Ingenuity Pathway Assistant.

Conflict of interest

None declared.

Abbreviations

3′ UTR	3′ untranslated region
ARE	AU-rich element adenylate(A)- and uridylate(U)-rich element
DMPK	Dystrophia myotonica protein kinase

GRE	GU-rich element, guanidine(G)- and uridylate(U)-rich element
m7GpppN cap	7-Methylguanosine cap
Met-tRNA	Methionine loaded onto transfer RNA
NFkB	Nuclear factor kappa-light chain enhancer of activated B cells
PTBP	Polypyrimidine tract binding protein
RRM	RNA-recognition motif
SRSF1	Serine/arginine-rich splicing factor
UPF1	Up-frameshift protein 1

Author details

Irina Vlasova-St. Louis* and Calandra Sagarsky

*Address all correspondence to: irinastl@umn.edu

Division of Infectious Diseases and International Medicine, Department of Medicine, Program in Infection and Immunity, University of Minnesota, Minneapolis, MN, USA

References

[1] de Klerk E, t Hoen PA. Alternative mRNA transcription, processing, and translation: Insights from RNA sequencing. Trends in Genetics. 2015;**31**(3):128-139

[2] Keene JD. Biological clocks and the coordination theory of RNA operons and regulons. Cold Spring Harbor Symposia on Quantitative Biology. 2007;**72**:157-165

[3] Moroy T, Heyd F. The impact of alternative splicing in vivo: Mouse models show the way. RNA. 2007;**13**(8):1155-1171

[4] Lee JE, Cooper TA. Pathogenic mechanisms of myotonic dystrophy. Biochemical Society Transactions. 2009;**37**(Pt 6):1281-1286

[5] Fabian MR, Sonenberg N, Filipowicz W. Regulation of mRNA translation and stability by microRNAs. Annual Review of Biochemistry. 2010;**79**:351-379

[6] Johnson EL, Robinson DG, Coller HA. Widespread changes in mRNA stability contribute to quiescence-specific gene expression patterns in a fibroblast model of quiescence. BMC Genomics. 2017;**18**(1):123

[7] Cook KB, Hughes TR, Morris QD. High-throughput characterization of protein-RNA interactions. Briefings in Functional Genomics. 2015;**14**(1):74-89

[8] Maeda K, Akira S. Regulation of mRNA stability by CCCH-type zinc-finger proteins in immune cells. International Immunology. 2017;**29**(4):149-155

[9] Chen CY, Xu N, Shyu AB. mRNA decay mediated by two distinct AU-rich elements from c-fos and granulocyte-macrophage colony-stimulating factor transcripts: Different deadenylation kinetics and uncoupling from translation. Molecular and Cellular Biology. 1995;**15**(10):5777-5788

[10] Vlasova IA, McNabb J, Raghavan A, Reilly C, Williams DA, Bohjanen KA, Bohjanen PR. Coordinate stabilization of growth-regulatory transcripts in T cell malignancies. Genomics. 2005;**86**(2):159-171

[11] Vlasova-St Louis I, Bohjanen PR. Coordinate regulation of mRNA decay networks by GU-rich elements and CELF1. Current Opinion in Genetics & Development. 2011;**21**(4): 444-451

[12] Blackinton JG, Keene JD. Functional coordination and HuR-mediated regulation of mRNA stability during T cell activation. Nucleic Acids Research. 2016;**44**(1):426-436

[13] Vlasova IA, Tahoe NM, Fan D, Larsson O, Rattenbacher B, Sternjohn JR, Vasdewani J, Karypis G, Reilly CS, Bitterman PB, Bohjanen PR. Conserved GU-rich elements mediate mRNA decay by binding to CUG-binding protein 1. Molecular Cell. 2008;**29**(2): 263-270

[14] Tenenbaum SA, Carson CC, Lager PJ, Keene JD. Identifying mRNA subsets in messenger ribonucleoprotein complexes by using cDNA arrays. Proceedings of the National Academy of Sciences of the United States of America. 2000;**97**(26):14085-14090

[15] Li YE, Xiao M, Shi B, Yang YT, Wang D, Wang F, Marcia M, Lu ZJ. Identification of high-confidence RNA regulatory elements by combinatorial classification of RNA-protein binding sites. Genome Biology. 2017;**18**(1):169

[16] Singh G, Ricci EP, Moore MJ. RIPiT-Seq: A high-throughput approach for footprinting RNA:Protein complexes. Methods. 2014;**65**(3):320-332

[17] Chi SW, Zang JB, Mele A, Darnell RB. Argonaute HITS-CLIP decodes microRNA-mRNA interaction maps. Nature. 2009;**460**(7254):479-486

[18] Licatalosi DD, Mele A, Fak JJ, Ule J, Kayikci M, Chi SW, Clark TA, Schweitzer AC, Blume JE, Wang X, Darnell JC, Darnell RB. HITS-CLIP yields genome-wide insights into brain alternative RNA processing. Nature. 2008;**456**(7221):464-469

[19] Hafner M, Landthaler M, Burger L, Khorshid M, Hausser J, Berninger P, Rothballer A, Ascano M, Jungkamp AC, Munschauer M, Ulrich A, Wardle GS, Dewell S, Zavolan M, Tuschl T. PAR-CliP – A method to identify transcriptome-wide the binding sites of RNA binding proteins. Journal of Visualized Experiments. 2010;(41)

[20] Keene JD, Komisarow JM, Friedersdorf MB. RIP-Chip: The isolation and identification of mRNAs, microRNAs and protein components of ribonucleoprotein complexes from cell extracts. Nature Protocols. 2006;**1**(1):302-307

[21] Jankowsky E, Harris ME. Mapping specificity landscapes of RNA-protein interactions by high throughput sequencing. Methods. 2017;**118–119**:111–118

[22] Nicholson CO, Friedersdorf MB, Bisogno LS, Keene JD. DO-RIP-seq to quantify RNA binding sites transcriptome-wide. Methods. 2017;**118-119**:16-23

[23] Shaw G, Kamen R, Pillars article: A conserved AU sequence from the 3′ untranslated region of GM-CSF mRNA mediates selective mRNA degradation. Cell. 1986;**46**:659–667, Journal of Immunology. 2012;**189**(1):5–13

[24] Raghavan A, Dhalla M, Bakheet T, Ogilvie RL, Vlasova IA, Khabar KS, Williams BR, Bohjanen PR. Patterns of coordinate down-regulation of ARE-containing transcripts following immune cell activation. Genomics. 2004;**84**(6):1002-1013

[25] Khabar KS, Bakheet T, Williams BR. AU-rich transient response transcripts in the human genome: Expressed sequence tag clustering and gene discovery approach. Genomics. 2005;**85**(2):165-175

[26] Peng SS, Chen CY, Shyu AB. Functional characterization of a non-AUUUA AU-rich element from the c-jun proto-oncogene mRNA: Evidence for a novel class of AU-rich elements. Molecular and Cellular Biology. 1996;**16**(4):1490-1499

[27] Antic D, Keene JD. Embryonic lethal abnormal visual RNA-binding proteins involved in growth, differentiation, and posttranscriptional gene expression. American Journal of Human Genetics. 1997;**61**(2):273-278

[28] Atasoy U, Curry SL, Lopez de Silanes I, Shyu AB, Casolaro V, Gorospe M, Stellato C. Regulation of eotaxin gene expression by TNF-alpha and IL-4 through mRNA stabilization: Involvement of the RNA-binding protein HuR. Journal of Immunology. 2003;**171**(8): 4369-4378

[29] Ogilvie RL, Abelson M, Hau HH, Vlasova I, Blackshear PJ, Bohjanen PR. Tristetraprolin down-regulates IL-2 gene expression through AU-rich element-mediated mRNA decay. Journal of Immunology. 2005;**174**(2):953-961

[30] Khabar KS, Dhalla M, Bakheet T, Sy C, al-Haj L. An integrated computational and laboratory approach for selective amplification of mRNAs containing the adenylate uridylate-rich element consensus sequence. Genome Research. 2002;**12**(6):985-995

[31] Ogilvie RL, Sternjohn JR, Rattenbacher B, Vlasova IA, Williams DA, Hau HH, Blackshear PJ, Bohjanen PR. Tristetraprolin mediates interferon-gamma mRNA decay. The Journal of Biological Chemistry. 2009;**284**(17):11216-11223

[32] Xu N, Chen CY, Shyu AB. Modulation of the fate of cytoplasmic mRNA by AU-rich elements: Key sequence features controlling mRNA deadenylation and decay. Molecular and Cellular Biology. 1997;**17**(8):4611-4621

[33] Bakheet T, Frevel M, Williams BR, Greer W, Khabar KS. ARED: Human AU-rich element-containing mRNA database reveals an unexpectedly diverse functional repertoire of encoded proteins. Nucleic Acids Research. 2001;**29**(1):246-254

[34] Graham R, Kyogoku C, Sigurdsson C, et al. Three functional variants of IFN regulatory factor 5 (IRF5) define risk and protective haplotypes for human lupus. Proceedings of the National Academy of Sciences of the United States of America. 2007;**104**(16):6758–6763

[35] Jacob CO, Hwang F, Lewis GD, Stall AM. Tumor necrosis factor alpha in murine systemic lupus erythematosus disease models: Implications for genetic predisposition and immune regulation. Cytokine. 1991;**3**(6):551-561

[36] Hodge DL, Berthet C, Coppola V, Kastenmuller W, Buschman MD, Schaughency PM, Shirota H, Scarzello AJ, Subleski JJ, Anver MR, Ortaldo JR, Lin F, Reynolds DA, Sanford ME, Kaldis P, Tessarollo L, Klinman DM, Young HA. IFN-gamma AU-rich element removal promotes chronic IFN-gamma expression and autoimmunity in mice. Journal of Autoimmunity. 2014;**53**:33-45

[37] Tebo J, Der S, Frevel M, Khabar KS, Williams BR, Hamilton TA. Heterogeneity in control of mRNA stability by AU-rich elements. Journal of Biological Chemistry. 2003;**278**(14): 12085-12093

[38] Al-Ahmadi W, Al-Ghamdi M, Al-Haj L, Al-Saif M, Khabar KS. Alternative polyadenylation variants of the RNA binding protein, HuR: Abundance, role of AU-rich elements and autoregulation. Nucleic Acids Research. 2009;**37**(11):3612-3624

[39] Lebedeva S, Jens M, Theil K, Schwanhausser B, Selbach M, Landthaler M, Rajewsky N. Transcriptome-wide analysis of regulatory interactions of the RNA-binding protein HuR. Molecular Cell. 2011;**43**(3):340-352

[40] Mukherjee N, Corcoran DL, Nusbaum JD, Reid DW, Georgiev S, Hafner M, Ascano M Jr, Tuschl T, Ohler U, Keene JD. Integrative regulatory mapping indicates that the RNA-binding protein HuR couples pre-mRNA processing and mRNA stability. Molecular Cell. 2011;**43**(3):327-339

[41] Yoon JH, De S, Srikantan S, Abdelmohsen K, Grammatikakis I, Kim J, Kim KM, Noh JH, White EJ, Martindale JL, Yang X, Kang MJ, Wood WH, 3rd, Noren Hooten N, Evans MK, Becker KG, Tripathi V, Prasanth KV, Wilson GM, Tuschl T, Ingolia NT, Hafner M, Gorospe M. PAR-CLIP analysis uncovers AUF1 impact on target RNA fate and genome integrity. Nature Communications. 2014;**5**:5248

[42] Vogel KU, Bell LS, Galloway A, Ahlfors H, Turner M. The RNA-binding proteins Zfp36l1 and Zfp36l2 enforce the thymic beta-selection checkpoint by limiting DNA damage response signaling and cell cycle progression. Journal of Immunology. 2016; **197**(7):2673-2685

[43] Vlasova-St Louis I, Bohjanen PR. Post-transcriptional regulation of cytokine signaling by AU-rich and GU-rich elements. Journal of Interferon & Cytokine Research. 2014;**34**(4): 233-241

[44] Vlasova-St Louis I, Bohjanen PR. Post-transcriptional regulation of cytokine and growth factor signaling in cancer. Cytokine & Growth Factor Reviews. 2017;**33**:83-93

[45] Kumagai Y, Vandenbon A, Teraguchi S, Akira S, Suzuki Y. Genome-wide map of RNA degradation kinetics patterns in dendritic cells after LPS stimulation facilitates identification of primary sequence and secondary structure motifs in mRNAs. BMC Genomics. 2016;**17**(Suppl 13):1032

[46] Vlasova IA, Bohjanen PR. Posttranscriptional regulation of gene networks by GU-rich elements and CELF proteins. RNA Biology. 2008;**5**(4):201-207

[47] Halees AS, Hitti E, Al-Saif M, Mahmoud L, Vlasova-St Louis IA, Beisang DJ, Bohjanen PR, Khabar K. Global assessment of GU-rich regulatory content and function in the human transcriptome. RNA Biology. 2011;**8**(4):681-691

[48] Rattenbacher B, Beisang D, Wiesner DL, Jeschke JC, von Hohenberg M, St Louis-Vlasova IA, Bohjanen PR. Analysis of CUGBP1 targets identifies GU-repeat sequences that mediate rapid mRNA decay, Molecular and Cellular Biology 2010;**30**(16):3970–3980

[49] Beisang D, Bohjanen P, Vlasova-St Louis I. CELF1, a multifunctional regulator of post-transcriptional networks. In: Abdelmohsen K, editor. Binding Protein. Croatia: InTech; 2012. pp. 181-206

[50] Le Tonqueze O, Gschloessl B, Namanda-Vanderbeken A, Legagneux V, Paillard L, Audic Y. Chromosome wide analysis of CUGBP1 binding sites identifies the tetraspanin CD9 mRNA as a target for CUGBP1-mediated down-regulation. Biochemical and Biophysical Research Communications. 2010;**394**(4):884-889

[51] Russo J, Lee JE, Lopez CM, Anderson J, Nguyen TP, Heck AM, Wilusz J, Wilusz CJ. The CELF1 RNA-binding protein regulates decay of signal recognition particle mRNAs and limits secretion in mouse myoblasts. PLoS One. 2017;**12**(1):e0170680

[52] Mori D, Sasagawa N, Kino Y, Ishiura S. Quantitative analysis of CUG-BP1 binding to RNA repeats. Journal of Biochemistry. 2008;**143**(3):377-383

[53] Marquis J, Paillard L, Audic Y, Cosson B, Danos O, Le Bec C, Osborne HB. CUG-BP1/CELF1 requires UGU-rich sequences for high-affinity binding. The Biochemical Journal. 2006;**400**(2):291-301

[54] Takahashi N, Sasagawa N, Suzuki K, Ishiura S. The CUG-binding protein binds specifically to UG dinucleotide repeats in a yeast three-hybrid system. Biochemical and Biophysical Research Communications. 2000;**277**(2):518-523

[55] Tollervey JR, Curk T, Rogelj B, Briese M, Cereda M, Kayikci M, Konig J, Hortobagyi T, Nishimura AL, Zupunski V, Patani R, Chandran S, Rot G, Zupan B, Shaw CE, Ule J. Characterizing the RNA targets and position-dependent splicing regulation by TDP-43. Nature Neuroscience. 2011;**14**(4):452-458

[56] Takeda JI, Masuda A, Ohno K. Six GU-rich (6GUR) FUS-binding motifs detected by normalization of CLIP-seq by nascent-seq. Gene. 2017;**618**:57-64

[57] Afroz T, Cienikova Z, Clery A, Allain FH. One, two, three, four! How multiple RRMs read the genome sequence. Methods in Enzymology. 2015;**558**:235-278

[58] Lee JE, Lee JY, Wilusz J, Tian B, Wilusz CJ. Systematic analysis of cis-elements in unstable mRNAs demonstrates that CUGBP1 is a key regulator of mRNA decay in muscle cells. PLoS One. 2010;**5**(6):e11201

[59] Beisang D, Rattenbacher B, Vlasova-St Louis IA, Bohjanen PR. Regulation of CUG-binding protein 1 (CUGBP1) binding to target transcripts upon T cell activation. The Journal of Biological Chemistry. 2012;**287**(2):950-960

[60] Bhardwaj A, Myers MP, Buratti E, Baralle FE. Characterizing TDP-43 interaction with its RNA targets. Nucleic Acids Research. 2013;**41**(9):5062-5074

[61] Bohjanen PR, Moua ML, Guo L, Taye A, Vlasova-St Louis IA. Altered CELF1 binding to target transcripts in malignant T cells. RNA. 2015;**21**(10):1757-1769

[62] Dembowski JA, Grabowski PJ. The CUGBP2 splicing factor regulates an ensemble of branchpoints from perimeter binding sites with implications for autoregulation. PLoS Genetics. 2009;**5**(8):e1000595

[63] Vlasova-St Louis I, Dickson AM, Bohjanen PR, Wilusz CJ. CELFish ways to modulate mRNA decay. Biochimica Et Biophysica Acta-Gene Regulatory Mechanisms. 2013; **1829**(6–7):695-707

[64] Daughters RS, Tuttle DL, Gao W, Ikeda Y, Moseley ML, Ebner TJ, Swanson MS, Ranum LP. RNA gain-of-function in spinocerebellar ataxia type 8. PLoS Genetics. 2009;**5**(8):e1000600

[65] Le Tonqueze O, Gschloessl B, Legagneux V, Paillard L, Audic Y. Identification of CELF1 RNA targets by CLIP-seq in human HeLa cells. Genomics Data. 2016;**8**:97-103

[66] Wang ET, Ward AJ, Cherone JM, Giudice J, Wang TT, Treacy DJ, Lambert NJ, Freese P, Saxena T, Cooper TA, Burge CB. Antagonistic regulation of mRNA expression and splicing by CELF and MBNL proteins. Genome Research. 2015;**25**(6):858-871

[67] Masuda A, Andersen HS, Doktor TK, Okamoto T, Ito M, Andresen BS, Ohno K. CUGBP1 and MBNL1 preferentially bind to 3′ UTRs and facilitate mRNA decay. Scientific Reports. 2012;**2**:209

[68] Pan Q, Shai O, Lee LJ, Frey BJ, Blencowe BJ. Deep surveying of alternative splicing complexity in the human transcriptome by high-throughput sequencing. Nature Genetics. 2008;**40**(12):1413-1415

[69] Wang ET, Sandberg R, Luo S, Khrebtukova I, Zhang L, Mayr C, Kingsmore SF, Schroth GP, Burge CB. Alternative isoform regulation in human tissue transcriptomes. Nature. 2008; **456**(7221):470-476

[70] Ladd AN, Cooper TA. Finding signals that regulate alternative splicing in the post-genomic era. Genome Biology. 2002;**3**(11):reviews0008

[71] Voelker RB, Berglund JA. A comprehensive computational characterization of conserved mammalian intronic sequences reveals conserved motifs associated with constitutive and alternative splicing. Genome Research. 2007;**17**(7):1023-1033

[72] Hu J, Lutz CS, Wilusz J, Tian B. Bioinformatic identification of candidate cis-regulatory elements involved in human mRNA polyadenylation. RNA. 2005;**11**(10):1485-1493

[73] Tian B, Hu J, Zhang H, Lutz CS. A large-scale analysis of mRNA polyadenylation of human and mouse genes. Nucleic Acids Research. 2005;**33**(1):201-212

[74] Bakheet T, Williams BR, Khabar KS. ARED 2.0: An update of AU-rich element mRNA database. Nucleic Acids Research. 2003;**31**(1):421-423

[75] Bakheet T, Williams BR, Khabar KS. ARED 3.0: The large and diverse AU-rich transcriptome. Nucleic Acids Research. 2006;**34**(Database issue):D111-D114

[76] Vlasova-St Louis I, Bohjanen PR. Feedback regulation of kinase Signaling pathways by AREs and GREs. Cell. 2016;**5**(1):1-14

[77] Fallmann J, Sedlyarov V, Tanzer A, Kovarik P, Hofacker IL. AREsite2: An enhanced database for the comprehensive investigation of AU/GU/U-rich elements. Nucleic Acids Research. 2016;**44**(D1):D90-D95

[78] Hitti E, Bakheet T, Al-Souhibani N, Moghrabi W, Al-Yahya S, Al-Ghamdi M, Al-Saif M, Shoukri MM, Lanczky A, Grepin R, Gyorffy B, Pages G, Khabar KS. Systematic analysis of AU-rich element expression in cancer reveals common functional clusters regulated by key RNA-binding proteins. Cancer Research. 2016;**76**(14):4068-4080

[79] Ohno K, Takeda JI, Masuda A. Rules and tools to predict the splicing effects of exonic and intronic mutations. Wiley Interdiscip Rev RNA. 2017. [Epub ahead of print]

[80] Chaudhury A, Cheema S, Fachini JM, Kongchan N, Lu G, Simon LM, Wang T, Mao S, Rosen DG, Ittmann MM, Hilsenbeck SG, Shaw CA, Neilson JR. CELF1 is a central node in post-transcriptional regulatory programmes underlying EMT. Nature Communications. 2016;**7**:13362

[81] Sandberg R, Neilson JR, Sarma A, Sharp PA, Burge CB. Proliferating cells express mRNAs with shortened 3′ untranslated regions and fewer microRNA target sites. Science. 2008;**320**(5883):1643-1647

[82] Chen CY, Shyu AB. Mechanisms of deadenylation-dependent decay. Wiley Interdisciplinary Reviews RNA. 2011;**2**(2):167-183

[83] Beisang D, Reilly C, Bohjanen PR. Alternative polyadenylation regulates CELF1/CUGBP1 target transcripts following T cell activation. Gene. 2014;**550**(1):93-100

[84] Mayr C. Evolution and biological roles of alternative 3' UTRs. Trends in Cell Biology. 2016;**26**(3):227-237

[85] Weng L, Li Y, Xie X, Shi Y. Poly(A) code analyses reveal key determinants for tissue-specific mRNA alternative polyadenylation. RNA. 2016;**22**(6):813-821

[86] Mayr C, Bartel DP. Widespread shortening of 3' UTRs by alternative cleavage and polyadenylation activates oncogenes in cancer cells. Cell. 2009;**138**(4):673-684

[87] Xiao MS, Zhang B, Li YS, Gao Q, Sun W, Chen W. Global analysis of regulatory divergence in the evolution of mouse alternative polyadenylation. Molecular Systems Biology. 2016;**12**(12):890

[88] Hoque M, Ji Z, Zheng D, Luo W, Li W, You B, Park JY, Yehia G, Tian B. Analysis of alternative cleavage and polyadenylation by 3′ region extraction and deep sequencing. Nature Methods. 2013;**10**(2):133-139

[89] Neve J, Patel R, Wang Z, Louey A, Furger AM. Cleavage and polyadenylation: Ending the message expands gene regulation. RNA Biology. 2017;**14**(7):865-890

[90] Phillips C, Pachikara N, Gunderson SI. U1A inhibits cleavage at the immunoglobulin M heavy-chain secretory poly(A) site by binding between the two downstream GU-rich regions. Molecular and Cellular Biology. 2004;**24**(14):6162-6171

[91] Li XQ, Du D. Motif types, motif locations and base composition patterns around the RNA polyadenylation site in microorganisms, plants and animals. BMC Evolutionary Biology. 2014;**14**:162

[92] Nazim M, Masuda A, Rahman MA, Nasrin F, Takeda JI, Ohe K, Ohkawara B, Ito M, Ohno K. Competitive regulation of alternative splicing and alternative polyadenylation by hnRNP H and CstF64 determines acetylcholinesterase isoforms. Nucleic Acids Research. 2017;**45**(3):1455-1468

[93] Yao C, Biesinger J, Wan J, Weng L, Xing Y, Xie X, Shi Y. Transcriptome-wide analyses of CstF64-RNA interactions in global regulation of mRNA alternative polyadenylation. Proceedings of the National Academy of Sciences of the United States of America. 2012;**109**(46):18773-18778

[94] Batra R, Charizanis K, Manchanda M, Mohan A, Li M, Finn DJ, Goodwin M, Zhang C, Sobczak K, Thornton CA, Swanson MS. Loss of MBNL leads to disruption of developmentally regulated alternative polyadenylation in RNA-mediated disease. Molecular Cell. 2014;**56**(2):311-322

[95] Huang C, Shi J, Guo Y, Huang W, Huang S, Ming S, Wu X, Zhang R, Ding J, Zhao W, Jia J, Huang X, Xiang AP, Shi Y, Yao C. A snoRNA modulates mRNA 3′ end processing and regulates the expression of a subset of mRNAs. Nucleic Acids Research. 2017;**45**(15):8647-8660

[96] Charlesworth A, Meijer HA, de Moor CH. Specificity factors in cytoplasmic polyadenylation, Wiley Interdisciplinary Reviews: RNA. 2013;**4**(4):437-461

[97] Shi Y, Manley JL. The end of the message: Multiple protein-RNA interactions define the mRNA polyadenylation site. Genes & Development. 2015;**29**(9):889-897

[98] Li W, Li W, Laishram RS, Hoque M, Ji Z, Tian B, Anderson RA. Distinct regulation of alternative polyadenylation and gene expression by nuclear poly(A) polymerases. Nucleic Acids Research. 2017;**45**(15):8930-8942

[99] Kashiwabara S, Nakanishi T, Kimura M, Baba T. Non-canonical poly(A) polymerase in mammalian gametogenesis. Biochimica et Biophysica Acta. 2008;**1779**(4):230-238

[100] Wang H, Li R, Zhou X, Xue L, Xu X, Liu B. Genome-wide analysis and functional characterization of the polyadenylation site in pigs using RNAseq data. Scientific Reports. 2016;**6**:36388

[101] Curinha A, Oliveira Braz S, Pereira-Castro I, Cruz A, Moreira A. Implications of polyadenylation in health and disease. Nucleus. 2014;**5**(6):508-519

[102] Tsuda K, Kuwasako K, Nagata T, Takahashi M, Kigawa T, Kobayashi N, Guntert P, Shirouzu M, Yokoyama S, Muto Y. Novel RNA recognition motif domain in the cytoplasmic polyadenylation element binding protein 3. Proteins. 2014;**82**(10):2879-2886

[103] Maillo C, Martin J, Sebastian D, Hernandez-Alvarez M, Garcia-Rocha M, Reina O, Zorzano A, Fernandez M, Mendez R. Circadian- and UPR-dependent control of CPEB4 mediates a translational response to counteract hepatic steatosis under ER stress. Nature Cell Biology. 2017;**19**(2):94-105

[104] Keller RW, Kuhn U, Aragon M, Bornikova L, Wahle E, Bear DG. The nuclear poly(A) binding protein, PABP2, forms an oligomeric particle covering the length of the poly(A) tail. Journal of Molecular Biology. 2000;**297**(3):569-583

[105] Kini HK, Silverman IM, Ji X, Gregory BD, Liebhaber SA. Cytoplasmic poly(A) binding protein-1 binds to genomically encoded sequences within mammalian mRNAs. RNA. 2016;**22**(1):61-74

[106] Wilkening S, Pelechano V, Steinmetz LM. Genome-wide identification of alternative polyadenylation events using 3'T-fill. Methods in Molecular Biology. 2016;**1358**:295-302

[107] Zheng D, Liu X, Tian B. 3'READS+, a sensitive and accurate method for 3′ end sequencing of polyadenylated RNA. RNA. 2016;**22**(10):1631-1639

[108] Subtelny AO, Eichhorn SW, Chen GR, Sive H, Bartel DP. Poly(A)-tail profiling reveals an embryonic switch in translational control. Nature. 2014;**508**(7494):66-71

[109] Park JE, Yi H, Kim Y, Chang H, Kim VN. Regulation of poly(A) tail and translation during the somatic cell cycle. Molecular Cell. 2016;**62**(3):462-471

[110] Yang Q, Allard P, Huang M, Zhang W, Clarke HJ. Proteasomal activity is required to initiate and to sustain translational activation of messenger RNA encoding the stem-loop-binding protein during meiotic maturation in mice. Biology of Reproduction. 2010; **82**(1):123-131

[111] Konig J, Zarnack K, Rot G, Curk T, Kayikci M, Zupan B, Turner DJ, Luscombe NM, Ule J. iCLIP reveals the function of hnRNP particles in splicing at individual nucleotide resolution. Nature Structural & Molecular Biology. 2010;**17**(7):909-915

[112] Zhu H, Zhou HL, Hasman RA, Lou H. Hu proteins regulate polyadenylation by blocking sites containing U-rich sequences. The Journal of Biological Chemistry. 2007; **282**(4):2203-2210

[113] Lim J, Ha M, Chang H, Kwon SC, Simanshu DK, Patel DJ, Kim VN. Uridylation by TUT4 and TUT7 marks mRNA for degradation. Cell. 2014;**159**(6):1365-1376

[114] Chang H, Lim J, Ha M, Kim VN. TAIL-seq: Genome-wide determination of poly(A) tail length and 3′ end modifications. Molecular Cell. 2014;**53**(6):1044-1052

[115] Morgan M, Much C, DiGiacomo M, Azzi C, Ivanova I, Vitsios DM, Pistolic J, Collier P, Moreira PN, Benes V, Enright AJ, O'Carroll D. mRNA 3′ uridylation and poly(A) tail length sculpt the mammalian maternal transcriptome. Nature. 2017;**548**(7667):347-351

[116] Saha S, Chakraborty A, Bandyopadhyay SS. Stabilization of oncostatin-M mRNA by binding of nucleolin to a GC-rich element in its 3'UTR. Journal of Cellular Biochemistry. 2016;**117**(4):988-999

[117] Chakraborty A, Mukherjee S, Saha S, De S, Sengupta Bandyopadhyay S. Phorbol-12-myristate-13-acetate-mediated stabilization of leukemia inhibitory factor (lif) mRNA: Involvement of Nucleolin and PCBP1. The Biochemical Journal. 2017;**474**(14):2349-2363

[118] Mendenhall EM, Koche RP, Truong T, Zhou VW, Issac B, Chi AS, Ku M, Bernstein BE. GC-rich sequence elements recruit PRC2 in mammalian ES cells. PLoS Genetics. 2010;**6**(12): e1001244

[119] Cho SJ, Jung YS, Chen X. Poly (C)-binding protein 1 regulates p63 expression through mRNA stability. PLoS One. 2013;**8**(8):e71724

[120] Xue Y, Zhou Y, Wu T, Zhu T, Ji X, Kwon YS, Zhang C, Yeo G, Black DL, Sun H, Fu XD, Zhang Y. Genome-wide analysis of PTB-RNA interactions reveals a strategy used by the general splicing repressor to modulate exon inclusion or skipping. Molecular Cell. 2009;**36**(6):996-1006

[121] Hwang CK, Wagley Y, Law PY, Wei LN, Loh HH. Phosphorylation of poly(rC) binding protein 1 (PCBP1) contributes to stabilization of mu opioid receptor (MOR) mRNA via interaction with AU-rich element RNA-binding protein 1 (AUF1) and poly a binding protein (PABP). Gene. 2017;**598**:113-130

[122] Kearse MG, Green KM, Krans A, Rodriguez CM, Linsalata AE, Goldstrohm AC, Todd PK. CGG repeat-associated non-AUG translation utilizes a cap-dependent scanning mechanism of initiation to produce toxic proteins. Molecular Cell. 2016;**62**(2):314-322

[123] Harkness RWt, Mittermaier AK. G-quadruplex dynamics. Biochimica et Biophysica Acta. 2017;**1865**(11):1544-1554

[124] Varizhuk A, Ischenko D, Tsvetkov V, Novikov R, Kulemin N, Kaluzhny D, Vlasenok M, Naumov V, Smirnov I, Pozmogova G. The expanding repertoire of G4 DNA structures. Biochimie. 2017;**135**:54-62

[125] Bolduc F, Garant JM, Allard F, Perreault JP. Irregular G-quadruplexes found in the untranslated regions of human mRNAs influence translation. The Journal of Biological Chemistry. 2016;**291**(41):21751-21760

[126] Ishiguro A, Kimura N, Watanabe Y, Watanabe S, Ishihama A. TDP-43 binds and transports G-quadruplex-containing mRNAs into neurites for local translation. Genes to Cells. 2016;**21**(5):466-481

[127] Fay MM, Lyons SM, Ivanov P. RNA G-Quadruplexes in biology: Principles and molecular mechanisms. Journal of Molecular Biology. 2017;**429**(14):2127-2147

[128] Kwok CK, Merrick CJ. G-Quadruplexes: Prediction, characterization, and biological application. Trends in Biotechnology. 2017

[129] Zheng KW, Xiao S, Liu JQ, Zhang JY, Hao YH, Tan Z. Co-transcriptional formation of DNA:RNA hybrid G-quadruplex and potential function as constitutional cis element for transcription control. Nucleic Acids Research. 2013;**41**(10):5533-5541

[130] Rouleau S, Glouzon JS, Brumwell A, Bisaillon M, Perreault JP. 3′ UTR G-quadruplexes regulate miRNA binding. RNA. 2017;**23**(8):1172-1179

[131] Lacerda R, Menezes J, Romao L. More than just scanning: The importance of cap-independent mRNA translation initiation for cellular stress response and cancer. Cellular and Molecular Life Sciences. 2017;**74**(9):1659-1680

[132] Wu TY, Hsieh CC, Hong JJ, Chen CY, Tsai YS. IRSS: A web-based tool for automatic layout and analysis of IRES secondary structure prediction and searching system in silico. BMC Bioinformatics. 2009;**10**:160

[133] Baird SD, Turcotte M, Korneluk RG, Holcik M. Searching for IRES. RNA. 2006;**12**(10):1755-1785

[134] Weingarten-Gabbay S, Elias-Kirma S, Nir R, Gritsenko AA, Stern-Ginossar N, Yakhini Z, Weinberger A, Segal E, Comparative g. Systematic discovery of cap-independent translation sequences in human and viral genomes. Science. 2016;**351**(6270):240-249

[135] Gritsenko AA, Weingarten-Gabbay S, Elias-Kirma S, Nir R, de Ridder D, Segal E. Sequence features of viral and human internal ribosome entry sites predictive of their activity, PLoS Computational Biology 2017;**13**(9):e1005734

[136] Terenin IM, Smirnova VV, Andreev DE, Dmitriev SE, Shatsky IN. A researcher's guide to the galaxy of IRESs. Cellular and Molecular Life Sciences. 2017;**74**(8):1431-1455

[137] Miles WO, Korenjak M, Griffiths LM, Dyer MA, Provero P, Dyson NJ. Post-transcriptional gene expression control by NANOS is up-regulated and functionally important in pRb-deficient cells. The EMBO Journal. 2014;**33**(19):2201-2215

[138] Morris AR, Mukherjee N, Keene JD. Ribonomic analysis of human Pum1 reveals cis-trans conservation across species despite evolution of diverse mRNA target sets. Molecular and Cellular Biology. 2008;**28**(12):4093-4103

[139] Galgano A, Forrer M, Jaskiewicz L, Kanitz A, Zavolan M, Gerber AP. Comparative analysis of mRNA targets for human PUF-family proteins suggests extensive interaction with the miRNA regulatory system. PLoS One. 2008;**3**(9):e3164

[140] Van Etten J, Schagat TL, Hrit J, Weidmann CA, Brumbaugh J, Coon JJ, Goldstrohm AC. Human Pumilio proteins recruit multiple deadenylases to efficiently repress messenger RNAs. The Journal of Biological Chemistry. 2012;**287**(43):36370-36383

[141] Geissler R, Grimson A. A position-specific 3'UTR sequence that accelerates mRNA decay. RNA Biology. 2016;**13**(11):1075-1077

[142] Wissink EM, Fogarty EA, Grimson A. High-throughput discovery of post-transcriptional cis-regulatory elements. BMC Genomics. 2016;**17**:177

[143] Hui J, Hung LH, Heiner M, Schreiner S, Neumuller N, Reither G, Haas SA, Bindereif A. Intronic CA-repeat and CA-rich elements: A new class of regulators of mammalian alternative splicing. The EMBO Journal. 2005;**24**(11):1988-1998

[144] Cereda M, Pozzoli U, Rot G, Juvan P, Schweitzer A, Clark T, Ule J. RNAmotifs: Prediction of multivalent RNA motifs that control alternative splicing. Genome Biology. 2014;**15**(1):R20

[145] Wainberg M, Alipanahi B, Frey B. Does conservation account for splicing patterns? BMC Genomics. 2016;**17**(1):787

[146] Samatanga B, Clery A, Barraud P, Allain FH, Jelesarov I. Comparative analyses of the thermodynamic RNA binding signatures of different types of RNA recognition motifs. Nucleic Acids Research. 2017;**45**(10):6037-6050

[147] Rogelj B, Easton LE, Bogu GK, Stanton LW, Rot G, Curk T, Zupan B, Sugimoto Y, Modic M, Haberman N, Tollervey J, Fujii R, Takumi T, Shaw CE, Ule J. Widespread binding of FUS along nascent RNA regulates alternative splicing in the brain. Scientific Reports. 2012;**2**:603

[148] Barbosa-Morais NL, Irimia M, Pan Q, Xiong HY, Gueroussov S, Lee LJ, Slobodeniuc V, Kutter C, Watt S, Colak R, Kim T, Misquitta-Ali CM, Wilson MD, Kim PM, Odom DT, Frey BJ, Blencowe BJ. The evolutionary landscape of alternative splicing in vertebrate species. Science. 2012;**338**(6114):1587-1593

[149] Ciafre SA, Galardi S. microRNAs and RNA-binding proteins: A complex network of interactions and reciprocal regulations in cancer. RNA Biology. 2013;**10**(6):935-942

[150] Jens M, Rajewsky N. Competition between target sites of regulators shapes post-transcriptional gene regulation. Nature Reviews. Genetics. 2015;**16**(2):113-126

[151] Jacobsen A, Wen J, Marks DS, Krogh A. Signatures of RNA binding proteins globally coupled to effective microRNA target sites. Genome Research. 2010;**20**(8):1010-1019

[152] Katoh T, Hojo H, Suzuki T. Destabilization of microRNAs in human cells by 3′ deadenylation mediated by PARN and CUGBP1. Nucleic Acids Research. 2015;**43**(15):7521-7534

[153] Oh M, Rhee S, Moon JH, Chae H, Lee S, Kang J, Kim S. Literature-based condition-specific miRNA-mRNA target prediction. PLoS One. 2017;**12**(3):e0174999

[154] Grimson A, Farh KK, Johnston WK, Garrett-Engele P, Lim LP, Bartel DP. MicroRNA targeting specificity in mammals: Determinants beyond seed pairing. Molecular Cell. 2007;**27**(1):91-105

[155] Van Peer G, De Paepe A, Stock M, Anckaert J, Volders PJ, Vandesompele J, De Baets B, Waegeman W. miSTAR: miRNA target prediction through modeling quantitative and qualitative miRNA binding site information in a stacked model structure. Nucleic Acids Research. 2017;**45**(7):e51

[156] Perbellini R, Greco S, Sarra-Ferraris G, Cardani R, Capogrossi MC, Meola G, Martelli F. Dysregulation and cellular mislocalization of specific miRNAs in myotonic dystrophy type 1. Neuromuscular Disorders. 2011;**21**(2):81-88

[157] Gambardella S, Rinaldi F, Lepore SM, Viola A, Loro E, Angelini C, Vergani L, Novelli G, Botta A. Overexpression of microRNA-206 in the skeletal muscle from myotonic dystrophy type 1 patients. Journal of Translational Medicine. 2010;**8**:48

[158] Rau F, Freyermuth F, Fugier C, Villemin JP, Fischer MC, Jost B, Dembele D, Gourdon G, Nicole A, Duboc D, Wahbi K, Day JW, Fujimura H, Takahashi MP, Auboeuf D, Dreumont N, Furling D, Charlet-Berguerand N. Misregulation of miR-1 processing is associated with heart defects in myotonic dystrophy. Nature Structural & Molecular Biology. 2011;**18**(7):840-845

[159] Erhard F, Dolken L, Jaskiewicz L, Zimmer R. PARma: Identification of microRNA target sites in AGO-PAR-CLIP data. Genome Biology. 2013;**14**(7):R79

[160] Derti A, Garrett-Engele P, Macisaac KD, Stevens RC, Sriram S, Chen R, Rohl CA, Johnson JM, Babak T. A quantitative atlas of polyadenylation in five mammals. Genome Research. 2012;**22**(6):1173-1183

[161] De S, Gorospe M. Bioinformatic tools for analysis of CLIP ribonucleoprotein data. Wiley Interdisciplinary Reviews RNA. 2017;**8**(4):1-14

[162] Jansen A, Gemayel R, Verstrepen KJ. Unstable microsatellite repeats facilitate rapid evolution of coding and regulatory sequences. Genome Dynamics. 2012;**7**:108-125

[163] Goodwin M, Swanson MS. RNA-binding protein misregulation in microsatellite expansion disorders. Advances in Experimental Medicine and Biology. 2014;**825**:353-388

[164] Ayhan F, Ikeda Y, Dalton JC, Day JW, Ranum LPW. Spinocerebellar ataxia type 8. In: Pagon RA, Adam MP, Ardinger HH, Wallace SE, Amemiya A, Bean LJH, Bird TD, Ledbetter N, Mefford HC, Smith RJH, Stephens K, editors. GeneReviews(R). Seattle: University of Washington; 1993. University of Washington, Seattle. GeneReviews is a registered trademark of the University of Washington, Seattle. All rights reserved, Seattle (WA)

[165] Meola G, Cardani R. Myotonic dystrophies: An update on clinical aspects, genetic, pathology, and molecular pathomechanisms. Biochimica et Biophysica Acta. 2015;**1852**(4):594-606

[166] Donnelly CJ, Zhang PW, Pham JT, Haeusler AR, Mistry NA, Vidensky S, Daley EL, Poth EM, Hoover B, Fines DM, Maragakis N, Tienari PJ, Petrucelli L, Traynor BJ, Wang J,

Rigo F, Bennett CF, Blackshaw S, Sattler R, Rothstein JD. RNA toxicity from the ALS/FTD C9ORF72 expansion is mitigated by antisense intervention. Neuron. 2013;**80**(2):415-428

[167] Banez-Coronel M, Ayhan F, Tarabochia AD, Zu T, Perez BA, Tusi SK, Pletnikova O, Borchelt DR, Ross CA, Margolis RL, Yachnis AT, Troncoso JC, Ranum LP. RAN translation in Huntington disease. Neuron. 2015;**88**(4):667-677

[168] Kong HE, Zhao J, Xu S, Jin P, Jin Y. Fragile X-associated tremor/ataxia syndrome: From molecular pathogenesis to development of therapeutics. Frontiers in Cellular Neuroscience. 2017;**11**:128

[169] Green KM, Linsalata AE, Todd PK. RAN translation-what makes it run? Brain Research. 2016;**1647**:30-42

[170] Cleary JD, Ranum LP. Repeat associated non-ATG (RAN) translation: New starts in microsatellite expansion disorders. Current Opinion in Genetics & Development. 2014;**26**:6-15

[171] Singh RK, Cooper TA. Pre-mRNA splicing in disease and therapeutics. Trends in Molecular Medicine. 2012;**18**(8):472-482

[172] van Agtmaal EL, Andre LM, Willemse M, Cumming SA, van Kessel IDG, van den Broek W, Gourdon G, Furling D, Mouly V, Monckton DG, Wansink DG, Wieringa B. CRISPR/Cas9-induced (CTGCAG)n repeat instability in the myotonic dystrophy type 1 locus: Implications for therapeutic genome editing, Molecular Therapy. 2017;**25**(1):24–43

[173] Popp MW, Maquat LE. Leveraging rules of nonsense-mediated mRNA decay for genome engineering and personalized medicine. Cell. 2016;**165**(6):1319-1322

[174] Turner M, Hodson D. Regulation of lymphocyte development and function by RNA-binding proteins. Current Opinion in Immunology. 2012;**24**(2):160-165

[175] Dassi E, Re A, Leo S, Tebaldi T, Pasini L, Peroni D, Quattrone A. AURA 2: Empowering discovery of post-transcriptional networks. Translation (Austin). 2014;**2**(1):e27738

[176] Keene JD. RNA regulons: Coordination of post-transcriptional events. Nature Reviews. Genetics. 2007;**8**(7):533-543

[177] Padgett RA. New connections between splicing and human disease. Trends in Genetics. 2012;**28**(4):147-154

[178] Babendure JR, Babendure JL, Ding JH, Tsien RY. Control of mammalian translation by mRNA structure near caps. RNA. 2006;**12**(5):851-861

[179] Wu B, Eliscovich C, Yoon YJ, Singer RH. Translation dynamics of single mRNAs in live cells and neurons. Science. 2016;**352**(6292):1430-1435

[180] Morisaki T, Lyon K, DeLuca KF, DeLuca JG, English BP, Zhang Z, Lavis LD, Grimm JB, Viswanathan S, Looger LL, Lionnet T, Stasevich TJ. Real-time quantification of single RNA translation dynamics in living cells. Science. 2016;**352**(6292):1425-1429

[181] Wang C, Han B, Zhou R, Zhuang X. Real-time imaging of translation on single mRNA transcripts in live cells. Cell. 2016;**165**(4):990-1001

[182] Shirokikh NE, Archer SK, Beilharz TH, Powell D, Preiss T. Translation complex profile sequencing to study the in vivo dynamics of mRNA-ribosome interactions during translation initiation, elongation and termination. Nature Protocols. 2017;**12**(4): 697-731

[183] Song J, Perreault JP, Topisirovic I, Richard S. RNA G-quadruplexes and their potential regulatory roles in translation. Translation (Austin). 2016;**4**(2):e1244031

[184] Kishore S, Jaskiewicz L, Burger L, Hausser J, Khorshid M, Zavolan M. A quantitative analysis of CLIP methods for identifying binding sites of RNA-binding proteins. Nature Methods. 2011;**8**(7):559-564

[185] Chen W, Hu XT, Shi QL, Zhang FB, He C. Silencing of Adrm1 by RNA interference suppresses proliferation of colorectal cancer cells. Zhonghua Zhong Liu Za Zhi. 2009; **31**(11):815-819

[186] Hafner M, Landthaler M, Burger L, Khorshid M, Hausser J, Berninger P, Rothballer A, Ascano Jr M, Jungkamp AC, Munschauer M, Ulrich A, Wardle GD, Dewell S, Zavolan M, Tuschl T. Transcriptome-wide identification of RNA-binding protein and microRNA target sites by PAR-CLIP. Cell. 2010;**141**(1):129–141

[187] Liu C, Rennie WA, Carmack CS, Kanoria S, Cheng J, Lu J, Ding Y. Effects of genetic variations on microRNA: Target interactions. Nucleic Acids Research. 2014;**42**(15):9543-9552

[188] Seok H, Ham J, Jang ES, Chi SW. MicroRNA target recognition: Insights from transcriptome-wide non-canonical interactions. Molecules and Cells. 2016;**39**(5):375-381

[189] Broughton JP, Pasquinelli AE. A tale of two sequences: MicroRNA-target chimeric reads. Genetics, Selection, Evolution. 2016;**48**:31

[190] Lemus-Diaz N, Boker KO, Rodriguez-Polo I, Mitter M, Preis J, Arlt M, Gruber J. Dissecting miRNA gene repression on single cell level with an advanced fluorescent reporter system. Scientific Reports. 2017;**7**:45197

Chapter 4

Influence of Endogenous Viral Sequences on Gene Expression

Kozue Sofuku and Tomoyuki Honda

Additional information is available at the end of the chapter

http://dx.doi.org/10.5772/intechopen.71864

Abstract

Endogenous viral elements (EVEs) are the heritable sequences present in eukaryotic genomes that have originated from viral nucleotide sequences. EVEs are subdivided into two groups, according to the presence or absence of long terminal repeats (LTRs). EVEs with LTRs are called endogenous retroviruses (ERVs), and they account for approximately 8% of the human genome. EVEs without LTRs seem to be related to non-reverse-transcribing RNA and DNA viruses, and recent studies have revealed that numerous vertebrate genomes contain these non-LTR EVEs. Such EVEs are proposed to play essential roles in gene expression. EVEs can regulate gene expression as *cis*-regulatory DNA and RNA elements. EVE-derived non-coding RNAs and/or proteins can also influence cell transcriptomes *in trans*. To maintain cell integrity, cells epigenetically silence the expression of most EVEs, making these elements generally biochemically inert. These epigenetic alterations around the EVE loci can also affect host transcriptomes. Here, we highlight the current knowledge available on the regulatory activities of ERVs and non-retroviral EVEs, especially the EVEs derived from bornaviruses, which are known as endogenous bornavirus-like elements (EBLs). Better knowledge of this area will improve our understanding of gene regulation and also the co-evolution of viruses and their hosts.

Keywords: endogenous viral sequences, retroviruses, bornavirus, long terminal repeats, co-evolution, genome

1. Introduction

Various viruses appear to have left heritable sequences originated from viral nucleotide sequences, called endogenous viral elements (EVEs), in eukaryotic genomes. EVEs are distinguished by the presence or absence of long terminal repeats (LTRs). EVEs with LTRs are called endogenous retroviruses (ERVs). The LTRs contain *cis*-regulatory sequences and RNA polymerase II (Pol II) promoters [1]. ERVs are formed by the integration of ancient retroviruses into the host genome during infection, and they account for around 8% of the human genome contents. Some ERV-derived genes that have been co-opted by the host play essential roles in biological processes, such as placentation in humans [2, 3]. On the other hand, recent studies have revealed that numerous vertebrate genomes also contain non-LTR EVEs, EVEs that have no LTRs [4–6]. Among these non-LTR EVEs, the bornavirus-derived EVEs (endogenous bornavirus-like elements (EBLs)), which have been relatively well studied, have provided clues about the biological significance of non-LTR EVEs in mammals [4, 7–11]. EBLs are the DNA sequences in vertebrate genomes (i.e., primates, rodents, and afrotherians) that are formed by the long interspersed nuclear element-1 (LINE-1)-mediated integration of viral sequences of an ancient non-retroviral RNA virus, bornavirus [4]. LINE-1, a host retrotransposon, encodes two proteins, ORF1p and ORF2p, which form LINE-1 ribonucleoprotein (RNP) together with LINE-1 RNA [12, 13]. ORF2p is known as endonuclease and reverse transcriptase in the LINE-1 retrotransposition, which is also used for retrotransposition of viral mRNAs of non-retroviral RNA viruses, thereby producing non-LTR EVEs. EBLs derived from the N, M, G, and L genes of bornaviruses, which are designated as EBLN, EBLM, EBLG, and EBLL, respectively, have been reported so far [14]. Although EBLs do not contain any cognate promoter sequences derived from bornavirus sequences, some EBLs are thought to influence gene expression.

EVEs use various mechanisms to regulate gene expression. First, genomic EVEs can regulate gene expression as *cis*-regulatory DNA elements. Second, EVEs produce non-coding RNAs and/or proteins that influence nearby genes and/or the global transcriptome *in trans*. Third, alterations in the epigenetic environment around the EVEs can also affect the transcriptome. In this review, we provide a brief overview of the regulatory activities (e.g., promoter activity and epigenetic regulation) of ERVs and EBLs in the context of gene expression regulation.

2. The influence of ERVs on gene expression

The exogenous retroviral genome contains the following genes: *gag,* which encodes the gene encoding retroviral structural proteins, *pol,* which encodes reverse transcriptase, protease, ribonuclease and integrase, and *env,* which encodes the envelope protein. The retrovirus viral genome also contains a primer-binding site (pbs) and the packaging signal (Ψ), both of which are important to the viral life cycle (**Figure 1A**). The reverse transcriptase encoded in the *pol* gene synthesizes viral DNA (proviral DNA) from the viral RNA, and the proviral DNA is then inserted into the host's genome which, when inherited in germ-line cells, become ERVs (**Figure 1B**). ERVs have been co-opted with the host and play essential roles in gene expression (**Figure 2**).

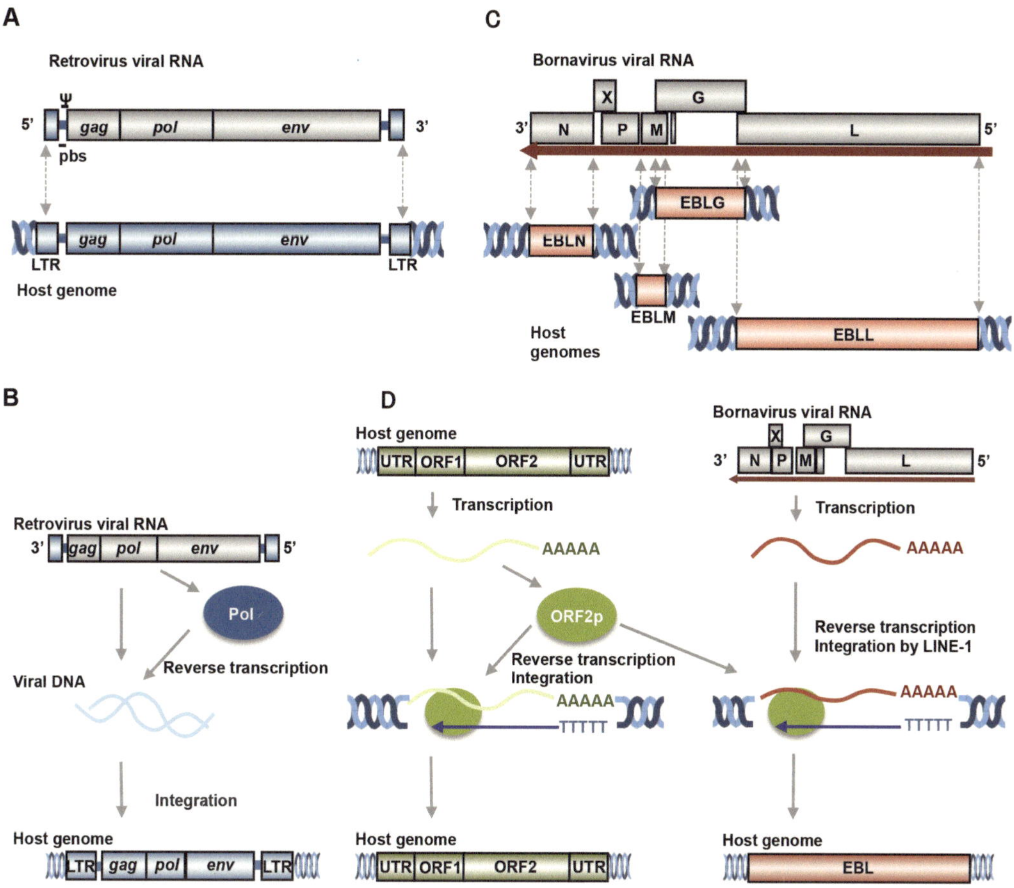

Figure 1. Summary of ERV and EBL structures and their biogenesis. (A) Structure of the retrovirus genome and ERV. LTR, the long terminal repeat; *gag*, the group-specific antigen gene; *pol*, the polymerase gene; *env*, the envelope gene; pbs, the primer-binding site; and Ψ, the packaging signal. (B) Mechanism of ERV biogenesis. Retrovirus reverse transcribes its RNA into a linear double-stranded DNA. The viral DNA is integrated into the host genome to form a provirus. (C) Structure of the bornavirus genome and EBLs. (D) Mechanism of LINE-1 retrotransposition and LINE-1-mediated EBL biogenesis. LINE-1 encodes two proteins, ORF1p and ORF2p. ORF2p encodes endonuclease and reverse transcriptase enzymes for the reverse transcription of LINE-1 RNA and genomic integration of its cDNA. ORF2p occasionally reverse transcribes other mRNAs *in trans*. EBLs seem to be generated from bornavirus mRNA in this manner.

2.1. Gene regulation by ERVs as regulatory DNAs

The LTRs of human ERVs (HERVs) have strong Pol II regulatory sequences [15, 16] and contain abundant transcription factor binding sites that function as promoters for HERV expression [17]. Although the full-length HERV is considered to have two LTRs, up to 85% of HERVs have undergone recombinatorial deletion [18], making most HERV loci solo LTRs. Solo LTRs can still serve as promoters in both the sense and antisense orientations and influence gene expression [19, 20].

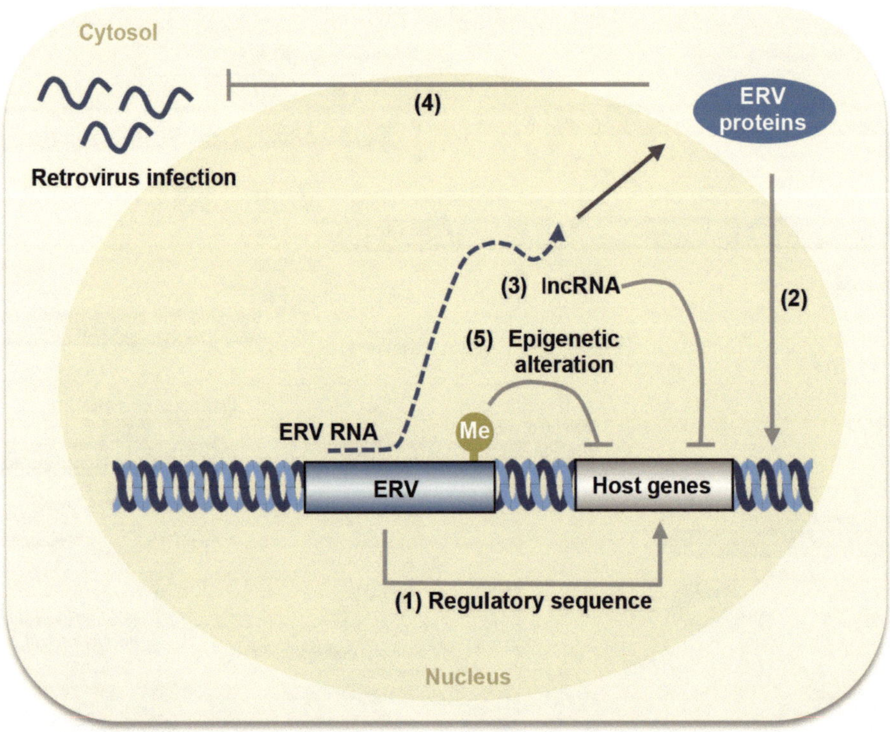

Figure 2. Influence of ERVs on gene expression. (1) ERVs function as *cis* or distal regulatory sequences. (2) ERV proteins may regulate the expression of host gene *in trans*. (3) ERV RNAs can work as lncRNAs to regulate the expression of the host genes. (4) ERV proteins may inhibit viral replication. (5) Epigenetic modifications that silence ERV expression can influence the expression of neighboring genes. The ochre circle (Me) indicates a central suppressive modification, DNA methylation, on the ERV locus.

For example, *IL2RB* and *NOS3* are genes whose expression in the placenta is solely related to the presence of LTR promoters [19]. Stem cell-specific LTR-derived promoters, such as mouse ERVK and human ERV1, control the expression of nuclear transcripts [21], whose expression is associated with maintenance of pluripotency. MER39 (an ERV1 class member) constitutes the promoter for human endometrial *Prl* [22]. MER41, another HERV, works as a *cis*-regulatory sequence of *AIM2* (a non-self DNA sensor), thereby regulating inflammatory responses [23]. The ERV-9 LTR is located near the 5′ end of the locus control region, around 40–70 kb upstream of the human fetal γ- and adult β-*globin* genes. LTR deletion was found to drastically suppress the β-*globin* gene and reactivate the γ-*globin* gene through a competitive mechanism involving *globin* gene switching [24]. Some lineage-specific ERVs, such as LTR19B and MER41, have dispersed numerous IFN-inducible enhancers in human genomes, thereby shaping the evolution of the transcriptional network underlying the interferon (IFN) response [23]. The expression of very long intergenic RNAs (vlincRNAs), which also control pluripotency, is driven by HERV LTR [25], suggesting a role for HERV LTRs in regulating the expression of not only protein-coding genes but also long non-coding RNAs (lncRNAs) [26].

2.2. Gene regulation by ERV proteins

The expression products of HERVs can also affect the physiological functioning and development of the host's tissues. For example, HERV-W (ERVWE1), HERV-FRD, and ERV-3 are three HERVs whose intact *env* genes are expressed as proteins in the human placenta [27–30]. HERV proteins play important roles in the proper formation of the placenta and are involved in the suppression of fetal tissue rejection [27, 31, 32]. The transmembrane envelope proteins of HERV-K, which modulate the expression of numerous cytokines, provide an example of gene expression regulation by a HERV protein [33]. HERVs may also be linked to a strategy used for inhibiting exogenous virus replication. For example, *Friend virus susceptibility 1* (*Fv1*), a mouse gene that originated from the *gag* gene of an ancient retrovirus, is known to restrict murine leukemia virus (MLV) at a stage after entry but before integration and formation of the provirus, thereby inhibiting viral replication [34, 35].

2.3. Gene regulation by HERV-driven lncRNAs

lincRNA-RoR is a large intergenic non-coding RNA driven by HERV-H [36]. lincRNA-RoR modulates reprograming and is indeed expressed at much higher levels in the embryonic stem cell line, H1-hESC, and human-induced pluripotent stem cells than in any other tissue or cell line [36, 37]. Knockdown of lincRNA-RoR affects the expression of other stem cell factors such as *KLF4*, *SOX2*, and *NANOG* [38, 39], resulting in an exit from the pluripotent state [37]. Together with vlincRNAs [25], HERV-driven lncRNAs can influence the transcriptome of the genes involved in pluripotency.

2.4. Gene regulation by epigenetic modification of ERVs

In addition to the abovementioned roles, LTRs are important sites for epigenetic modifications that restrict HERV in the human genome. DNA methylation, which is carried out by DNA methyltransferases, histone methylation, and histone deacetylation are the major host mechanisms used for gene silencing [10, 11]. Indeed, HERVs are heavily methylated in normal tissues [42]. By contrast, histone deacetylation alone is not sufficient to repress HERV expression. Rather, histone deacetylation in combination with other epigenetic modifications, particularly DNA methylation, is required for sufficient silencing of HERVs [43]. Furthermore, histone demethylation, which is carried out by lysine-specific histone demethylases (KDMs), also silences HERV expression [44, 45]. All these epigenetic alterations to ERV loci can affect the expression of nearby genes. For example, MuERV-L/MERVL, a mouse ERV, is repressed by a KDM1A-mediated epigenetic modification [45]. Some zygotic genome activation (ZGA) genes use an LTR of MERVL as a promoter or contain an MERVL element within 5 kb of their transcriptional start sites [45]. These ERV-linked ZGA genes become de-repressed in KDM1A mutant cells, which coincide with an expanded cell fate potential [45]. Thus, KDM1A recruitment to the MERVL LTRs seems to alter the chromatin structure around the loci, which in turn suppresses the expression of ERV-linked ZGA genes during early mammalian embryonic development.

2.5. Possible links between ERVs and human diseases

The recent studies on ERVs have revealed possible interactions between ERVs and their hosts with the potential to contribute to the development of diseases such as cancer and neurologic diseases. For example, the HERV expression is upregulated in various types of cancers [46–48]. Many HERV LTR regions, such as LTR10 and MER61, have a near-perfect p53 DNA binding site [49]. The tumor suppressor protein p53 is a sequence-specific transcription factor, which regulates genes of diverse biological pathways [50]. Thus, ERVs may regulate carcinogenesis via the p53 pathway. *CSF1R* gene, an oncogene, is activated by a demethylated MaLR LTR [51]. LTR-driven CSF1R is expressed aberrantly in anaplastic large cell lymphoma [51], suggesting that ERV LTRs may also directly contribute to tumor growth via activation of oncogenes. HERVs have also involved in neurological and psychiatric diseases. For example, the expression levels of HERV-H are significantly higher in patients with attention deficit hyperactivity disorder (ADHD) compared with healthy controls [52]. Furthermore, the HERV-W env mRNA expression is selectively upregulated in brain tissue from patients with multiple sclerosis compared with controls [53]. Although links between the upregulation of ERVs and these diseases are reported, the contribution of upregulated ERVs to the disease development is still unclear and further studies are clearly required for demonstrating it.

3. The influence of nonretroviral EVEs on gene expression

EBLs are the only nonretroviral RNA virus-derived EVEs found in the human genome. EBLs seem to be generated from bornavirus mRNA in a LINE1-dependent manner (**Figure 1C** and **D**). Thus, they are a unique form of a processed pseudogene, which is derived from the sequences of an exogenous virus but not endogenous sequences, and they evidence the mechanism of retrotransposon-mediated RNA-to-DNA information flow from the virus to the host [4]. In the human genome, seven EBLNs (hsEBLN-1 to hsEBLN-7) and one EBLG have been identified to date [4–6]. All seven hsEBLNs are expressed as RNAs in at least one tissue, suggesting the possibility of a biological function for these EBLs [9].

3.1. Gene regulation by EBLN RNAs

hsEBLN-1 is one of the most studied EBLs in the human genome. Because no natural selection of hsEBLN-1 and its orthologues is detected [54], hsEBLN-1 is thought to function as a DNA element or non-coding RNA, or even to have lost its function (**Figure 3**). He et al. reported that 1067 and 2004 genes are up- and downregulated, respectively, after knockdown of hsEBLN-1 RNA in human oligodendroglia cells [55]. The top 10 most upregulated genes were *PI3, RND3, BLZF1, SOD2, EPGN, SBSN, INSIG1, OSMR, CREB3L2,* and *MSMO1*, and the top 10 most downregulated genes were *KRTAP2–4, FLRT2, DIDO1, FAT4, ESCO2, ZNF804A, SUV420H1, ZC3H4, YAE1D1,* and *NCOA5*. Gene ontology revealed that hsEBLN-1 may regulate the expression of genes related to the cell cycle, the mitogen-activated protein kinase pathway, p53 signaling, and apoptosis [55].

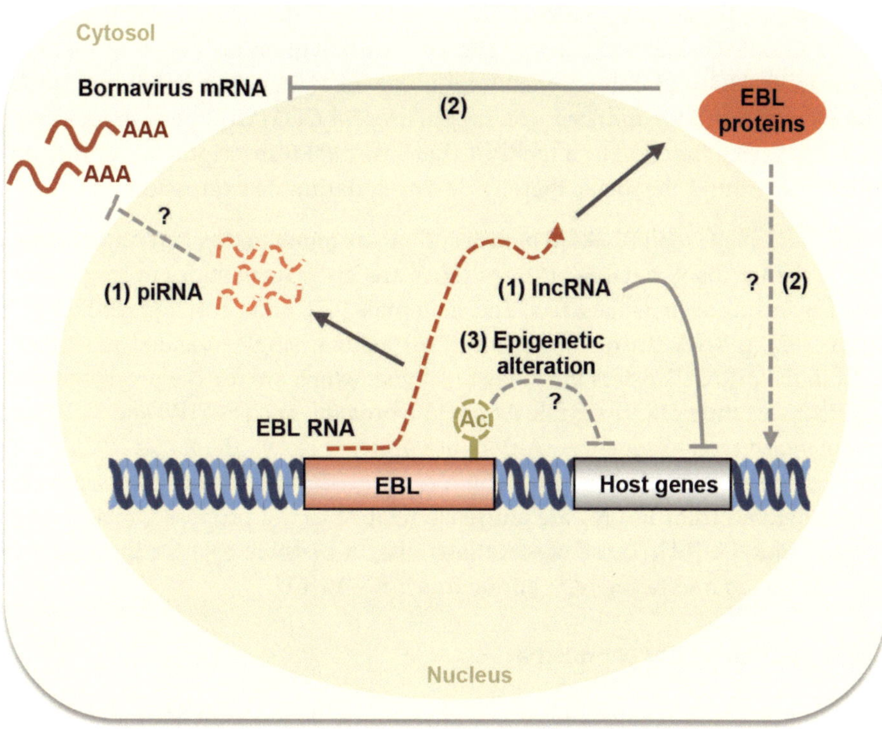

Figure 3. Influence of EBLs on gene expression. (1) An EBL-derived lncRNA regulates the expression of a neighboring gene. piRNAs derived from EBLs may have the potential to provide antiviral responses against bornaviruses. (2) An EBL protein inhibits bornavirus transcription. Likewise, some EBL proteins may possibly regulate host gene expression. (3) Alteration of the epigenetic environment to restrain the EBL expression may influence the expression of neighboring genes. The ochre broken line circle (Ac) indicates deacetylation of the EBL locus.

Unlike ERVs, EBLs are thought not to be transposable themselves. Nevertheless, the hsEBLN-1 locus is silenced by several epigenetic blocks, dominantly histone deacetylation and DNA methylation, similar to the case of human immunodeficiency virus (HIV) provirus silencing [9, 56, 57]. This contrasts with the silencing mechanism of ERVs because, as described above, DNA methylation but not histone deacetylation plays a major role [58]. Thus, the silencing mechanisms for the hsEBLN-1 locus might be more similar to those of exogenous retroviruses than to those of ERVs. This epigenetic alteration around hsEBLN integration may affect the epigenetic status of its neighboring loci and, consequently, the expression of nearby genes. Histone deacetylase (HDAC) inhibitor treatment did not affect transcription of the *COMMD3* gene in mouse and rat cells, which have no EBLN sequence at the locus syntenic to the hsEBLN-1 locus, whereas the treatment led to decreased transcription of *COMMD3* orthologues in human and monkey cells, which have the EBLN sequence at the locus. *COMMD3* belongs to the copper metabolism gene MURR1 domain-containing (COMMD) family. COMMD proteins have a structurally conserved COMM domain, and they are all able to interact with different NF-κB subunits [59]. Because one of the central roles of NF-κB is induction of proinflammatory mediators like cytokines, chemokines, and adhesion molecules, EBLN-1 may regulate immune responses indirectly through the COMMD3-NF-κB pathway [59, 60]. Moreover, suppression of the hsEBLN-1 RNA induced by HDAC inhibitor treatment using siRNA against hsEBLN-1 RNA eliminated the HDAC inhibitor-induced downregulation of *COMMD3* gene expression. Thus, hsEBLN-1 RNA may function as a lncRNA that scaffolds transcriptional repressors of the *COMMD3* gene around the locus, thereby downregulating its expression.

Several EBLN-derived small RNAs in mouse and rat are annotated as PIWI-interacting RNAs (piRNAs) in the GenBank database [61]. piRNAs are 25–33 nucleotides in length, are found in diverse organisms such as flies, fish, and mammals [62], and protect germ-line cells from transposons [62]. piRNA clusters are transcribed as long single-stranded precursor RNAs derived from the piRNA clusters in the host genome, which are further processed into small mature piRNAs. Mature piRNAs guide Argonaute proteins, such as PIWI and MIWI proteins, to complementary target sequences. Argonaute proteins cleave the target RNAs, suppressing their expression. piRNAs are also known to epigenetically silence the target gene loci. All piRNAs derived from EBLNs are antisense relative to the proposed ancient bornaviral nucleoprotein mRNA [61]. These observations offer a possible role for the EBLN-derived piRNA-like RNAs in interfering with bornavirus mRNAs [61].

3.2. Gene regulation by EBLN proteins

Among the human EBLNs, hsEBLN-1 and hsEBLN-2 have maintained long open reading frames with the potential to code for proteins of 366 and 225 amino acids, respectively. Indeed, some studies have reported that hsEBLN-1 proteins were detected in particular cell lines [63]. Moreover, Kobayashi et al. reported that EBLNs encode functional proteins in afrotherians [10]. Therefore, it is still possible that EBLN proteins regulate gene expression *in trans*. Furthermore, EBLNs may potentially inhibit the replication of related exogenous viruses, similarly to certain ERVs. EBLN from the thirteen-lined ground squirrel (*Ictidomys tridecemlineatus*) genome, named itEBLN, is associated with bornavirus RNPs and inhibits bornavirus polymerase activity [7].

4. Conclusions

The researches on gene regulation by EVEs have provided us with important knowledge about the evolution of regulatory sequences in the genome [5, 64]. Although integrated viral sequences are usually eliminated from the host genome, some eventually reach fixation and form EVEs. Such EVEs are not merely genetic parasites; rather, they introduce useful genetic novelties to the genome. In this article, we briefly reviewed two types of EVEs, ERVs and the non-LTR EVEs, EBLs. ERVs provide novel regulatory sequences and sites for epigenetic regulation. Transcripts derived from ERVs can also function as lncRNAs or protein-coding mRNAs, which may regulate gene expression. In particular, ERV-related transcripts are often associated with pluripotency. EBLs might also function as regulatory DNA elements such as promoters and enhancers. They are transcribed in one tissue at least, suggesting that

EBL transcripts may function as lncRNAs or protein-coding mRNAs. Consistently, we have shown the evidence for the roles of EBL transcripts as lncRNA molecules in gene expression. In particular, several EBLs are associated with antiviral responses against related viruses. Additionally, both ERVs and EBLs regulate not only host gene expression, but related viral gene expression also. Further extensive studies on EVEs will augment our understanding of their biological significance in gene expression and their involvement in the co-evolution of viruses and mammals.

Acknowledgements

The preparation of this article was supported in part by the Japan Society for the Promotion of Science (JSPS) KAKENHI grant numbers JP24115709, JP25115508, JP25860336 (TH), MEXT KAKENHI grant number 15K08496 (TH), and grants from the Takeda Science Foundation, Senri Life Science Foundation, and The Shimizu Foundation for Immunology and Neuroscience grant for 2015 (TH). We thank Sandra Cheesman for editing a draft of this manuscript.

Abbreviations

EVE	endogenous viral element
LTR	long terminal repeat
ERV	endogenous retrovirus
Pol II	RNA polymerase II
EBL	endogenous bornavirus like element
LINE-1	long interspersed nuclear element-1
RNP	ribonucleoprotein complex
HERV	human endogenous retrovirus
lncRNA	long non-coding RNA
MLV	murine leukemia virus
KDM	lysine-specific histone demethylase
ZGA	zygotic genome activation
ADHD	attention-deficit hyperactivity disorder
HIV	human immunodeficiency virus

HDAC	histone deacetylase
siRNA	small interfering RNA
piRNA	PIWI-interacting RNA

Author details

Kozue Sofuku and Tomoyuki Honda*

*Address all correspondence to: thonda@virus.med.osaka-u.ac.jp

Division of Virology, Department of Microbiology and Immunology, Graduate School of Medicine, Osaka University, Osaka, Japan

References

[1] Mager DL, Stoye JP. Mammalian endogenous retroviruses. Microbiology Spectrum. 2015; **3**:1-20

[2] Dupressoir A, Vernochet C, Bawa O, Harper F, Pierron G, Opolon P, et al. Syncytin-A knockout mice demonstrate the critical role in placentation of a fusogenic, endogenous retrovirus-derived, envelope gene. Proceedings of the National Academy of Sciences of the United States of America. 2009;**106**:12127-12132

[3] McCoy JM, Mi S, Lee X, Li X, Veldman GM, Finnerty H, et al. Syncytin is a captive retroviral envelope protein involved in human placentalmorphogenesis. Nature. 2000; **403**:785-789

[4] Horie M, Honda T, Suzuki Y, Kobayashi Y, Daito T, Oshida T, et al. Endogenous non-retroviral RNA virus elements in mammalian genomes. Nature. 2010;**463**:84-87

[5] Katzourakis A, Gifford RJ. Endogenous viral elements in animal genomes. PLoS Genetics. 2010;**6**:e1001191

[6] Belyi VA, Levine AJ, Skalka AM. Unexpected inheritance: Multiple integrations of ancient bornavirus and ebolavirus/marburgvirus sequences in vertebrate genomes. PLoS Pathogens. 2010;**6**:e1001030

[7] Fujino K, Horie M, Honda T, Merriman DK, Tomonaga K. Inhibition of Borna disease virus replication by an endogenous bornavirus-like element in the ground squirrel genome. Proceedings of the National Academy of Sciences of the United States of America. 2014;**111**:13175-13180

[8] Parrish NF, Tomonaga K. Endogenized viral sequences in mammals. Current Opinion in Microbiology. 2016;**31**:176-183

[9] Sofuku K, Parrish NF, Honda T, Tomonaga K. Transcription profiling demonstrates epigenetic control of non-retroviral RNA virus-derived elements in the human genome. Cell Reports. 2015;**12**:1548-1554

[10] Kobayashi Y, Horie M, Nakano A, Murata K, Itou T, Suzuki Y. Exaptation of Bornavirus-like nucleoprotein elements in Afrotherians. PLoS Pathogens. 2016;**12**:e1005785

[11] Honda T, Tomonaga K. Endogenous non-retroviral RNA virus elements evidence a novel type of antiviral immunity. Mobile Genetic Elements. 2016;**6**:e1165785

[12] Feng Q, Moran JV, Kazazian HH, Boeke JD. Human L1 retrotransposon encodes a conserved endonuclease required for retrotransposition. Cell. 1996;**87**:905-916

[13] Martin SL. The ORF1 protein encoded by LINE-1: Structure and function during L1 retrotransposition. Journal of Biomedicine & Biotechnology. 2006;**2006**:45621

[14] Horie M. The biological significance of bornavirus-derived genes in mammals. Current Opinion in Virology. 2017;**25**:1-6

[15] Criscione SW, Zhang Y, Thompson W, Sedivy JM, Neretti N. Transcriptional landscape of repetitive elements in normal and cancer human cells. BMC Genomics. 2014;**15**:1-17

[16] Thompson PJ, Macfarlan TS, Lorincz MC. Long terminal repeats: From parasitic elements to building blocks of the transcriptional regulatory repertoire. Molecular Cell. 2016;**62**:766-776

[17] Manghera M, Douville RN. Endogenous retrovirus-K promoter: A landing strip for inflammatory transcription factors? Retrovirology. 2013;**10**:16

[18] Belshaw R, Watson J, Katzourakis A, Howe A, Woolven-Allen J, Burt A, et al. Rate of recombinational deletion among human endogenous retroviruses. Journal of Virology. 2007;**81**:9437-9442

[19] Cohen CJ, Lock WM, Mager DL. Endogenous retroviral LTRs as promoters for human genes: A critical assessment. Gene. 2009;**448**:105-114

[20] Dunn CA, Romanish MT, Gutierrez LE, van de Lagemaat LN, Mager DL. Transcription of two human genes from a bidirectional endogenous retrovirus promoter. Gene. 2006; **366**:335-342

[21] Fort A, Hashimoto K, Yamada D, Salimullah M, Keya CA, Saxena A, et al. Deep transcriptome profiling of mammalian stem cells supports a regulatory role for retrotransposons in pluripotency maintenance. Nature Genetics. 2014;**46**:558-566

[22] Emera D, Casola C, Lynch VJ, Wildman DE, Agnew D, Wagner GP. Convergent evolution of endometrial prolactin expression in primates, mice, and elephants through the independent recruitment of transposable elements. Molecular Biology and Evolution. 2012;**29**:239-247

[23] Chuong EB, Elde NC, Feschotte C. Regulatory evolution of innate immunity through co-option of endogenous retroviruses. Science. 2016;**351**:1083-1087

[24] Tuan D, Pi W. Human β-globin gene locus, ERV-9 LTR retrotransposon interacts with and activates β-but not γ-globin gene. Blood. 2014;**124**:2686

[25] St Laurent G, Shtokalo D, Dong B, Tackett MR, Fan X, Lazorthes S, et al. VlincRNAs controlled by retroviral elements are a hallmark of pluripotency and cancer. Genome Biology. 2013;**14**:R73

[26] Hurst T, Magiorkinis G. Epigenetic control of human endogenous retrovirus expression: Focus on regulation of long-terminal repeats (LTRs). Virus. 2017;**9**:130

[27] Black SG, Arnaud F, Palmarini M, Spencer TE. Endogenous retroviruses in trophoblast differentiation and placental development. American Journal of Reproductive Immunology. 2010;**64**:255-264

[28] de Parseval N, Lazar V, Casella J-F, Benit L, Heidmann T. Survey of human genes of retroviral origin: Identification and transcriptome of the genes with coding capacity for complete envelope proteins. Journal of Virology. 2003;**77**:10414-10422

[29] Blond JL, Lavillette D, Cheynet V, Bouton O, Oriol G, Chapel-Fernandes S, et al. An envelope glycoprotein of the human endogenous retrovirus HERV-W is expressed in the human placenta and fuses cells expressing the type D mammalian retrovirus receptor. Journal of Virology. 2000;**74**:3321-3329

[30] Venables PJW. Abundance of an endogenous Retrovial envelope protein in placental Trophoblasts suggests a biological function. Virology. 1995;**221**:589-592

[31] Li F, Nellåker C, Yolken RH, Karlsson H. A systematic evaluation of expression of HERV-W elements; influence of genomic context, viral structure and orientation. BMC Genomics. 2011;**12**:22

[32] Dupressoir A, Heidmann T. Syncytins-retroviral envelope genes captured for the benefit of placental development. Medecine. Sciences. 2011;**27**:163-169

[33] Morozov VA, Dao Thi VL, Denner J. The Transmembrane protein of the human endogenous retrovirus - K (HERV-K) modulates cytokine release and gene expression. PLoS One. 2013;**8**:e70399

[34] Stoye JP. Fv1, the mouse retrovirus resistance gene. Revue Scientifique et Technique. 1998;**17**:269-277

[35] Best S, Le Tissier P, Towers G, Stoye JP. Positional cloning of the mouse retrovirus restriction gene Fv1. Nature. 1996;**382**:826-829

[36] Kelley DR, Rinn JL. Transposable elements reveal a stem cell specific class of long non-coding RNAs. Genome Biology. 2012;**13**:R107

[37] Loewer S, Cabili MN, Guttman M, Loh Y-H, Thomas K, Park IH, et al. Large intergenic non-coding RNA-RoR modulates reprogramming of human induced pluripotent stem cells. Nature Genetics. 2010;**42**:1113-1117

[38] Wang Y, Xu Z, Jiang J, Xu C, Kang J, Xiao L, et al. Endogenous miRNA sponge lincRNA-RoR regulates Oct4, Nanog, and Sox2 in human embryonic stem cell self-renewal. Developmental Cell. 2013;**25**:69-80

[39] Feng S, Yao J, Chen Y, Geng P, Zhang H, Ma X, et al. Expression and functional role of rReprogramming-related long noncoding RNA (lincRNA-ROR) in Glioma. Journal of Molecular Neuroscience. 2015;**56**:623-630

[40] Kazanets A, Shorstova T, Hilmi K, Marques M, Witcher M. Epigenetic silencing of tumor suppressor genes: Paradigms, puzzles, and potential. Biochimica et Biophysica Acta - Reviews on Cancer. 2016;**1865**:275-288

[41] Williams SA, Chen L-F, Kwon H, Ruiz-Jarabo CM, Verdin E, Greene WC. NF-κB p50 promotes HIV latency through HDAC recruitment and repression of transcriptional initiation. The EMBO Journal. 2006;**25**:139-149

[42] Szpakowski S, Sun X, Lage JM, Dyer A, Rubinstein J, Kowalski D, Sasaki C, Costa J, Lizardi PM. Loss of epigenetic silencing in tumors preferentially affects primate-specific retroelements. Gene. 2009;**448**:151-167

[43] Lavie L, Kitova M, Maldener E, Meese E, Mayer J. CpG methylation directly regulates transcriptional activity of the human endogenous retrovirus family HERV-K(HML-2). Journal of Virology. 2005;**79**:876-883

[44] Shi Y, Lan F, Matson C, Mulligan P, Whetstine JR, Cole PA, et al. Histone demethylation mediated by the nuclear amine oxidase homolog LSD1. Cell. 2004;**119**:941-953

[45] Macfarlan TS, Gifford WD, Agarwal S, Driscoll S, Lettieri K, Wang J, et al. Endogenous retroviruses and neighboring genes are coordinately repressed by LSD1/KDM1A. Genes and Development. 2011;**25**:594-607

[46] Cegolon L, Salata C, Weiderpass E, Vineis P, Palù G, Mastrangelo G. Human endogenous retroviruses and cancer prevention: Evidence and prospects. BMC Cancer. 2013;**13**:4

[47] Kassiotis G. Endogenous retroviruses and the development of cancer. Journal of Immunology. 2014;**192**:1343-1349

[48] Katoh I. Impacts of endogenous retroviruses on tumorigenesis, immunity, stem cells, and research safety. Frontiers in Oncology. 2014;**4**:66

[49] Wang T, Zeng J, Lowe CB, Sellers RG, Salama SR, Yang M, et al. Species-specific endogenous retroviruses shape the transcriptional network of the human tumor suppressor protein p53. Proceedings of the National Academy of Sciences of the United States of America. 2007;**104**:18613

[50] Levine AJ. p53, the cellular gatekeeper for growth and division. Cell. 1997;**88**:323-331

[51] Lamprecht B, Walter K, Kreher S, Kumar R, Hummel M, Lenze D, et al. Derepression of an endogenous long terminal repeat activates the CSF1R proto-oncogene in human lymphoma. Nature Medicine. 2010;**16**:571-579

[52] Balestrieri E, Pitzianti M, Matteucci C, D'Agati E, Sorrentino R, Baratta A, et al. Human endogenous retroviruses and ADHD. The World Journal of Biological Psychiatry. 2014;**15**:499-504

[53] Antony JM, van Marle G, Opii W, Butterfield DA, Mallet F, Yong VW, et al. Human endogenous retrovirus glycoprotein–mediated induction of redox reactants causes oligodendrocyte death and demyelination. Nature Neuroscience. 2004;**7**:1088-1095

[54] Kobayashi Y, Horie M, Tomonaga K, Suzuki Y. No evidence for natural selection on endogenous borna-like nucleoprotein elements after the divergence of Old World and New World monkeys. PloS One. 2011;**6**:e24403

[55] He P, Sun L, Zhu D, Zhang H, Zhang L, Guo Y, et al. Knock-down of endogenous Bornavirus-like nucleoprotein 1 inhibits cell growth and induces apoptosis in human oligodendroglia Cells. International Journal of Molecular Sciences. 2016;**17**:435

[56] Blazkova J, Trejbalova K, Gondois-Rey F, Halfon P, Philibert P, Guiguen A, et al. CpG methylation controls reactivation of HIV from latency. PLoS Pathogens. 2009;**5**:e1000554

[57] Nabel G, Baltimore D. An inducible transcription factor activates expression of human immunodeficiency virus in T cells. Nature. 1987;**326**:711-713

[58] Matsui T, Leung D, Miyashita H, Maksakova IA, Miyachi H, Kimura H, et al. Proviral silencing in embryonic stem cells requires the histone methyltransferase ESET. Nature. 2010;**464**:927-931

[59] Burstein E, Hoberg JE, Wilkinson AS, Rumble JM, Csomos RA, Komarck CM, et al. COMMD proteins, a novel family of structural and functional homologs of MURR1. Journal of Biological Chemistry. 2005;**280**:22222-22232

[60] Bartuzi P, Hofker MH, Van de Sluis B. Tuning NF-κB activity: A touch of COMMD proteins. Biochimica et Biophysica Acta - Molecular Basis of Disease. 2013;**1832**:2315-2321

[61] Parrish NF, Fujino K, Shiromoto Y, Iwasaki YW, Ha H, Xing J, et al. piRNAs derived from ancient viral processed pseudogenes as transgenerational sequence-specific immune memory in mammals. RNA. 2015;**21**:1691-1703

[62] Meister G. Argonaute proteins: Functional insights and emerging roles. Nature Reviews Genetics. 2013;**14**:447-459

[63] Myers KN, Barone G, Ganesh A, Staples CJ, Howard AE, Beveridge RD, et al. The bornavirus-derived human protein EBLN1 promotes efficient cell cycle transit, microtubule organisation and genome stability. Scientific Reports. 2016;**6**:35548

[64] Weiss RA, Griffiths D, Villesen P, Aagaard L. The discovery of endogenous retroviruses. Retrovirology. 2006;**3**:67

Chapter 5

Cross-Talk Categorisations in Data-Driven Models of Signalling Networks: A System-Level View

A.K.M. Azad, Alfons Lawen and Jonathan M. Keith

Additional information is available at the end of the chapter

http://dx.doi.org/10.5772/intechopen.72408

Abstract

Data-driven models of signalling networks are becoming increasingly important in systems biology in order to reflect the dynamic patterns of signalling activities in a context-specific manner. State-of-the-art approaches for categorising and detecting signalling cross-talks may not be suitable for such models since they rely on static topologies of cell signalling networks and prior biological knowledge. In this chapter, we review state-of-the-art approaches that categorise all possible cross-talks in signalling networks and propose a novel categorisation specific to data-driven network models. Considering such models as undirected networks, we propose two categories of signalling cross-talks between any two given signalling pathways. In a Type-I cross-talk, a signalling link $\{g_i, g_j\}$ connects two signalling pathways, where g_i and g_j are signalling nodes that belong to two distinct pathways. In a Type-II cross-talk, two signalling links $\{g_i, g_j\}$ and $\{g_j, g_k\}$ meet at the intersection of two signalling pathways at a shared signalling node g_j. We compared our categorisation approach with others and found that all the types of cross-talks defined by those approaches can be mapped to Type-I and Type-II cross-talks when underlying signalling activities are considered as non-causal relationships. Next, we provided a simple but intuitive algorithm called *XDaMoSiN* (cross-talks in data-driven models of signalling networks) to detect both Type-I and Type-II cross-talks between any two given signalling pathways in a data-driven network model. By detecting cross-talks in such network models, our approach can be used to analyse and decipher latent mechanisms of various cell phenotypes, such as cancer or acquired drug resistance, that may evolve due to the highly adaptable and dynamic nature of signal transduction networks.

Keywords: signalling cross-talks, data-driven models, signalling network, cancer signalling, signal re-wiring, acquired drug resistance

1. Introduction

A signal transduction network is a collection of all cell signalling pathways where each pathway is a series of biochemical events, transmitting input signals from receptor proteins to intracellular target proteins (e.g., transcription factors). The outcomes mediated by signalling pathways include various cellular activities such as cell growth, proliferation, differentiation, migration, adhesion, and apoptosis [1, 2]. Interactions among distinct signalling pathways are called signalling cross-talks and may also play vital roles in mediating or modulating cellular activities [3] under different disease-related cell conditions such as cancer and acquired drug resistance.

Models of signal transduction networks often take a qualitative approach that relies on prior biological knowledge obtained from experimental findings in various cell lines [4, 5]. However, the pattern of cell signalling activities is not static and can vary in different cell lines [4, 5]. Moreover, different cell lines for which the underlying network architectures of signalling activities are conserved may yield different responses even in similar experimental settings [5]. In the same cell, different ligands can produce different signalling connections [5, 6]. Moreover, different drugs and different treatment conditions may also induce different signalling dependencies and thus create a dynamic re-wiring in the signalling network topology [6–8]. Therefore, understanding a signalling network topology demands a data-driven modelling approach in order to reflect its context-specific nature in a particular cell type, and a particular experimental configuration. Here, data-driven models of signalling networks are models in which network edges are inferred solely based on signalling data [4] using machine learning approaches such as least square regression [9], Bayesian networks [10–12], and time-lag correlation [13]. In contrast, static models of signalling networks are based on canonical signalling mechanisms obtained from the literature [4]. Recent advancements in high-throughput data generation techniques facilitate the quantification of signalling responses, thereby producing large volumes of data measuring protein abundances and activities [4].

Detecting signalling cross-talks using data-driven models of signalling networks is an important task in systems biology since such cross-talks may reveal novel mechanistic details underlying perturbed cellular conditions. Receptor tyrosine kinase (RTK) heterodimerisation is one of the forms of signalling cross-talks (also known as receptor function cross-talks) [14], which has been reported to be involved in the processes of tumourigenesis and developing acquired drug resistance in many cancers [6]. Usually, epidermal growth factor receptor (EGFR) strongly activates extracellular signal-regulated kinase (ERK) signalling, but it is also a weak activator of the phosphatidylinositol 3-kinase (PI3K) signalling pathway. Interestingly, when EGFR cross-talks with human epidermal growth factor receptor 2 (HER2) through heterodimerisation, it activates both signalling pathways significantly [15], thereby contributing tumourigenesis by stimulating proliferation and preventing cell death [6]. In another example, the RTK expression of AXL was found to be a mechanism of acquired resistance to EGFR inhibitors [16], and AXL is found to be transactivated by EGFR through heterodimerisation (cross-talk) [6].

In this chapter, we review existing approaches that have been used in the literature to categorise cross-talks in signalling networks. However, all these methods are limited in application to *static* models of signalling networks and cannot be used to categorise cross-talks when the types of signalling activities (e.g., reaction, catalysis, or inhibition) are not known. We therefore introduce a novel cross-talk categorisation for a *single cell* model to resolve such issues. We also compare our categorisation with the existing approaches. Finally, we present an algorithm to computationally detect all signalling cross-talks that are included in our proposed categorisation. Natarajan et al. [17] reported that a global analysis of both known and novel cross-talks can reveal system-level insights into context-dependent signalling: many ligand stimuli converge on a relatively small number of signalling molecules to produce unique responses. Thus, we hypothesise that our approach will be useful to elucidate similar novel system-level aspects of signalling networks derived from context-specific signalling data through the identification of cross-talks.

1.1. Existing methods for categorising cross-talks

Only a few studies have attempted to categorise types or modes of cross-talks between two signalling pathways [6, 14, 18]. In reviewing signalling cross-talks between transforming growth factor-β/bone morphogenic protein (TGF-β/BMP) and other signalling pathways, Guo and Wang [18] distinguished three different modes of signalling cross-talks. According to that study, two pathways: $pathway_1$ and $pathway_2$ cross-talk when (1) some component of $pathway_1$ physically interacts with some component of $pathway_2$ (*Mode-A*), (2) some component of $pathway_2$ plays a role as an enzymatic or transcriptional target of some component of $pathway_2$ (*Mode-B*), or (3) signals from $pathway_1$ modulate or compete for a key modulator or mediator protein that is shared between $pathway_1$ and $pathway_2$ (*Mode-C*).

Donaldson and Calder [14] proposed five types of signalling cross-talk between any two signalling pathways: $pathway_1$ and $pathway_2$. They are as follows:

- **Signal-flow cross-talk**: an alternative reaction that enhances the signalling in $pathway_1$ by producing, or catalysing, or inhibiting the production of a protein mediated by the signalling of $pathway_2$. For example, there exists signal-flow cross-talk between mitogen-activated protein kinase (MAPK) and integrin signalling pathways [19], where the increased rate of activation of some key protein in the integrin pathway is mediated by signalling through the MAPK pathway.
- **Receptor function cross-talk**: an alternative reaction to activate/inhibit the receptor of $pathway_1$ by some enzyme of $pathway_2$ without the need of a ligand (a protein that activates a receptor protein). For example, oestrogen receptor may become activated without the need of oestrogen ligand by other signalling pathways [20].
- **Gene expression cross-talk**: a component (typically, a protein) of $pathway_1$ inhibits or modifies the transcription or protein production of genes in $pathway_2$. For example, transcription factor glucocorticoid receptor (GR) of hormone signalling pathways translocates to the nucleus and inhibits the transcriptional activities of the transcription factor nuclear factor-κB (NF-κB) that is activated in response to inflammatory stimuli and environmental stressors [21].
- **Substrate availability cross-talk**: $pathway_1$ and $pathway_2$ share a protein (or a set of proteins) and both of the pathways compete for the activation of that shared protein(s). For example,

two MAPK pathways in the yeast *S. cerevisiae* that share mitogen-activated protein kinase kinase kinase (MAPKKK) protein STE11 (Sterility gene 11) and possess homologous mitogen-activated protein kinase kinase (MAPKK) and MAPK proteins compete for the activation of the MAPK cascade [22].

- **Intracellular communication cross-talk**: the gene products of $pathway_1$ act as ligands for the receptor of $pathway_2$. For example, TGF-β and Wnt (Wingless-related integration site) signalling regulate the production of ligands of one another [18].

Donaldson and Calder [14] also reviewed some computational models that deal with cross-talks between specific pathways including MAPK pathway, AKT pathways, and protein kinase C (PKC) pathways. These models [22–24] use ordinary differential equations (ODEs) where the notion of the cross-talk was a part of the system of equations without any explicit way of detecting or categorising them [14].

Kolch et al. [6] described three types of cross-talks such as heterodimerisation between signalling proteins, node sharing, and competition for nodes. Signalling protein heterodimerisation is a biochemical process where a protein complex is formed by two different macromolecules, and RTK heterodimerisation is a common example of this type of cross-talk [6]. For example, EGFR heterodimerisation with ErbB2 (erythroblastic leukaemia viral oncogene B2 also known as HER2) or ErbB3 (erythroblastic leukaemia viral oncogene B3) (also known as HER3, human epidermal growth factor receptor 3) activates both ERK and PI3K signalling pathways [15] and thereby mediates proliferation and cell survival signals in tumourigenesis [6]. In another example, the transactivation of AXL (an RTK) is caused by EGFR heterodimerisation, and the expression of AXL was found to be a mechanism of resistance to EGFR inhibitors [16].

An example of node (i.e. protein) sharing cross-talk is the scaffolding protein (a protein that binds with multiple members of a signalling pathway) GRB2-associated binding partner (GAB), which is shared by two signalling pathways: EGFR and insulin receptor (IR) pathways [25]. Lastly, an example of cross-talk in the form of competition for nodes (i.e. proteins) was recently identified, consisting of a switch-like coordination between proliferation and apoptotic signalling through rapidly accelerated fibrosarcoma (RAF)-ERK signalling and mammalian STE20-like protein kinase (MST2) signalling [26]. In mammalian cells, rapidly accelerated fibrosarcoma1 (RAF1) inhibits MST2-induced apoptosis (promotes proliferation) [27], whereas Ras association domain-containing protein 1A (RASSF1A) activates MST2 (promotes apoptosis) [28]. Romano et al. [26] showed that this signalling coordination is switch-like, since MST2 binds mutually exclusively with its inhibitor RAF1 and activator RASSF1A by changing its binding affinities from low to high.

Identifying the above cross-talk categories requires prior biological knowledge of the nature of signalling links. An essentially *static* model of signal transduction networks is thus assumed. However, in data-driven models of signalling networks, connectivity among signalling nodes may differ from cell to cell [6]. In order to reveal novel signalling dynamics in cell-specific, ligand-specific, or treatment-specific contextual data, we define a novel cross-talk categorisation in the following section.

2. Methods

2.1. Proposed cross-talk categorisation in data-driven networks

2.1.1. *Approaches for inferring data-driven signalling networks*

Although our main focus in this chapter is to propose a cross-talk categorisation, here we briefly mention some approaches that fit data-driven models of signalling networks to quantitative signalling datasets. Some high-throughput proteomics techniques that quantitatively measure phosphorylation activities of phosphoproteins (signalling proteins) include mass spectrometry, flow-cytometry, ribonucleic acid interference (RNAi) screening, and reverse-phase protein array (RPPA) [13, 29]. Apart from proteomics data, some approaches use gene expression measurements of phosphoproteins as a proxy for protein expression (i.e. protein activity) [30–32] in order to fit data-driven models of signalling networks. However, inference methods include modelling both causal [9–12, 29, 33] and non-causal (simple correlations) relationships [13, 34] among phosphoproteins. To identify causal relationships in a signalling network topology, various approaches have been applied such as least square regression [9], various models on Bayesian networks [10–12] and dynamic Bayesian networks [29], and maximum entropy [33]. Correlation-based approaches include measuring the simple Pearson correlation [34] and time-lag correlation [13]. The rationale behind applying such simple correlation-based approaches to infer signalling network structure is that individual signals may co-vary with respect to one another [4]. **Figure 1** presents a schematic diagram of a possible framework that can use our proposed novel cross-talk categorisation algorithm to find cross-talks in data-driven models of signalling networks.

2.1.2. *Proposed cross-talk categorisation*

In order to generalise our cross-talk categorisation for both causal and non-causal network models, we consider a signalling network as an undirected network. Let $G(V,E)$ be an undirected graph that represents an entire signalling network containing a set of signalling pathways, where V is a set of n signalling components (typically proteins or protein complexes, denoted g_i, for $i = 1, 2, \ldots, n$) and E is a set of *unordered* pairs of signalling components of the form $\{g_i, g_j\}$ representing signalling links inferred from data. We propose two types of signalling cross-talks between any two signalling pathways, denoted $pathway_1$ and $pathway_2$, which is shown in **Figure 2**. Here, a pathway is defined merely as a list of signalling components, usually obtained from databases such as KEGG [35], WikiPathways [36], and Reactome [37].

2.1.2.1. *Type-I cross-talk*

$\{g_i, g_j\} \in E$ is a Type-I cross-talk between $pathway_1$ and $pathway_2$ if $(g_i \in pathway_1 \wedge g_j \in pathway_2) \wedge (g_i \notin pathway_2 \wedge g_j \notin pathway_1)$.

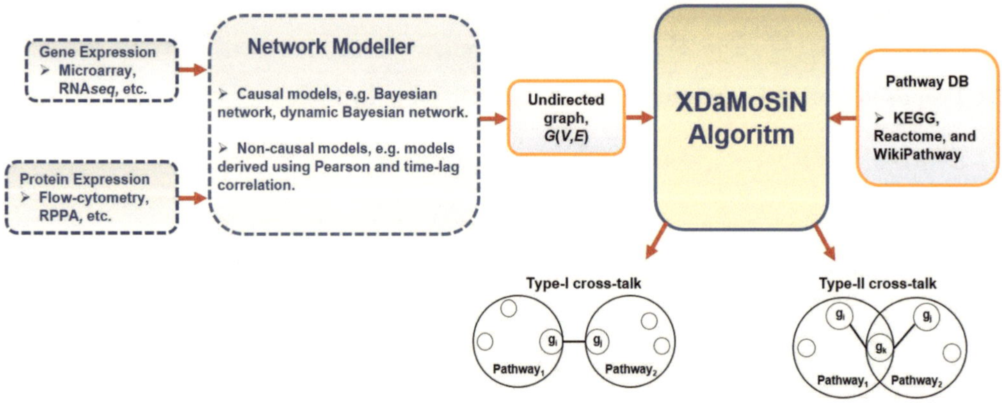

Figure 1. A schematic diagram of a possible framework that can use our algorithm to find cross-talks in data-driven model of signalling networks. This algorithm takes two inputs: (a) an undirected graph, $G(V,E)$ and (b) a pathway database. Approaches to generate data-driven models of signalling networks (details are skipped in this chapter) can use various types of data including gene and protein expression data.

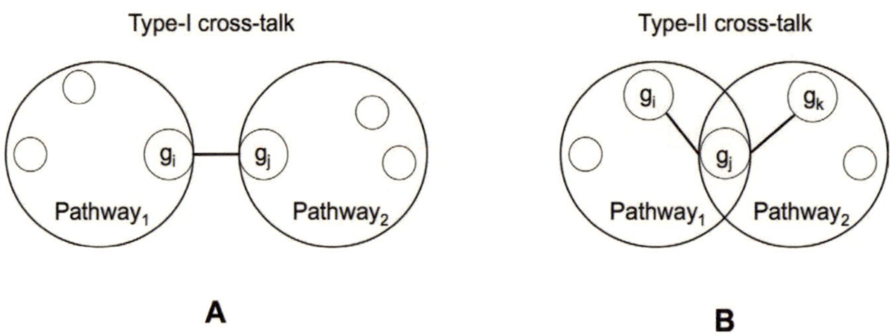

Figure 2. Proposed categorisations of signalling cross-talks, Type-I (A) and Type-II (B). Here, each of the pathways is a collection of signalling nodes (typically proteins or protein complexes). A Type-I cross-talk is a signalling link $\{g_i, g_j\}$ that connects two signalling pathways where neither of the two pathways contains both signalling nodes, g_i and g_j. A Type-II signalling cross-talk is a pair of signalling links $\{g_i, g_j\}$ and $\{g_j, g_k\}$ residing at the intersection of two signalling pathways with a shared node g_j.

2.1.2.2. Type-II cross-talk

$\{g_i, g_j\} \in E \wedge \{g_j, g_k\} \in E$ is a Type-II cross-talk between $pathway_1$ and $pathway_2$ if $(g_i \in pathway_1 \wedge g_j \in pathway_1) \wedge (g_j \in pathway_2 \wedge g_k \in pathway_2)$.

2.2. An algorithm for detecting proposed cross-talks

In **Figure 3**, we present a simple but intuitive algorithm for identifying Type-I and Type-II cross-talks in data-driven signalling network models. We refer to our algorithm as XDaMoSiN (cross-talk in data-driven models of signalling network). Note that our approach considers data-driven models of signalling networks as undirected networks in order to generalise our categorisation for both causal and non-causal network models. The only assumption we make here is that pathway annotations of signalling pathways are known from pathway databases such as KEGG [35], Reactome [37], and WikiPathways [36]. In these annotations, a pathway is defined as a list of signalling nodes. Note that the signalling links among these nodes are modelled using data-driven relationships. Therefore, a data-driven model of a signalling network is defined as where *V* is a list of *n* signalling nodes and *E* is a list of signalling links $\{g_i, g_j\}$ inferred from data. This algorithm takes two inputs: *G* (the network) and *PathwayDB* (a pathway database) and produces two outputs: *Type_I_crosstalk* and *Type_II_crosstalk*, which are two lists containing all Type-I and Type-II cross-talks (**Figure 3**). Here, we consider *PathwayDB* as a list, where each element in that list is also a list, containing signalling nodes in a particular pathway, and is indexed by the corresponding pathway ID (typically, the pathway name).

In the first part of the algorithm, we find all the Type-I cross-talks among all the pathways in *PathwayDB*. At first, we initialise the list *Type_I_crosstalk*, which collects all such Type-I

```
XDaMoSiN (G,PathwayDB)
/* Part#1 : Find  Type − I  crosstalks */
  Type_I_crosstalk ← ∅
  for each link {g_i, g_j} ∈ E
    List_i ← ∅
    List_j ← ∅
    for each pathway_id ∈ PathwayDB
      List_p ← FindList(PathwayDB, pathway_id)
      if g_i ∈ List_p
        List_i ← List_i ∪ {pathway_id}
      end if
      if g_j ∈ List_p
        List_j ← List_j ∪ {pathway_id}
      end if
    end for
    if List_i \ List_j is not ∅ and List_j \ List_i is not ∅
      Type_I_crosstalk ← Type_I_crosstalk ∪ {{g_i, g_j}}
    end if
  end for

/* Part#2 : Find  Type − II  crosstalks */
  Type_II_crosstalk ← ∅
  for each g_j ∈ V
    L_j ← ∅
    for each pathway_id ∈ PathwayDB
      L_p ← FindList(PathwayDB, pathway_id)
      for each g_i ∈ L_p
        if {g_i, g_j} ∈ E and {g_i, g_j} ⊂ L_p
          L_j ← L_j ∪ (pathway_id, g_i)
        end if
      end for
    end for
    for each pair (pathway_id_1, g_i) ∈ L_j
      for each pair (pathway_id_2, g_k) ∈ L_j
        if pathway_id_1 is not pathway_id_2
          Type_II_crosstalk ← Type_II_crosstalk ∪ {{g_i, g_j} ∧ {g_j, g_k}}
        end if
      end for
    end for
  end for
```

Figure 3. The pseudocode for XDaMoSiN algorithm.

cross-talks. Then we check each signalling link $\{g_i, g_j\} \in E$ to determine whether it plays a role as Type-I cross-talk. Here, we loop through all pathways and save pathway IDs that contain g_i or g_j, individually. For this purpose, we maintain two intermediate lists, called $List_i$ and $List_j$, respectively. If $List_i$ contains some pathway IDs that are not in $List_j$, and *vice versa*, then we identify $\{g_i, g_j\}$ as a Type-I cross-talk. Note, we assume here that an intermediate function called *FindList(PathwayDB, pathway_id)* exists, which constructs a list of signalling nodes in a particular pathway with ID: *pathway_id* in the *PathwayDB*.

In the second part of the algorithm, we find all Type-II cross-talks. First, we examine each signalling node g_j individually, to determine whether it is shared by more than one pathway and has incident signalling link(s) (from E) in those pathways. For this purpose, for each signalling node g_j, we construct an intermediate list, called L_j. This list collects ordered pairs of information: (1) each incident signalling node g_i in $\{g_i, g_j\} \in E$ that is contained in a pathway labelled *pathway_id* and (2) the *pathway_id* itself. Next, for any combination of pairs in the list L_j, such as (*pathway_id_1*,g_i) and (*pathway_id_2*,g_k), if *pathway_id_1* and *pathway_id_2* are different, then we define $\{g_i, g_j\} \wedge \{g_j, g_k\}$ as a Type-II cross-talk between *pathway_id_1* and *pathway_id_2*.

3. Results

3.1. Type-I and Type-II cross-talks include cross-talks from other state-of-the-art categorisations

We compare the cross-talk categorisation approaches, including our proposed methods, in **Figure 4**. This comparison reveals an interesting aspect of these categorisations: *cross-talks between any two pathways can be identified when their corresponding causal relationships are ignored,* that is, considering the signalling network as an undirected network only. At the same time, we note that our approach can include all types of cross-talks defined by other categorisation.

Type-I cross-talks can represent *signal-flow cross-talks, receptor function cross-talks,* and *gene-expression cross-talks* from Donaldson and Calder [14], *Mode-A* and *Mode-B* cross-talks from Guo and Wang [18], and cross-talk of signalling protein heterodimerisation from Kolch et al. [6]. In a cross-talking pair $\{g_i, g_j\}$ in each of these categories, one signalling component g_i belongs to one pathway and g_j belongs to another pathway, or vice versa, but mutually exclusively (**Figure 4**). Again, Type-II cross-talks represent the cross-talk types of *substrate availability* and *intracellular communications* from Donaldson and Calder [14], *Mode-C* cross-talks from Guo and Wang [18], and *signalling node sharing* and *competition for nodes* from Kolch et al. [6], since in all of these categories, there exists a shared component between $pathway_1$ and $pathway_2$ for which the other components of those individual pathways compete for modification or activation of that shared component (**Figure 4**).

Moreover, Donaldson and Calder [14] reported that their categorisation comprehensively covered all possible types of signalling cross-talks in a single cell model. Since Type-I and Type-II cross-talks include all cross-talks from Donaldson and Calder [**Figure 4**], we claim that our categorisation is also comprehensive. Moreover, Donaldson and Calder made a claim that their

http://dx.doi.org/10.5772/intechopen.72408

Proposed Categorisation	Related Study		
	Donaldson et al.	Guo et al.	Kolch et al.
1) *Type-I cross-talk*: $\{g_i, g_j\} \in E$ s.t. $(g_i \in pathway_1 \wedge$ $g_j \in pathway_2) \bigwedge$ $(g_i \notin pathway_2 \wedge$ $g_j \notin pathway_1)$	1) *Signal-flow cross-talk*: An alternate reaction to activate a protein 'Y' through an enzyme 'X' 2) *Receptor function cross-talk*: An alternate reaction to activate a receptor 'R' by an enzyme 'X' 3) *Gene expression cross-talk*: Activate/Inhibit the expression of a gene 'g' by a protein 'Y'	1) *Mode-A*: Components of one pathway physically interact with components of another pathway 2) *Mode-B*: Components of one pathway are enzymatic or transcriptional targets of components of another pathway	1) *Heterodimerisation between signalling proteins*: Two different signalling proteins from two different signalling pathways bind with each other
2) *Type-II cross-talk*: $\{g_i, g_j\} \in E \wedge$ $\{g_j, g_k\} \in E$ s.t. $(g_i \in pathway_1 \wedge$ $g_j \in pathway_1) \bigwedge$ $(g_j \in pathway_2 \wedge$ $g_k \in pathway_2)$	4) *Substrate availability cross-talk*: Pathways compete for activation of a shared protein 'Y' 5) *Intra-cellular communication cross-talk*: Output of the expression of a gene 'g' of a pathway acts as ligand of another pathway	3) *Mode-C*: One pathway modulates or competes for a key modulator or mediator of another	1) *Signalling node sharing*: A signalling node that is shared by two different signalling pathways. 2) *Competition for nodes*: Competing protein interactions coordinately regulate a signalling node mutually exclusively

Figure 4. Comparative categorisations of signalling cross-talks. Here, $\{g_i, g_j, g_k\} \in V\$$, V and E are the set of signalling components and signalling links, respectively.

approach can be useful for detecting cross-talks in data-driven models of signalling networks. However, we note that their proposed algorithm (see the appendix of [14]) was based on qualitative logic only, and is not explicit how that could be used for dealing with network models derived from *high-throughput* quantitative signalling data such as mass spectometry and RPPA data. Moreover, since they used modular architecture of signal propagation (receptor function, three-stage cascade, and gene expression [14]) in detecting all signalling cross-talks, their approach is not suitable for models derived from gene expression data only. There are some studies [30–32] that attempted to infer signalling network topology using gene expression as a proxy for signalling protein activities, since gene expression data are usually cheaper to generate and are possible to produce in large scale [32].

4. Discussion and conclusion

The data-driven modelling of signalling networks and the detection of cross-talks in those models provide effective ways to elucidate novel mechanisms of perturbed signalling activities in various disease conditions such as cancer and drug resistance. In this chapter, we reviewed some state-of-the-art approaches that categorise signalling cross-talks and identified a limitation of their applicability to data-driven models, since they rely on a static topology of signalling networks. Here, we propose a novel cross-talk categorisation (Type-I and Type-II) that can not only be applicable to data-driven models but also generalises all types of cross-talks defined by other approaches. We also presented a simple but intuitive algorithm for detecting Type-I and Type-II cross-talks between any two signalling pathways.

In combination with other computational and statistical methodologies, our approach is useful in systems biology to generate novel but biologically plausible hypotheses in a data-dependent manner.

The notion of cross-talking is inherently present in biological systems, which might involve interactions between/among signalling and regulatory pathway activities. Yamaguchi et al. [38] reported that in acquired resistance, RTK-mediated signalling pathways cross-talk with downstream *effector* pathways via altering the activities of effector proteins including transcription factors and enzymes and thus causes the dysregulation in the expression of multiple target gene, specially involved in growth and cell survival processes. Therefore, in addition to the signalling cross-talks, it is also important to efficiently find cross-talks between/among signalling and regulatory pathways as well. Although this chapter primarily focuses on the signalling cross-talks only, our definition of data-driven models biological systems as undirected graphs and the categorisations of Type-I and Type-II cross-talks can be generalised. Thus, our proposed algorithm will be able to identify cross-talks among any set of pathways including cell signalling and regulatory pathways.

Author details

A.K.M. Azad[1*], Alfons Lawen[2] and Jonathan M. Keith[3]

*Address all correspondence to: a.azad@monash.edu

1 Clayton School of IT, Faculty of IT, Monash University, Clayton, VIC, Australia

2 Department of Biochemistry and Molecular Biology, School of Biomedical Sciences, Monash University, Clayton, VIC, Australia

3 School of Mathematical Science, Monash University, Clayton, VIC, Australia

References

[1] Brivanlou AH, Darnell JE. Signal transduction and the control of gene expression. Science. 2002;**295**(5556):813-818

[2] Sarkar S, Mandal M. Growth factor receptors and apoptosis regulators: Signalling pathways, prognosis, chemosensitivity and treatment outcomes of breast cancer. Breast Cancer (Auckl.). 2009;**3**:47-60

[3] Ding S, Chamberlain M, McLaren A, Goh L, Duncan I, Wolf CR. Cross-talk between signalling pathways and the multidrug resistant protein MDR-1. British Journal of Cancer. 2001;**85**(8):1175-1184

[4] Janes KA, Yaffe MB. Data-driven modelling of signal-transduction networks. Nature Reviews. Molecular Cell Biology. 2006;**7**(11):820-828

[5] Schoeberl B, Pace E, Howard S, Garantcharova V, Kudla A, Sorger PK, Nielsen UB. A data-driven computational model of the ErbB receptor signaling network. Conference Proceedings: Annual International Conference of the IEEE Engineering in Medicine and Biology Society. 2006;**1**:53-54

[6] Kolch W, Halasz M, Granovskaya M, Kholodenko BN. The dynamic control of signal transduction networks in cancer cells. Nature Reviews. Cancer. 2015;**15**(9):515-527

[7] Santos SD, Verveer PJ, Bastiaens PI. Growth factor-induced MAPK network topology shapes Erk response determining PC-12 cell fate. Nature Cell Biology. 2007;**9**(3):324-330

[8] Von Kriegsheim A, Baiocchi D, Birtwistle M, Sumpton D, Bienvenut W, Morrice N, Yamada K, Lamond A, Kalna G, Orton R, Gilbert D, Kolch W. Cell fate decisions are specified by the dynamic ERK interactome. Nature Cell Biology. 2009;**11**(12): 1458-1464

[9] Janes KA, Kelly JR, Gaudet S, Albeck JG, Sorger PK, Lauffenburger DA. Cue-signal-response analysis of TNF-induced apoptosis by partial least squares regression of dynamic multivariate data. Journal of Computational Biology. 2004;**11**(4):544-561

[10] Woolf PJ, Prudhomme W, Daheron L, Daley GQ, Lauffenburger DA. Bayesian analysis of signaling networks governing embryonic stem cell fate decisions. Bioinformatics. 2005;**21**(6):741-753

[11] Sachs K, Perez O, Pe'er D, Lauffenburger DA, Nolan GP. Causal protein-signaling networks derived from multiparameter single-cell data. Science. 2005;**308**(5721):523-529

[12] Sachs K, Itani S, Carlisle J, Nolan GP, Pe'er D, Lauffenburger DA. Learning signaling network structures with sparsely distributed data. Journal of Computational Biology. 2009;**16**(2):201-212

[13] Santra T, Kholodenko B, Kolch W. An integrated Bayesian framework for identifying phosphorylation networks in stimulated cells. Advances in Experimental Medicine and Biology. 2012;**736**:59-80

[14] Donaldson R, Calder M. Modular modelling of signalling pathways and their cross-talk. Theoretical Computer Science. 2012;**456**:30-50

[15] Birtwistle MR, Hatakeyama M, Yumoto N, Ogunnaike BA, Hoek JB, Kholodenko BN. Ligand-dependent responses of the ErbB signaling network: Experimental and modeling analyses. Molecular Systems Biology. 2007;**3**:144

[16] Meyer AS, Miller MA, Gertler FB, Lauffenburger DA. The receptor AXL diversifies EGFR signaling and limits the response to EGFR-targeted inhibitors in triple-negative breast cancer cells. Science Signaling. 2013;**6**(287):ra66

[17] Natarajan M, Lin K-M, Hsueh RC, Sternweis PC, Ranganathan R. A global analysis of cross-talk in a mammalian cellular signalling network. Nature Cell Biology. 2006;**8**(6): 571-580

[18] Guo X, Wang XF. Signalling cross-talk between TGF-beta/BMP and other pathways. Cell Research. 2009;**19**(1):71-88

[19] Schwartz MA, Ginsberg MH. Networks and crosstalk: Integrin signalling spreads. Nature Cell Biology. 2002;**4**(4):E65-E68

[20] Katzenellenbogen BS. Estrogen receptors: Bioactivities and interactions with cell signaling pathways. Biology of Reproduction. 1996;**54**(2):287-293

[21] De Bosscher K, Vanden Berghe W, Haegeman G. Cross-talk between nuclear receptors and nuclear factor kappaB. Oncogene. 2006;**25**(51):6868-6886

[22] McClean MN, Mody A, Broach JR, Ramanathan S. Cross-talk and decision making in MAP kinase pathways. Nature Genetics. 2007;**39**(3):409-414

[23] Hatakeyama M, Kimura S, Naka T, Kawasaki T, Yumoto N, Ichikawa M, Kim JH, Saito K, Saeki M, Shirouzu M, Yokoyama S, Konagaya A. A computational model on the modulation of mitogen-activated protein kinase (MAPK) and Akt pathways in heregulin-induced ErbB signalling. The Biochemical Journal. 2003;**373**(Pt 2):451-463

[24] Sreenath SN, Soebiyanto R, Mesarovic MD, Wolkenhauer O. Coordination of crosstalk between MAPK-PKC pathways: An exploratory study. IET Systems Biology. 2007;**1**(1):33-40

[25] Borisov N, Aksamitiene E, Kiyatkin A, Legewie S, Berkhout J, Maiwald T, Kaimachnikov NP, Timmer J, Hoek JB, Kholodenko BN. Systems-level interactions between insulin-EGF networks amplify mitogenic signaling. Molecular Systems Biology. 2009;**5**:256

[26] Romano D, Nguyen LK, Matallanas D, Halasz M, Doherty C, Kholodenko BN, Kolch W. Protein interaction switches coordinate Raf-1 and MST2/Hippo signalling. Nature Cell Biology. 2014;**16**(7):673-684

[27] O'Neill E, Rushworth L, Baccarini M, Kolch W. Role of the kinase MST2 in suppression of apoptosis by the proto-oncogene product Raf-1. Science. 2004;**306**(5705):2267-2270

[28] Matallanas D, Romano D, Yee K, Meissl K, Kucerova L, Piazzolla D, Baccarini M, Vass JK, Kolch W, O'neill E. RASSF1A elicits apoptosis through an MST2 pathway directing proapoptotic transcription by the p73 tumor suppressor protein. Molecular Cell. 2007;**27**(6):962-975

[29] Hill SM, Lu Y, Molina J, Heiser LM, Spellman PT, Speed TP, Gray JW, Mills GB, Mukherjee S. Bayesian inference of signalling network topology in a cancer cell line. Bioinformatics. 2012;**28**(21):2804-2810

[30] Amadoz A, Sebastian-Leon P, Vidal E, Salavert F, Dopazo J. Using activation status of signaling pathways as mechanism-based biomarkers to predict drug sensitivity. Scientific Reports. 2015;**5**:18494

[31] Sebastian-Leon P, Carbonell J, Salavert F, Sanchez R, Medina I, Dopazo J. Inferring the functional effect of gene expression changes in signaling pathways. Nucleic Acids Research. 2013;**41**(Web Server issue):W213-W217

[32] Neapolitan R, Xue D, Jiang X. Modeling the altered expression levels of genes on signaling pathways in tumors as causal bayesian networks. Cancer Informatics. 2014;**13**:77-84

[33] Locasale JW, Wolf-Yadlin A. Maximum entropy reconstructions of dynamic signaling networks from quantitative proteomics data. PLoS One. 2009;**4**(8):e6522

[34] Imami K, Sugiyama N, Imamura H, Wakabayashi M, Tomita M, Taniguchi M, Ueno T, Toi M, Ishihama Y. Temporal profiling of lapatinib-suppressed phosphorylation signals in EGFR/HER2 pathways. Molecular & Cellular Proteomics. 2012;**11**(12):1741-1757

[35] Kanehisa M. The KEGG database. Novartis Foundation Symposium. 2002;**247**:91-101

[36] Kelder T, van Iersel MP, Hanspers K, Kutmon M, Conklin BR, Evelo CT, Pico AR. WikiPathways: Building research communities on biological pathways. Nucleic Acids Research. 2012;**40**(Database issue):D1301-D1307

[37] Croft D, Mundo AF, Haw R, Milacic M, Weiser J, Wu G, Caudy M, Garapati P, Gillespie M, Kamdar MR, Jassal B, Jupe S, Matthews L, May B, Palatnik S, Rothfels K, Shamovsky V, Song H, Williams M, Birney E, Hermjakob H, Stein L, D'Eustachio P. The Reactome pathway knowledgebase. Nucleic Acids Research. 2014;**42**(Database issue):D472-D477

[38] Yamaguchi H, Chang SS, Hsu JL, Hung MC. Signaling cross-talk in the resistance to HER family receptor targeted therapy. Oncogene. 2014;**33**(9):1073-1081

Section 3

Non-Coding RNAs and Degradation of RNAs

Chapter 6

Interplay between Transcription and RNA Degradation

Toshimichi Yamada, Masami Nagahama and
Nobuyoshi Akimitsu

Additional information is available at the end of the chapter

http://dx.doi.org/10.5772/intechopen.71862

Abstract

Amount of mRNA depends on the both the rates of mRNA transcription in the nucleus and mRNA degradation in the cytoplasm. Although each of the processes was studied independently, recent studies demonstrated the interplay between transcription and mRNA degradation in various cellular processes, such as cell-cycle, cellular differentiation, and stress responses. In this review, we discuss the benefit of the interplay in the gene expressions and the mechanisms how these two processes are coupled. We also review recent genome-wide methods to measure the rates of transcription and degradation.

Keywords: RNA degradation, transcription factor, RNA binding proteins, synthegradase, RNA buffering, mRNA imprinting, NGS

1. Introduction

Gene expression involves multiple processes such as the transcription, translation, and degradation of messenger RNAs (mRNAs). Each of these processes was studied independently. In the nucleus, RNA polymerase II (RNAPII) and various transcription factors are recruited to the promoter of protein-coding genes to initiate transcription [1, 2]. Nascent mRNA is co-transcriptionally capped at 5′-end [3, 4], spliced [5], and matured at the 3′-end [6] (**Figure 1**). During these post-transcriptional modifications, every transcript is associated with various RNA-binding proteins (RBPs), forming large ribonucleoprotein complexes (mRNPs). This mRNP assembly process is subject to quality control by nuclear surveillance mechanisms [7, 8]. After the quality control, mRNPs are transported to cytoplasm.

In the cytoplasm, the translationally inactive mRNPs would accumulate in P bodies or stress granules where mRNPs are degraded [9, 10] (**Figure 2**). Degradation of the cytoplasmic

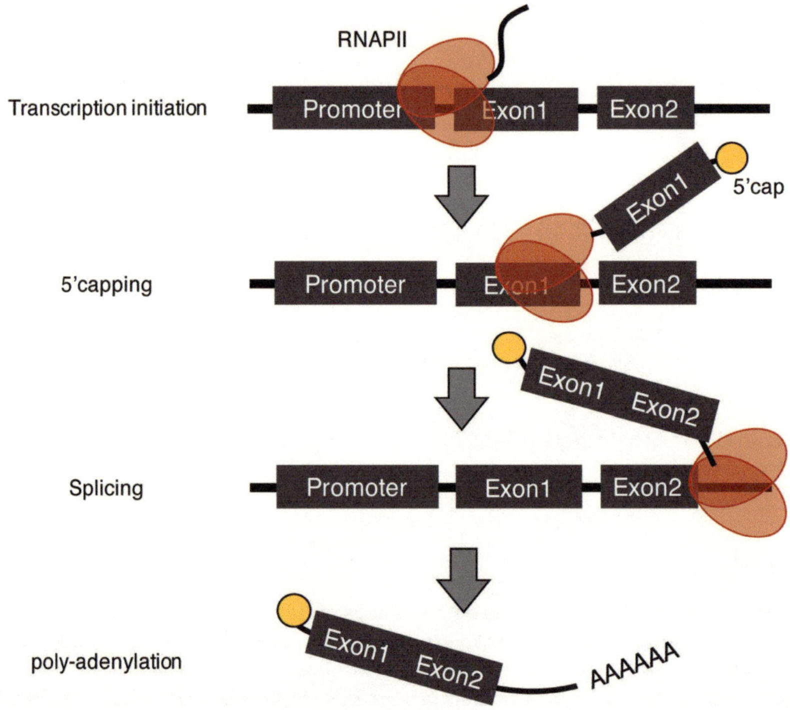

Figure 1. Scheme of co-transcriptional mRNA processing. An m^{7}G cap (a circle) is added co-transcriptionally to the 5′end of the nascent RNA. During the elongation, introns are removed by splicing machinery. Cleavage and polyadenylation are mediated after the transcription to form mature transcripts.

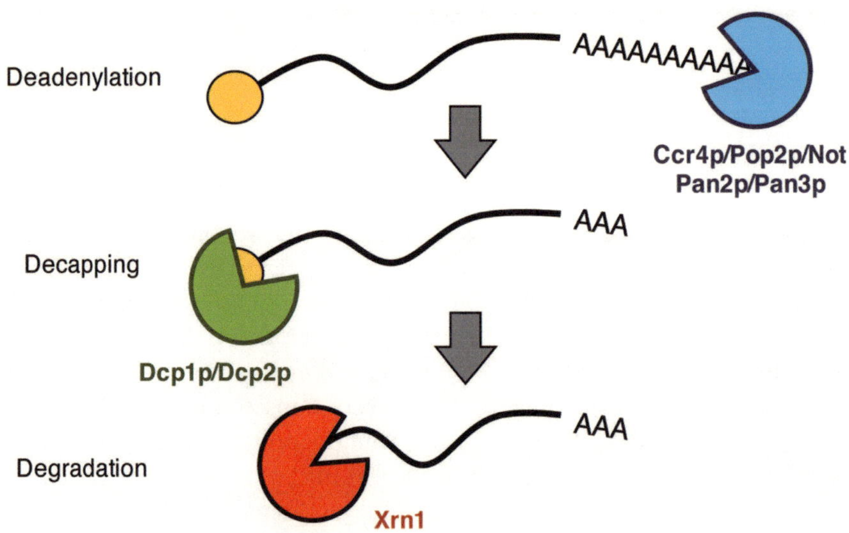

Figure 2. The 5′ → 3′ degradation pathway exonuclease-mediated decay begins with shortening of Pan2/Pan3 or CCR4-not complexes. After the decapping of 5′cap structure (a circle), the body of mRNA is degraded with 5′-to-3′polarity by XRN1.

Names in yeast	Human homologs	Function
Ccr4p	hCCR4	Carbon catabolite repressor 4. Catalytic subunits of the complex
Pop2p	CNOT7/CNOT8	Also known as Caf1 (Ccr4 associated factor 1). Related to RNase D family
Not	CNOT1	Negative on TATA. A large scaffolding protein
Pan2p	PAN2	PolyA nuclease2. Contains a nuclease domain of the RNase D
Pan3p	PAN3	PolyA nuclease3. Co-factor of Pan2
Dcp1p	DCP1A/DCP1B	Decapping protein1, Co-activator
Dcp2p	DCP2	Decapping protein2. Catalytically active decapping enzyme
Pat1p	PAT1A/PAT1B	Recruit Lsm1-7 to P-bodies to trigger decapping
Lsm1-7p	LSM 1-7	Seven Sm-like proteins. Deadenylation-dependent mRNA decapping factors
Dhh1p	RCX/p54	DEAD box helicase. ATP-dependent RNA helicase in mRNA decapping
Xrn1p	XRN1/XRN2	Major 5′-3′ Exoribonuclease1, requiring 5′ monophosphate

Table 1. Yeast RNA degradation factors and its human homologs.

mRNA is initiated by shortening of the poly(A) tail, which is called deadenylation. In yeast, this deadenylation is catalyzed either by Ccr4p/Pop2p/Not complex or by the Pan2p/Pan3p complex [11, 12]. After the deadenylation, the 5′-cap structure was removed by the concerted action of the decapping complex, Dcp1p/Dcp2p, which is stimulated by Pat1p, the Lsm1-7p, and Dhh1p [13, 14]. The decapping reaction exposes the 5′-monophosphate of the terminal residue, promoting the 5′ → 3′ degradation pathway by the major cytoplasmic exoribonuclease Xrn1p [15] (**Table 1**).

The life of mRNA seems to be straightforward. However, recent studies have shown evidence of the interplay between transcription and degradation: transcription rate is regulated by decay factor; degradation rate is regulated by transcription factor and even by some promoters. This complex network enables cells to shape appropriate gene expression profiles during cell cycle processes, cellular differentiation, stress and immune responses [16–18].

2. Biological processes coupling transcription and decay

The functional connection between the transcription and degradation of mRNA shapes the characteristic patterns of gene expression. In this section, we introduce several examples of the coordination between transcription and degradation in various biological processes.

To respond to environmental cues, cells must switch their steady level of gene expression in a rapid and transient mode. This sharp rise of mRNAs can be efficiently achieved if the stabilization of transcripts enhances their transcription rates. An example for such functional coupling is observed in osmotic stress in *S. cerevisiae*. With mild osmotic stress (0.4 M NaCl), 121 mRNAs belonging to the functional groups "stress response" and "trehalose production" increase both transcription rates and stability [19]. The study of oxidative stress (0.5 mM H_2O_2) in fission yeast revealed a major role of transcriptional up-regulation in the stress, but also showed the first minutes after stress induction as a critical time for mRNA degradation to support the control rapid gene regulation by transcription [20]. In contrast to oxidative stress, a moderate heat shock induced a global trend for mRNA stabilization, whereas transcription rate contributed only a transient increase immediately upon stress [21]. The difference observed in these studies suggested the interplay between transcription and degradation is carefully regulated in the cells. Indeed, Shalem et al. demonstrated that alternative modes of such interplay determine the kinetics of the transcriptome in response to stress. They subjected yeast to two stresses; oxidative stress and DNA damage. In oxidative stress, many genes show fast response followed by relaxation, resulting in a quick and transient response, whereas in the DNA damage experiment, the response is slow and long enduring. Measurement of the genome-wide decay profile showed condition-specific changes in decay rates. In the transient response, most induced genes were destabilized, exhibiting counteraction between transcription and degradation. This interplay profile can reconcile a high steady-state level with short response time among induced genes. In contrast, slow repression response was achieved by destabilization of the transcripts [22].

As abnormal gene expression is deleterious to living cells, it is critical to maintain steady levels of mRNA; hence, mRNA levels are said to be "buffered". When genome-wide transcription was attenuated by mutating RNAPII of *S. cerevisiae*, the cells maintain a steady level of the transcripts by decreasing their decay rates [23]. This study also revealed that buffering of mRNA levels required the RNA exonuclease Xrn1. Conversely, impairing mRNA degradation by deleting deadenylase subunits of the Ccr4-Not complex caused the decrease in both degradation and synthesis rates [24]. This mutual feedback maintains the steady levels of mRNAs and establishes a cellular mRNA surveillance network. It is mysterious that the synthesis-decay feedback exists despite the separation of mRNA synthesis and degradation into nuclear and cytoplasmic compartments. One possible model was proposed by Haimovich et al. [25]. They showed that the components related to mRNA degradations shuttle between cytoplasm and the nucleus, in a manner dependent on proper mRNA degradation. In the nucleus, they associated with chromatin and regulated transcription rate.

Cross talk between mRNA synthesis and decay can also be gene specific. In budding yeast, stability of core histone mRNAs is temporally co-regulated with their transcription during the cell cycle. Entry into S phase showed rapid increase in their transcription, followed by a prompt decrease in their abundance right after exiting the S phase [26–28]. Similar to histone mRNAs, there should be numerous genes of which expression levels are regulated in a cell-cycle-dependent manner. By using DNA microarrays, Spellman et al. found that about 800 genes are cell cycle regulated, which correspond to 10% of all protein-coding genes in yeast genome [29]. The mechanism for how cells coordinate the characteristic and integrated expression pattern during cell-cycle is not fully understood.

Interestingly, a functional coupling between the transcription and degradation was exploited by herpes virus [30]. Gamma-herpesviruses encode a cytoplasmic endonuclease, SOX, which cleaves cellular mRNAs. These cleaved fragments are subsequently degraded by the cellular exonuclease Xrn1. This accelerated decay triggered the repression of RNAPII transcription rate. The findings suggest that mammalian cells can sense broad alternation in RNA degradation. It is not the initial cleavages by SOX that are detected, but rather the increased activity of cellular Xrn1 that generates a transcriptional response. Furthermore, the viral mRNAs escaped the degradation induced transcriptional repression, and this escape requires Xrn1. The opposing roles for Xrn1 in the host and viral transcriptional response may indicate that herpesviruses have evolved to benefit from this intrinsic feedback mechanism.

3. Mechanism underlying coupling transcription and decay

The mechanism underlying transcription in the nucleus affects mRNA decay in the cytoplasm and vice versa is intensively studied in *S. cerevisiae*. The regulation of mRNA decay mediated by the transcription is categorized into *cis*-acting elements and *trans*-activating factors. *Cis*-acting elements directly regulate the mRNA decay by interacting with RNA binding proteins and/or decay factors [31, 32]. *trans*-activating factors are recruited onto the mRNA during its transcription. This interaction is maintained in cytoplasm, regulating the stability of the mRNA. In contrast, there are only a few examples for regulation of the transcription by mRNA decay, and this is still under intense investigation.

3.1. *cis*-acting elements

mRNA contains 5′ untranslated region (UTR) and 3′UTR outside the coding region. These two UTR regulate the fate of mRNAs. Here we discuss how the transcription of 3′UTR regulates its length, and thus causes the modification of mRNA stability.

3.1.1. 3′UTR

The turnover of an mRNA is mostly regulated by *cis*-acting elements located in the 3′UTR [33], such as AU-rich elements (AREs) [34, 35], GU-rich elements [36], PUF response elements [37], miRNA binding sites [38, 39], and the poly(A) tail [40]. In principle, the length of 3′UTR affect the stability of mRNA because longer 3′UTR would contain more *cis*-acting elements compared with short 3′UTR (**Figure 3**). Eukaryotic cells control the length of 3′UTR with alternative polyadenylation [41, 42]. Genome-wide polyadenylation maps were established by several RNA-seq studies. Direct RNA sequencing (DRS) technology provided a comprehensive view of global polyadenylation events in human and yeast, and estimated that 72% of yeast genes and more than half of human genes show alternative polyadenylation patterns [43]. Moreover, 3′ region extraction and deep sequencing (3′READS) was used to comprehensively map polyadenylation sites in the mouse genome [44]. 3′READS revealed that about 80% of mRNA and 66% of long noncoding RNA undergo alternative polyadenylation. Importantly, 3′READS found a global trend of up-regulation

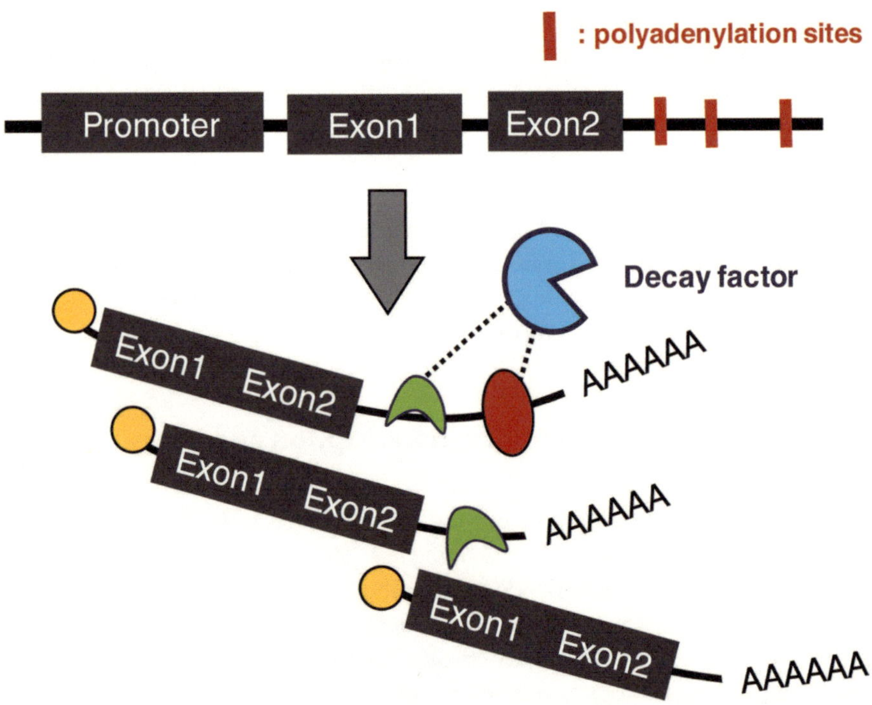

Figure 3. Alternative polyadenylation affects 3′UTR lengths. Longer UTRs allow more RBPs to associate with the mRNA (indicated by arrowhead and ellipse, respectively). The RBPs regulate the mRNA stability by recruiting decay factor.

of isoforms using promoter-distal polyadenylation sites in development and differentiation, suggesting that the RNA degradation pathway will be reconstructed globally through the development. These two studies, however, lack quantitative analysis of mRNA stability and 3′UTR length modification by alternative polyadenylation. Geisberg et al. developed a method to measure mRNA half-lives of mRNA isoform in yeast [45]. Based on clusters of isoforms with different half-lives, they identified hundreds of sequences responsible for mRNA stabilization. Specifically, the poly(U) sequence was found to be the stabilizing element.

3.1.2. Promoter regulates mRNA stability

Surprisingly, several reports showed that promoter regions also affect mRNA degradation after the mRNA leaves the nucleus. The first report of promoter-regulated mRNA stability was published in 1993. This study showed that swapping of the β-globin promoter in HeLa cells to that of the Herpes simplex virus 1 thymidine kinase (HSV1-TK) stabilizes a nonsense mutation in the mRNA, while this effect was not observed with the replacement for the CMV promoter [46]. A problem in this study was that the authors cannot rule out the possibility that different amounts of mature β-globin mRNAs may be caused by the different efficiencies of the splicing. This problem can be avoided by targeting genes without introns.

In 2011, two studies in the *S. cerevisiae* demonstrated clearly that promoters and associated *cis*-acting elements coordinate their transcription and decay (**Figure 4**). A conventional yeast promoter consists of a core element and an upstream activating sequence (UAS). Promoter swapping of native UAS of the *RPL30* gene with that of the *ACT1* gene increased the stability of *RPL30* mRNA significantly [47]. A *cis*-element, comprising two Rap1p-binding sites, and Rap1p itself are necessary and sufficient to induce stabilization of the transcript. Moreover, Rap1p stimulates both synthesis and decay of endogenous transcripts. Thus, this study proposed that interaction of Rap1p with the target promoter affects the composition of mRNP, resulting in modification of the mRNA degradation rate. Considering that Rap1p has an effect in coupling transcription with mRNA decay, this study also introduced a concept called "synthegradase". They also estimated at least 150 yeast genes would be regulated by synthegradases during optimal proliferation conditions. Notably, this number is likely to increase with different environmental conditions.

A second example is the study about cell cycle-regulated decay in yeast cells using single molecule fluorescence *in situ* hybridization (FISH) [48]. Promoter swapping of *SWI5* and *CLB2* genes with *ACT1* made their stability close to *ACT1*. This study also showed that the mitotic exit network protein Dbf2p accounts for the coordinated decay of the transcripts. Chromatin immunoprecipitation and RNA immunoprecipitation of Dbf2p showed that Dbf2p interacts with both the transcript promoter and mRNA, suggesting that this protein is recruited to the promoter and then subsequently stalled on the mRNA. As Dbf2 can interact with the Ccr4-Not complex [49], this promoter-regulated decay may manifest through the regulation of deadenylation.

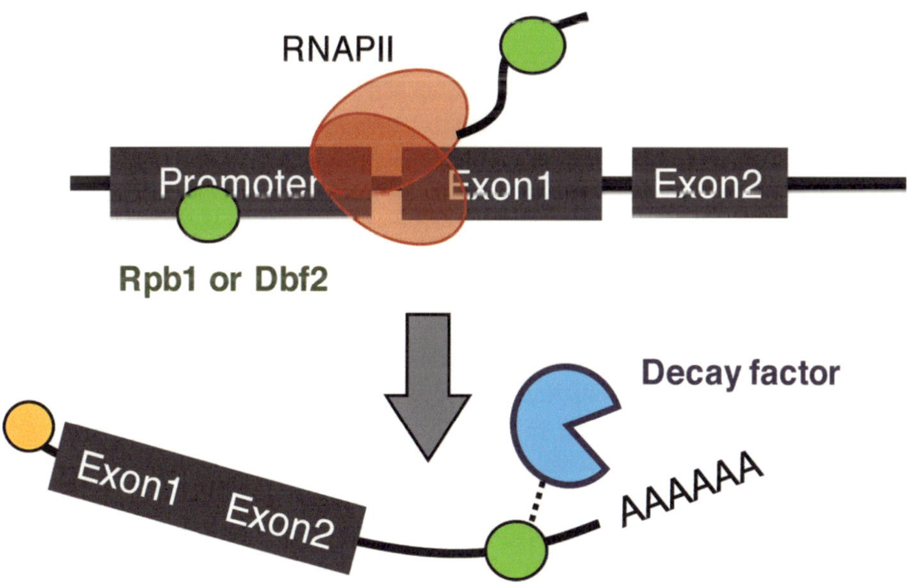

Figure 4. Promoter-regulating degradation. Transcription factor such as Rpb1 or Dbf2 (a circle on the promoter) binds to transcripts. After the export into the cytoplasm, the transcription factors in cytoplasm recruit decay factor to promote RNA degradation.

Although these two works are focused on specific genes, Dori-Bachash et al. extended to the genome-wide scale [50]. They demonstrated that swapping UAS between two yeast species affected both transcription and degradation. Adjacent yeast genes sharing a common promoter displayed similar mRNA decay rates, which also indicated that promoters couple transcription and degradation. Notably, similar coordination between transcription and degradation were found in mouse and human models. Because the diverse genes and regulatory elements were associated with promoter-regulated coordination, this phenomenon could be generated by genome-wide mechanisms of gene regulation.

3.2. *trans*-acting proteins

trans-acting proteins are recruited onto the mRNA during transcription, and affect post-transcriptional regulation after mRNA is exported to nucleoplasm. This process is termed "mRNA imprinting", which confers classical genetic information flexibility [51]. This mRNA imprinting lasts throughout the mRNA lifetime and is required for proper post-transcriptional regulation. Here, we focus how mRNA imprinting regulates the degradation rate.

3.2.1. *Rpb4 and Rpb7*

To date, the best characterized *trans*-acting proteins are two subunits of the core RNAPII, Rpb4p and Rpb7p. Rpb4p and Rpb7p associate with the core polymerase as a heterodimer. Two studies provided evidence that the nascent pre-mRNA emerging from the active site of RNAPII interacts with Rpb7p [52, 53]. Moreover, Rpb4/7p shuttle between the nucleus and the cytoplasm [54], suggesting that this heterodimer influences mRNA physiology in the cytoplasm. These facts suggest that Rpb4/7p would be imprinted on the mRNA. Several pieces of experimental results revealed that Rpb4/7p promotes the mRNA decay [55, 56]: both Rpb4p and Rpb7p affected the deadenylation step; both Rpb4p and Rpb7p interact with the mRNA decapping components of the Pat1p-Lsm1-7p complex; and Rpb4p and Rpb7p localized to cytoplasmic P-bodies where mRNA is degraded. In this manner, Rpb4/7p would link the activity of the basal transcription apparatus with that of the mRNA degradation machinery [57].

3.2.2. *Snf1*

Snf1p is the yeast ortholog of human AMP-activated protein kinase (AMPK) involved in diverse stress environments [58–60]. Recent studies also revealed that Snf1p is related to post-transcriptional regulation. Culturing yeast in glucose-containing growth medium represses Snf1-dependent transcription of target genes and promotes mRNA degradation of the corresponding mRNAs, which is called glucose-induced decay of mRNA [61, 62]. In low glucose concentrations, Snf1 activates the transcription of glucose-induced genes required for energy metabolism. In contrast, when glucose concentration is high, termination of transcription and activation of the degradation of the glucose-induced transcripts occur, resulting in rapid reduction of mRNA levels. Braun et al. fused nonglucose-responsive genes *MAP2* and *IDP2* to the *ADH2* promoter. This promoter swapping caused a significant destabilization of these mRNAs, indicating that the *ADH2* promoter alone is responsible for glucose-induced mRNA decay [63]. To understand the molecular mechanism of Snf1-dependent decay, quantitative mass spectrometry was used to identify proteins phosphorylated in a Snf1-dependent manner [64]. This phosphoproteomic analysis identified 210 Snf1-dependent phosphopeptides in 145 proteins. Notably, mRNA decay factors, such as Eap1p, Ccr4p, Dhh1p, and Xrn1p were the targets of Snf1p-dependent phosphorylation. As expected, mutation of three Snf1-dependent phosphorylation sites in Xrn1 reduced glucose-induced mRNA decay. Therefore, Snf1p-dependent transcription and decay of glucose-specific mRNAs could be activated by triggering the cytoplasmic decay factors.

3.3. mRNA decay factors modulating transcription

Currently, two mRNA decay factors are proposed to regulate the transcription: Ccr4p/Pop2p/Not complex (deadenylase) and Xrn1p (exoribonuclease). Ccr4p/Pop2p/Not complex is deadenylase, catalyzing the initial deadenylation step of polyadenylated mRNAs prior to their decapping. Historically, Ccr4p, the major catalytic subunit, was initially discovered as an activator of transcription [65, 66], rather than deadenylase [67]. Other studies showed that Not proteins repress the transcription of TATA-less promoter [68, 69]. Furthermore, the Ccr4/Not complex was involved in transcription elongation by interacting with RNAPII [25, 70]. Although numerous studies indicate the bifunctional aspect of Ccr4p/Pop2p/Not complex in posttranscriptional regulation, no study, to our knowledge, has focused on the cross-talk between mRNA synthesis and degradation. To reveal the whole picture of the complex, further investigations are necessary.

Xrn1 targets cytoplasmic RNA substrates marked by a decapped 5′ monophosphate for further 5′-to′3′ degradation [71–73]. In 2013, two studies revealed the functional role of Xrn1p in the crosstalk between transcription and degradation. Haimovich et al. performed serial experiments that suggest the direct role of Xrn1 in transcription [25]. First, Xrn1p shuttled between the cytoplasm and the nucleus in a manner dependent on mRNA degradation. Second, GRO-seq data demonstrated that the densities of active Pol II are affected by deleting Xrn1p or by mutating its active site. A similar result was also confirmed by single-cell FISH. Third, the whole-genome-binding feature of Xrn1p showed that Xrn1p binds to promoters of genes of which transcription is highly affected by Xrn1p disruption, suggesting that promoter binding is a transcriptional function. Fourth, inhibition of Xrn1p accumulated transcriptionally incompetent Pol II at the nascent mRNAs. This result suggested that Xrn1p functions in transcription elongation. Therefore, the researchers concluded that Xrn1 is an essential factor for mRNA synthesis-degradation coupling, and referred to Xrn1p as "synthegradosome." The report published by Sun et al. showed that depletion of Xrn1p caused a global activation of mRNA transcription monitored by comparative dynamic transcriptome analysis (cDTA) [23]. They also searched for nuclear factors, which repress mRNA transcription by Xrn1, and identified transcription repressor Nrg1 as the downstream of Xrn1. Increase in mRNA degradation rates are compensated by an increase in mRNA transcription, suggesting that overall mRNA levels are "buffered". This study showed that Xrn1p was required for the RNA buffering. As summarized above, the two studies reached different conclusions regarding the consequences of deleting or inactivating Xrn1p. From these results, we may conclude that Xrn1p is related to coupling mRNA synthesis and degradation; however, the mechanism of this interplay is still unresolved.

4. Direct measurements for transcription and degradation rates at the genome-wide level

The difficulty in studying the interplay between transcription and degradation is in measuring the kinetics of the processes, especially at the genome-wide level. Recent advances in RNA-seq technologies enable us to determine the rate of transcription and/or degradation.

4.1. BRIC-seq

RNA stabilities are measured by the decrease in RNA after inhibiting transcription [74–76]. However, transcription affects degradation rates, as discussed previously, which obscure the native half-lives of transcripts. Tani et al. developed an inhibitor-free method termed 5′ Bromo-uridine (BrU) Immunoprecipitation Chase-deep sequencing analysis (BRIC-seq) [77, 78]. BRIC-seq applies BrU for metabolic labeling of endogenous transcripts. After removing BrU from the medium, total RNAs are then isolated from the cells at sequential time points. BrUs-labeled RNAs are purified through immunopurification by using BrU antibody. The half-life of each transcript is calculated from the decreasing amount of BrU-RNA measured by RNA-seq (**Figure 5**).

4.2. GRO-seq, PRO-seq, NET-seq

Global Run-On sequencing (GRO-seq) was developed to measure transcription rate. GRO-seq maps the genome-wide positions, amounts and orientation of transcriptionally engaged RNAP [79, 80]. In GRO-seq, transcription is inhibited in living cells, and then reinitiated in isolated nuclei under conditions that allow labeling of nascent transcripts (nuclear run-on) with BrU. Capturing nascent transcripts from active RNAP provides a direct synthesis rate of the transcription. Similar to GRO-seq, precision nuclear run-on sequencing (PRO-seq) maps the location of active RNAP at base pair resolution [81]. PRO-seq uses biotin-labeled NTP (biotin-NTP) during the nuclear run-on procedure. Addition of only one of the four biotin NTPs restricts RNAP to incorporating a single or a few identical bases, resulting in sequence reads that have the same 3′ end base within each library. Native elongating transcript sequencing (NET-seq) can also obtain a nascent transcription profile with single-nucleotide resolution [82–84]. In NET-seq, nascent RNA was detected in the active site of RNAP by immunoprecipitation of FLAG-tagged RNAP.

4.3. 4sU-seq and TT-seq

Here we would like to introduce two methods that can determine the kinetics of both transcription and degradation. These two technologies will advance the study of the

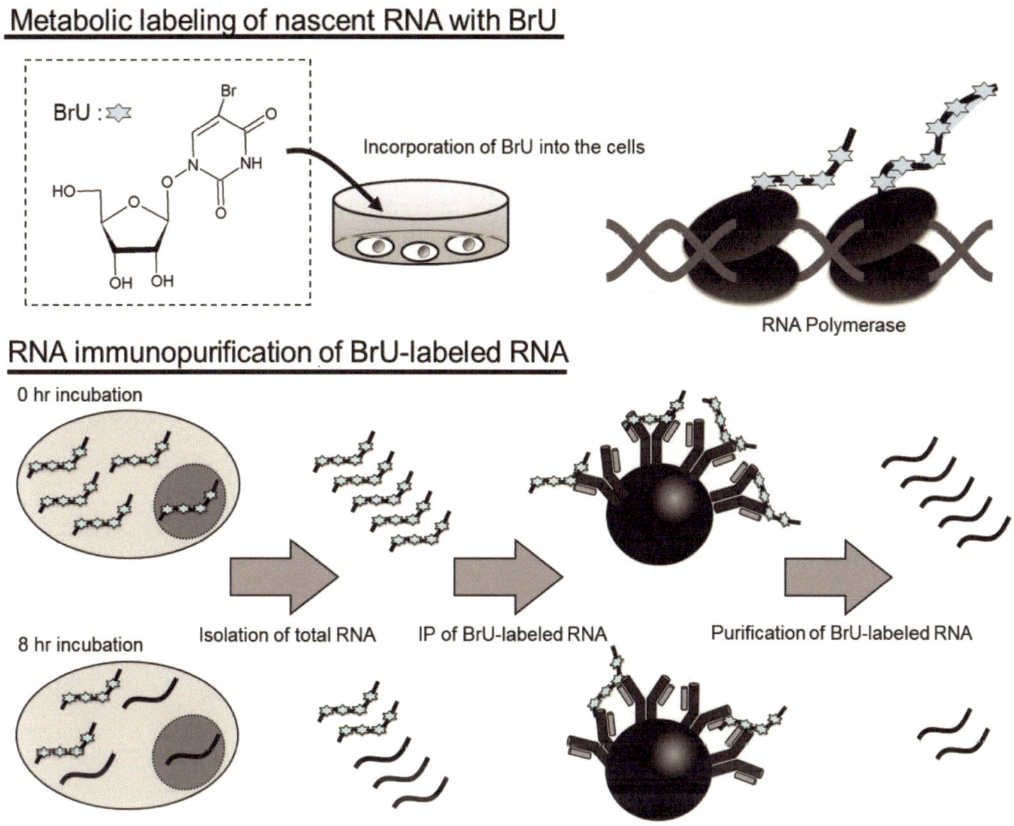

Figure 5. Overview of the BRIC-seq protocol.

interplay between transcription and degradation. Rabani et al. combined pulse labeling of mRNA with 4sU and computational modeling to estimate RNA transcription and degradation rates [85]. Newly transcribed RNA (4sU-labeled RNA) contains nascent RNA transcribed during the labeling pulse. When the labeling time is sufficiently short, the 4sU-labeled RNA is still in the nucleus, reflecting the average transcription rate. A computational model separates the RNA levels into transcription and degradation, and thus estimates the degradation rates from the experimental results of total RNA level and transcription rate.

The disadvantage of 4sU-seq is that it fails to map transcripts uniformly, because only a short 3′ region of nascent transcripts is labeled with 4sU, and long pre-existing 5′ regions dominate the RNA-seq data. To overcome this 5′ bias, transient transcriptome sequencing (TT-seq) fragments the 4sU-RNA before isolation. This fragmentation permits the immunoprecipitation of only newly transcribed 4sU-RNA fragments. Notably, TT-seq monitors RNA synthesis, whereas GRO-seq, PRO-seq, and NET-seq detect RNAs attached to RNAPs. Furthermore, TT-seq can determine transcription termination sites because TT-seq detected transient RNA downstream of the polyadenylation site.

5. Conclusion

The balance between mRNA transcription and decay determines the mRNA levels, which is a key aspect in the gene regulation. The study of interplay between transcription and decay is only the beginning. Our knowledge is still limited to the specific signaling pathway in yeast. As described in chapter 4, genome-wide analysis of transcription and decay will provide a comprehensive view of the interplay. Moreover, it will be critically important to verify the coupling of transcription and decay in mammalian system because mammalian cells contain numerous RBPs with defined roles in mRNA decay. It would be interesting to determine whether any of these RBPs also regulate transcription. It is a well-known fact that aberrant regulation of gene expression causes serious diseases. Therefore, studying the interplay between transcription and decay in mammalian cells will be beneficial for understanding diseases with defects in RNA expression levels.

Author details

Toshimichi Yamada[1], Masami Nagahama[1] and Nobuyoshi Akimitsu[2*]

*Address all correspondence to: akimitsu@ric.u-tokyo.ac.jp

1 Meiji Pharmaceutical University, Tokyo, Japan

2 Isotope Science Center, The University of Tokyo, Japan

References

[1] Koleske, Young. An RNA polymerase II holoenzyme responsive to activators. Nature. 1994;**368**(6470):466-469. DOI: 10.1038/368466a0

[2] Orphanides G, Lagrange T, Reinberg D. The general transcription factors of RNA polymerase II. Genes & Development. 1996;**10**:2657-2683

[3] Shuman. Structure, mechanism, and evolution of the mRNA capping apparatus. Progress in Nucleic Acid Research and Molecular Biology. 2001;**66**:1-40

[4] Shatkin AJ. Capping of eucaryotic mRNAs. Cell. 1976;**9**(4):645-653. DOI: 10.1016/0092-8674(76)90128-8

[5] Matera G, Wang Z. A day in the life of the spliceosome. Nature Reviews Molecular Cell Biology. 2014;**15**(2):108-121. DOI: 10.1038/nrm3742

[6] Sarkar N. Polyadenylation of mRNA in prokaryotes. Annual Review of Biochemistry. 1997;**66**:173-197. DOI: 10.1146/annurev.biochem.66.1.173

[7] Jensen T, Dower K, Libri D, Rosbash M. Early formation of mRNP license for export or quality control? Molecular Cell. 2003;**11**(5):1129-1138. DOI: 10.1016/S1097-2765(03)00191-6

[8] Stutz F, Izaurralde E. The interplay of nuclear mRNP assembly, mRNA surveillance and export. Trends in Cell Biology. 2003;**13**(6):319-327. DOI: 10.1016/S0962-8924(03)00106-5

[9] Balagopal V, Parker R. Polysomes, P bodies and stress granules: States and fates of eukaryotic mRNAs. Current Opinion in Cell Biology. 2009;**21**(3):403 408. DOI: 10.1016/j.ceb.2009.03.005

[10] Decker C, Parker R. P-bodies and stress granules: Possible roles in the control of translation and mRNA degradation. Cold Spring Harbor Perspectives in Biology. 2012;**4**(9):a012286. DOI: 10.1101/cshperspect.a012286

[11] Collart M. Global control of gene expression in yeast by the Ccr4-not complex. Gene. 2003;**313**:1-16. DOI: 10.1016/S0378-1119(03)00672-3

[12] Schäfer I, Rode M, Bonneau F, Schüssler S, Conti E. The structure of the Pan2–Pan3 core complex reveals cross-talk between deadenylase and pseudokinase. Nature Structural & Molecular Biology. 2014;**21**(7):591-598. DOI: 10.1038/nsmb.2834

[13] Song M-G, Li Y, Kiledjian M. Multiple mRNA decapping enzymes in mammalian cells. Molecular Cell. 2010;**40**(3):423-432. DOI: 10.1016/j.molcel.2010.10.010

[14] Arribas-Layton M, Wu D, Lykke-Andersen J, Song H. Structural and functional control of the eukaryotic mRNA decapping machinery. Biochimica et Biophysica Acta (BBA) - Gene Regulatory Mechanisms. 2013;**1829**(6-7):580-589. DOI: 10.1016/j.bbagrm.2012.12.006

[15] Medina D et al. Cytoplasmic 5′-3′ exonuclease Xrn1p is also a genome-wide transcription factor in yeast. Frontiers in Genetics. 2014;**5**:1. DOI: 10.3389/fgene.2014.00001

[16] Haimovich G, Choder M, Singer R, Trcek T. The fate of the messenger is pre-determined: A new model for regulation of gene expression. Biochimica et Biophysica Acta (BBA) - Gene Regulatory Mechanisms. 2013;**1829**(6-7):643-653. DOI: 10.1016/j.bbagrm.2013.01.004

[17] Braun, Young. Coupling mRNA synthesis and decay. Molecular and Cellular Biology. 2014;**34**(22):4078-4087. DOI: 10.1128/MCB.00535-14

[18] Das S, Sarkar D, Das B. The interplay between transcription and mRNA degradation in *Saccharomyces cerevisiae*. Microbial Cell. 2017;**4**(7):212-228. DOI: 10.15698/mic2017.07.580

[19] Romero-Santacreu L, Moreno J, Pérez-Ortín JEE, Alepuz P. Specific and global regulation of mRNA stability during osmotic stress in *Saccharomyces cerevisiae*. RNA. 2009; **15**:1110-1120

[20] Marguerat S, Lawler K, Brazma A, Bähler J. Contributions of transcription and mRNA decay to gene expression dynamics of fission yeast in response to oxidative stress. RNA Biology. 2014;**11**:702-714

[21] Castells-Roca L, García-Martínez J, Moreno J. Heat shock response in yeast involves changes in both transcription rates and mRNA stabilities. PLoS One. 2011;**6**(2):e17272. DOI: 10.1371/journal.pone.0017272

[22] Shalem O, Dahan O, Levo M. Transient transcriptional responses to stress are generated by opposing effects of mRNA production and degradation. Molecular Systems Biology. 2008;**4**:223. DOI: 10.1038/msb.2008.59

[23] Sun M, Schwalb B, Pirkl N, Maier KC, Schenk A. Global analysis of eukaryotic mRNA degradation reveals Xrn1-dependent buffering of transcript levels. Molecular Cell. 2013;**52**(1):52-62. DOI: 10.1016/j.molcel.2013.09.010

[24] Sun M, Schwalb B, Schulz D, Pirkl N, Etzold S. Comparative dynamic transcriptome analysis (cDTA) reveals mutual feedback between mRNA synthesis and degradation. Genome Research. 2012;**22**(7):1350-1359. DOI: 10.1101/gr.130161.111

[25] Haimovich G, Medina DA, Causse SZ, Garber M. Gene expression is circular: Factors for mRNA degradation also foster mRNA synthesis. Cell. 2013;**153**(5):1000-1011. DOI: 10.1016/j.cell.2013.05.012

[26] Marzluff WF, Wagner EJ, Duronio RJ. Metabolism and regulation of canonical histone mRNAs: Life without a poly (a) tail. Nature Reviews Genetics. 2008;**9**(11):843-854. DOI: 10.1038/nrg2438

[27] Hereford LM, Osley MA, Ludwig JR, McLaughlin CS. Cell-cycle regulation of yeast histone mRNA. Cell. 1981;**24**(2):367-375. DOI: 10.1016/0092-8674(81)90326-3

[28] Marzluff WF, Duronio RJ. Histone mRNA expression: Multiple levels of cell cycle regulation and important developmental consequences. Current Opinion in Cell Biology. 2002;**4**(6):692-699. DOI: 10.1016/S0955-0674(02)00387-3

[29] Spellman PT, Sherlock G, Zhang MQ. Comprehensive identification of cell cycle–regulated genes of the yeast *Saccharomyces cerevisiae* by microarray hybridization. Molecular Biology of the Cell. 1998;**9**(12):3273-3297. DOI: 10.1091/mbc.9.12.3273

[30] Abernathy E, Gilbertson S, Alla R, Glaunsinger B. Viral nucleases induce an mRNA degradation-transcription feedback loop in mammalian cells. Cell Host & Microbe. 2015;**18**(2):243-253. DOI: 10.1016/j.chom.2015.06.019

[31] Garneau NL, Wilusz J. The highways and byways of mRNA decay. Nature Reviews. Molecular Cell Biology. 2007;**8**(2):113-126. DOI: 10.1038/nrm2104

[32] Xie X, Lu J, Kulbokas EJ, Golub TR, Mootha V. Systematic discovery of regulatory motifs in human promoters and 3′ UTRs by comparison of several mammals. Nature. 2005;**434**(7031):338-345. DOI: 10.1038/nature03441

[33] Jackson RJ, Standart N. Do the poly (a) tail and 3′ untranslated region control mRNA translation? Cell. 1990;**62**(1):15-24. DOI: 10.1016/0092-8674(90)90235-7

[34] Chen C, Shyu AB. AU-rich elements: Characterization and importance in mRNA degradation. Trends in Biochemical Sciences. 1995;**20**(11):465-470. DOI: 10.1016/S0968-0004(00)89102-1

[35] Jing Q, Huang S, Guth S, Zarubin T, Motoyama A. Involvement of microRNA in AU-rich element-mediated mRNA instability. Cell. 2005;**120**(5):623-634. DOI: 10.1016/j.cell.2004.12.038

[36] Kim HH, Gorospe M. GU-rich RNA: Expanding CUGBP1 function, broadening mRNA turnover. Molecular Cell. 2008;**29**(2):151-152. DOI: 10.1016/j.molcel.2008.01.005

[37] Wickens M, Bernstein DS, Kimble J, Parker R. A PUF family portrait: 3′ UTR regulation as a way of life. Trends in Genetics. 2002;**18**(3):150-157. DOI: 10.1016/S0168-9525(01)02616-6

[38] Huntzinger E, Izaurralde E. Gene silencing by microRNAs: Contributions of translational repression and mRNA decay. Nature Reviews Genetics. 2011;**12**(2):99-110. DOI: 10.1038/nrg2936

[39] Lai EC, Micro RNA. Are complementary to 3′ UTR sequence motifs that mediate negative post-transcriptional regulation. Nature Genetics. 2002;**30**(4):363-364. DOI: 10.1038/ng865

[40] Dreyfus M, Régnier P. The poly (a) tail of mRNAs: Bodyguard in eukaryotes, scavenger in bacteria. Cell. 2002;**111**(5):611-613. DOI: 10.1016/S0092-8674(02)01137-6

[41] Giammartino DD, Nishida K, Manley JL. Mechanisms and consequences of alternative polyadenylation. Molecular Cell. 2011;**43**(6):853-866. DOI: 10.1016/j.molcel.2011.08.017

[42] Lutz CS, Moreira A. Alternative mRNA polyadenylation in eukaryotes: An effective regulator of gene expression. Wiley interdisciplinary reviews. RNA. 2011;**2**(1):23-31. DOI: 10.1002/wrna.47

[43] Ozsolak F, Kapranov P, Foissac S, Kim SW. Comprehensive polyadenylation site maps in yeast and human reveal pervasive alternative polyadenylation. Cell. 2010;**143**(6):1018-1029. DOI: 10.1016/j.cell.2010.11.020

[44] Hoque M et al. Analysis of alternative cleavage and polyadenylation by 3′ region extraction and deep sequencing. Nature Methods. 2013;**10**(2):133-139. DOI: 10.1038/nmeth.2288

[45] Geisberg JV, Moqtaderi Z, Fan X, Ozsolak F, Struhl K. Global analysis of mRNA isoform half-lives reveals stabilizing and destabilizing elements in yeast. Cell. 2014;**156**(4):812-824. DOI: 10.1016/j.cell.2013.12.026

[46] Enssle J, Kugler W, Hentze MW. Determination of mRNA fate by different RNA polymerase II promoters. Proceedings of the National Academy of Science in U.S.A. 1993;**90**(21):10091-10095

[47] Bregman A, Avraham-Kelbert M, Barkai O, Duek L. Promoter elements regulate cytoplasmic mRNA decay. Cell. 2011;**147**(7):1473-1483. DOI: 10.1016/j.cell.2011.12.005

[48] Trcek T, Larson DR, Moldón A, Query CC, Singer RH. Single-molecule mRNA decay measurements reveal promoter-regulated mRNA stability in yeast. Cell. 2011;**147**(7):1473-1483. DOI: 10.1016/j.cell.2011.12.005

[49] Liu HY, Toyn JH, Chiang YC, Draper MP. DBF2, a cell cycle-regulated protein kinase, is physically and functionally associated with the CCR4 transcriptional regulatory complex. The EMBO Journal. 1997;**16**(17):5289-5298. DOI: 10.1093/emboj/16.17.5289

[50] Dori-Bachash M, Shalem O. Widespread promoter-mediated coordination of transcription and mRNA degradation. Genome Biology. 2012;**13**(12):R114. DOI: 10.1186/gb-2012-13-12-r114

[51] Choder M. mRNA imprinting: Additional level in the regulation of gene expression. Cellular Logistics. 2011;**1**(1):37-40. DOI: 10.4161/cl.1.1.14465

[52] Újvári A, Luse DS. RNA emerging from the active site of RNA polymerase II interacts with the Rpb7 subunit. Nature Structural & Molecular Biology. 2006;**13**(1):49-54. DOI: 10.1038/nsmb1026

[53] Chen CY, Chang CC, Yen CF. Mapping RNA exit channel on transcribing RNA polymerase II by FRET analysis. Proceedings of the National Academy of Science in U.S.A. 2009;**106**(1):127-132. DOI: 10.1073/pnas.0811689106

[54] Selitrennik M, Duek L, Lotan R, Choder M. Nucleocytoplasmic shuttling of the Rpb4p and Rpb7p subunits of Saccharomyces Cerevisiae RNA polymerase II by two pathways. Eukaryotic Cell. 2006;**5**(12):2092-2103. DOI: 10.1128/EC.00288-06

[55] Lotan R, Goler-Baron V, Duek L, Haimovich G. The Rpb7p subunit of yeast RNA polymerase II plays roles in the two major cytoplasmic mRNA decay mechanisms. The Journal of Cell Biology. 2007;**178**(7):1133-1143. DOI: 10.1083/jcb.200701165

[56] Lotan R, Bar-On VG, Harel-Sharvit L. The RNA polymerase II subunit Rpb4p mediates decay of a specific class of mRNAs. Genes & Development. 2005;**19**(24):3004-3016

[57] Goler-Baron V, Selitrennik M, Barkai O. Transcription in the nucleus and mRNA decay in the cytoplasm are coupled processes. Genes & Development. 2008;**22**(15):2022-2027. DOI: 10.1101/gad.473608

[58] Dichtl B, Stevens A, Tollervey D. Lithium toxicity in yeast is due to the inhibition of RNA processing enzymes. The EMBO Journal. 1997;**16**(23):7184-7195. DOI: 10.1093/emboj/16.23.7184

[59] Portillo F, Mulet JM, Serrano R. A role for the non-phosphorylated form of yeast Snf1: Tolerance to toxic cations and activation of potassium transport. FEBS Letters. 2005;**579**(2):512-516. DOI: 10.1016/j.febslet.2004.12.019

[60] DeRisi J, Iyer V, Brown P. Exploring the metabolic and genetic control of gene expression on a genomic scale. Science. 1997;**278**(5338):680-686. DOI: 10.1126/science.278.5338.680

[61] Cereghino, Atencio, Saghbini, Beiner, Scheffler. Glucose-dependent turnover of the mRNAs encoding succinate dehydrogenase peptides in *Saccharomyces cerevisiae*: Sequence elements in the 5′ untranslated region of the Ip mRNA play a dominant role. Molecular Biology of the Cell. 1995;**6**(9):1125-1143. DOI: 10.1091/mbc.6.9.1125

[62] Scheffler I, de la Cruz B, Prieto S. Control of mRNA turnover as a mechanism of glucose repression in *Saccharomyces cerevisiae*. The International Journal of Biochemistry & Cell Biology. 1998;**30**(11):1175-1193. DOI: 10.1016/S1357-2725(98)00086-7

[63] Braun KA, Dombek KM, Young ET. Snf1-dependent transcription confers glucose-induced decay upon the mRNA product. Molecular and Cellular Biology. 2016;**36**(4): 628-644. DOI: 10.1128/MCB.00436-15

[64] Braun KA, Vaga S, Dombek KM, Fang F. Phosphoproteomic analysis identifies proteins involved in transcription-coupled mRNA decay as targets of Snf1 signaling. Science Signaling. 2014;**7**(333):ra64. DOI: 10.1126/scisignal.2005000

[65] Denis CL. Identification of new genes involved in the regulation of yeast alcohol dehydrogenase II. Genetics. 1984;**108**(4):833-844

[66] Draper MP, Liu HY, Nelsbach AH. CCR4 is a glucose-regulated transcription factor whose leucine-rich repeat binds several proteins important for placing CCR4 in its proper promoter context. Molecular and Cellular Biology. 1994;**14**(7):4522-4531

[67] Tucker M, Valencia-Sanchez MA, Staples RR, Chen J. The transcription factor associated Ccr4 and Caf1 proteins are components of the major cytoplasmic mRNA deadenylase in Saccharomyces Cerevisiae. Cell. 2001;**104**(3):377-386. DOI: 10.1016/S0092-8674(01)00225-2

[68] Collart MA, Struhl K. NOT1 (CDC39), NOT2 (CDC36), NOT3, and NOT4 encode a global-negative regulator of transcription that differentially affects TATA-element utilization. Genes & Development. 1994;**8**:525-537. DOI: 10.1101/gad.8.5.525

[69] Collart MA. The NOT, SPT3, and MOT1 genes functionally interact to regulate transcription at core promoters. Molecular and Cellular Biology. 1996;**16**(12):6668-6676. DOI: 10.1128/MCB.16.12.6668

[70] Denis CL, Chiang YC, Cui Y, Chen J. Genetic evidence supports a role for the yeast CCR4-NOT complex in transcriptional elongation. Genetics. 2001;**158**(2):627-634

[71] Nagarajan VK, Jones CI, Newbury SF, Green PJ. XRN 5 3 exoribonucleases: Structure, mechanisms and functions. Biochimica et Biophysica Acta (BBA)-Gene Regulatory Mechanisms. 2013;**1829**:590-603. DOI: 10.1016/j.bbagrm.2013.03.005

[72] Chang JH, Xiang S, Xiang K, Manley JL. Structural and biochemical studies of the 5′→ 3′ exoribonuclease Xrn1. Nature Structural & Molecular Biology. 2011;**8**(3):270-276. DOI: 10.1038/nsmb.1984

[73] Jinek M, Coyle SM, Doudna JA. Coupled 5′ nucleotide recognition and processivity in Xrn1-mediated mRNA decay. Molecular Cell. 2011;**41**(5):600-608. DOI: 10.1016/j.molcel.2011.02.004

[74] Molin C, Jauhiainen A, Warringer J, Nerman O, Sunnerhagen P. mRNA stability changes precede changes in steady-state mRNA amounts during hyperosmotic stress. RNA. 2009;**15**(4):600-614. DOI: 10.1261/rna.1403509

[75] Chen C-Y, Ezzeddine N, Shyu A-B, Messenger RNA. Half-life measurements in mammalian cells. Methods in Enzymology. 2008;**448**:335-357. DOI: 10.1016/s0076-6879(08)02617-7

[76] Grigull J, Mnaimneh S, Pootoolal J, Robinson M, Hughes T. Genome-wide analysis of mRNA stability using transcription inhibitors and microarrays reveals posttranscriptional control of ribosome biogenesis factors. Molecular and Cellular Biology. 2004;**24**(12):5534-5547. DOI: 10.1128/MCB.24.12.5534-5547.2004

[77] Imamachi N et al. BRIC-seq: A genome-wide approach for determining RNA stability in mammalian cells. Methods. 2014;**67**(1):55-63. DOI: 10.1016/j.ymeth.2013.07.014

[78] Tani H et al. Genome-wide determination of RNA stability reveals hundreds of short-lived noncoding transcripts in mammals. Genome Research. 2012;**22**(5):947-956. DOI: 10.1101/gr.130559.111

[79] Gardini A. Global run-on sequencing (GRO-Seq). Enhancer RNAs: Methods and Protocols. 2017;**1468**:111-120. DOI: 10.1007/978-1-4939-4035-6_9

[80] Core LJ, Waterfall JJ, Lis JT. Nascent RNA sequencing reveals widespread pausing and divergent initiation at human promoters. Science. 2008;**322**(5909):1845-1848. DOI: 10.1126/science.1162228

[81] Kwak H, Fuda NJ, Core LJ, Lis JT. Precise maps of RNA polymerase reveal how promoters direct initiation and pausing. Science. 2013;**339**(6122):950-953. DOI: 10.1126/science.1229386

[82] Mayer A et al. Native elongating transcript sequencing reveals human transcriptional activity at nucleotide resolution. Cell. 2015;**161**(3):541-554. DOI: 10.1016/j.cell.2015.03.010

[83] Churchman LS, Weissman JS. Nascent transcript sequencing visualizes transcription at nucleotide resolution. Nature. 2011;**469**(7330):368-373. DOI: 10.1038/nature09652

[84] Nojima T, Gomes T, Grosso A, Kimura H, Dye MJ. Mammalian NET-seq reveals genome-wide nascent transcription coupled to RNA processing. Cell. 2015;**161**(3):526-540. DOI: 10.1016/j.cell.2015.03.02

[85] Rabani M, Levin JZ, Fan L, Adiconis X. Metabolic labeling of RNA uncovers principles of RNA production and degradation dynamics in mammalian cells. Nature Biotechnology. 2011;**29**(5):436-442. DOI: 10.1038/nbt.1861

Chapter 7

Post-Transcriptional Control of RNA Expression in Cancer

Carlos DeOcesano-Pereira,
Fernando Janczur Velloso,
Ana Claudia Oliveira Carreira,
Carolina Simões Pires Ribeiro,
Sheila Maria Brochado Winnischofer,
Mari Cleide Sogayar and Marina Trombetta-Lima

Additional information is available at the end of the chapter

http://dx.doi.org/10.5772/intechopen.71861

Abstract

Approximately 80% of the human genome contains functional DNA, including protein coding genes, non-protein coding regulatory DNA elements and non-coding RNAs (ncRNAs). An altered transcriptional signature is not only a cause, but also a consequence of the characteristics known as the hallmarks of cancer, such as sustained proliferation, replicative immortality, evasion of growth suppression and apoptotic signals, angiogenesis, invasion, metastasis, evasion of immune destruction and metabolic re-wiring. Post-transcriptional events play a major role in determining this signature, which is evidenced by the fact that alternative RNA splicing takes place in more than half of the human genes, and, among protein coding genes, more than 60% contain at least one conserved miRNA binding site. In this chapter, we will discuss the involvement of post-transcriptional events, such as RNA processing, the action of non-coding RNAs and RNA decay in cancer development, and how their machinery may be used in cancer diagnosis and treatment.

Keywords: post-transcriptional control, splicing, microRNAs, long non-coding RNAs, mRNA decay

1. Introduction

The word cancer defines a group of diverse diseases, which share unique traits. Tumor cells display mechanisms of sustained proliferation, replicative immortality, evasion of growth suppression and apoptotic signals, angiogenesis, invasion, metastasis, evasion of immune destruction and metabolic re-wiring [1]. These characteristics represent a great challenge to cancer treatment being both a cause and a consequence of an abnormal gene expression profile. Efforts to understand the consequences of these different expression profiles and the mechanisms underlying them contribute to clarify cancer biology and, consequently, to predict response to and optimization of therapeutic approaches [2–4].

There are several layers of gene expression modulation including epigenetics, transcriptional modulation, RNA expression control, translational regulation and post-translational modifications. All these mechanisms work in an orchestrated manner leading to specific expression signatures and phenotypes. In this chapter, we focus on RNA expression control mechanisms, which take place after RNA polymerase recognition of the gene promoter and start of RNA synthesis, discussing their implications to malignant transformation and cancer progression.

2. mRNA processing

RNA processing takes place after the start of transcription, resulting in a mature mRNA which is able to fulfill its function. This process comprises: 5′-Cap addition, splicing and poly(A) addition. RNA splicing is a process in which portions of the pre-RNA, denominated introns, are excised and the remaining portions (exons) are bound to form the mature RNA. Both *cis* and *trans* elements act to recognize exon/intron boundaries and/or to orchestrate the splicing machinery, the spliceosome, a complex of five small nuclear ribonucleoprotein particles (snRNP) and 100–200 non-snRNP proteins which catalyze the splicing reaction [5–7]. Recognition of the intron/exon boundaries is context-dependent; as a result, a single gene can originate several mature RNAs and, therefore, several proteins with independent or even opposite functions. This alternative splicing (AS) occurs by recognition of the alternative donor or acceptor splice sites, exon inclusion or exclusion, intron incorporation or combinatory mechanisms as mutually exclusive exons and so on. AS stands out as a major source for transcripts and proteins variability, occurring in approximately 59% of human genes [8] and almost 95% of the multi-exon genes [9]. Splicing factor genes are commonly mutated in different types of cancer and several splice variants have already been implicated in cancer development [10].

The splicing profile of a certain tissue changes dramatically when compared with malignant cells with their normal counterparts [11–13]. This difference may result from mutations or single-nucleotide polymorphisms (SNPs) on acceptor, donor splice sites, enhancing or silencing sequences which lead to alterations in the exon/intron boundary recognition; or due to deregulated expression or change of function mutation in a *trans* regulator (reviewed in [14, 15]). Serine-rich protein (SRP) and heterologous nuclear ribonuclear particle (hnRNP) are two protein families which are classically involved in splicing modulation by interacting with intronic or exonic enhancer or silencer sequences [16, 17]. The SRSF1 member of the SRP family is one of the most well characterized splice factor, being described as up-regulated in lung [18] and breast cancers [19, 20]. In the breast cancer model, SRSF1 association to a sequence near to a donor splice site usually promotes exon inclusion, while its association in the vicinities of an acceptor splice site leads to exon skipping or inclusion [20]. Important cancer-related gene transcripts, such as Casp9 [21], CD44 [22] and VEGF [23], are among SRSF1 known targets.

Cell survival outcome is a perfect example of the influence of AS in basic cellular mechanisms, with alternative isoforms of several apoptotic-related gene transcripts displaying opposite roles, when compared to their canonical variant, shifting the cell status from apoptosis-prone to the survival state (reviewed in [24]). Upon an apoptotic stimulus, cytochrome C is released from the mitochondria and forms a complex with Apaf-1. The N-terminal portion of Apaf-1 interacts with the N-terminal pro-domain of pro-caspase-9, leading to Caspase-9 activation, which, in turn, activates the Caspase-3 and -7 effector proteases (reviewed in [25]). Caspase-9, a key player in this process, has an alternative-splicing variant in which exclusion of the exon cassette 3, 4, 5 and 6 leads to a protein isoform which lacks part of its large subunit. This Caspase-9b isoform retains the domain which interacts with Apaf-1, but lacks the Caspase-9 catalytic site, thus acting like a dominant negative and inhibiting the apoptotic pathway [26, 27]. The ratio between these two isoforms modulates the propensity of the cells to respond to death stimuli, altering their chemo-sensitivity and, potentially, the treatment's outcome. Interestingly, while Akt mediates exclusion of the exon cassette via phosphorylation of the RNA splicing factor SRp30a [28]; in this case, SRSF1 interacts with an intronic enhancer site at intron 6 favoring the exon cassette inclusion, which renders the cells more sensitive to chemotherapeutic agents as the combined therapy with daunorubicin and erlotinib [21]. Taking into account that SRSF1 is upregulated in non-small cell lung cancer cells, this case exemplifies the complexity of splicing as an expression regulator and how it can be explored to optimize therapy efficacy.

Another great source of transcripts variability is alternative polyadenylation (APA), since approximately 30% of human mRNAs display alternative polyadenylation sites [29]. Polyadenylation occurs in almost every mammalian transcript, a process in which an endonucleolytic cleavage is catalyzed by polyadenylation machinery proteins, immediately followed by polyadenylation (200 300 nucleotides, on average, in humans) of the 3′ end by poly(A) polymerases (reviewed in [30]). The resulting alternative transcripts will have different sizes, depending on the localization of the alternative poly(A) site, originating alternative 3′-untranslated regions (3′-UTR). Also, more rarely, when polyadenylation occurs inside the open reading frame region, it may originate truncated forms of the translated protein [31]. The 3′-UTR is extremely important to transcripts stability, localization and regulation by *trans* elements (such as miRNAs and RNA binding proteins), topics to be further discussed in this chapter and which have great implications for cancer development.

A shift in the polyadenylation global pattern occurs in tumor cells, with the proximal poly(A) sites being favored, when compared to their normal counterparts [29]. Also, highly proliferative murine T lymphocytes favor shorter 3′-UTRs, which is also observed in colorectal cancer, but only for certain groups of genes, including those involved in cell cycle, nucleic acid-binding and processing factors. It has been proposed that such shortening would restrict miRNA modulation over the transcripts, increasing their expression [32, 33]. Such a mechanism is observed upon treatment of ER^+ breast cancer cells with the proliferation stimulant 17β-estradiol. This treatment leads to APA of the *CD6* transcript, which is essential for the start of DNA replication, originating a shorter 3′-UTR. The generated *CD6* variant is resistant to repression dependent on its 3′-UTR and is more efficiently translated, correlating with a higher rate of BrdU incorporation by the cells [34].

Curiously, mammalian RNAs can also be post-transcriptionally modified through a process called RNA editing. Well-known cases are the RNA editing enzymes adenosine and cytidine deaminases, which catalyze the conversion of adenine into inosine and of cytosine into uracil, respectively [35]. Adenosine deaminases acting on RNA (ADAR) enzymes act on double-stranded RNA regions, usually the secondary structure of a single mRNA molecule. Through a hydrolytic deamination at C6, ADAR enzymes catalyze adenine conversion into inosine, which pairs with cytosine. Cytidine deaminases are much more specific and different members of the APOBEC3 family are transcriptionally regulated by p53 [36]. Altered RNA editing signatures were found in different types of tumors, such as glioblastoma [37], breast [38] and gastric cancers [39, 40]. If located at a coding region, these editing events may cause a missense mutation. One example is ADAR-1 editing of the *Antizyme Inhibitor 1* (*AZIN1*), which leads to a serine-to-glycine substitution at residue 367 [41]. AZIN1 is an inactive homolog of ornithine decarboxylase (ODC) that competitively binds to antizymes [42]. ADAR-1 editing increases AZIN1 affinity to antizyme, leading to a decrease in ODC antizyme-mediated degradation and promoting polyamines biosynthesis, with consequent cell proliferation and a more aggressive behavior in hepatocellular carcinoma cells [41]. Although editing on consensus splicing sites are rare, ADAR enzymes alter the global splicing pattern of the cell by editing splicing regulatory *cis* elements and, possibly, indirectly, by altering the activity of *trans* elements [43, 44].

The interaction of transcripts with long non-coding RNAs (lncRNAs) and microRNAs are important post-transcriptional regulatory mechanisms which will be further addressed in this chapter. RNA edition adds a layer of complexity to this apparatus. It is estimated that over 70% of potential editing sites within long non-coding RNAs may lead to changes in their secondary structure, a feature which is crucial for its target recognition [45]. If the editing takes place in a precursor miRNA, it can lead to alterations in its biosynthesis and target recognition, increasing their range of action [46–48]. Alterations in the mRNA 3′-UTR may alter its recognition by a specific miRNA or lncRNA [37, 40, 47]. Furthermore, RNA editing may also modulate RNA expression by regulating RNA decay. This is exemplified by the ADAR-1 interaction with the RNA binding protein HuR, which promotes HuR binding to the target transcript, increasing its stability [49].

3. miRNAs

Several RNA-based mechanisms evolved in eukaryotes to modulate gene expression or suppress invading material. In animals, the small non-coding RNAs (18–30 nucleotides) are subdivided into three major classes, namely microRNA (miRNA), small interfering RNA (siRNA) and PIWI-interacting RNA (piRNA). The main purpose of piRNAs are suggested to be silencing of transposable elements in germline cells [45], siRNAs and miRNAs seem to have evolved from an antiviral defense system into an ubiquitous gene expression modulation mechanism [46, 47]. Originally identified in *Caenorhabditis elegans* [48], miRNAs are the dominating class of small RNAs in most somatic tissues, being highly conserved and repressing the expression of target genes by inhibiting mRNAs translation and/or stability [49, 50]. The latest update of the human miRNA database lists 2588 mature miRNAs, processed out of 1881 precursors [51]. miRNA genes are originally transcribed by RNA polymerase II (Pol II) as a long (typically over 1 kb) primary transcript (pri-miRNA) bearing hairpins, in which miRNA sequences are embedded [52]. Hairpins are cropped by the Drosha nuclear RNase III liberating the stem-loop shaped ~65 nucleotide long precursor miRNA (pre-miRNA) [53]. Upon exporting to the cytoplasm through Exportin 5 (EXP5), pre-miRNAs are cleaved by DICER near the terminal loop, liberating a small RNA duplex [54]. This duplex is subsequently loaded onto RNA-induced silencing complex (RISC), RNP effector complexes containing Argonaut (AGO) proteins. Finally, unwinding of the RNA duplex allows the final single-stranded miRNA to act as a guide for the effector complex [55]. Specific targeting is accomplished by base pairing between mRNA and miRNA, as miRNAs usually guide RISC to 3′UTR regions in target protein-coding transcripts [56], recruiting proteins that lead to target RNA degradation, deadenylation or decay [53]. However, miRNAs may also interact with 5′UTR and coding sequence (CDS) regions, culminating in a range of effects, from translational activation to repression.

More than 60% of human protein-coding genes contain at least one conserved miRNA-binding site [57], encompassing every major cellular functional pathway. Therefore, miRNAs biogenesis needs to be under tight temporal and spatial control, and their deregulation is evidently associated with a wide range of human diseases, including cancer [58]. The first instance of the direct involvement of a miRNA in cancer was uncovered in 2002. A critical region at chromosome 13q14, frequently deleted in chronic lymphocytic leukemia (CLL), was shown to harbor miRNA genes miR-15a and miR-16-1. About 70% of CLL cases have null or reduced expression of these miRNAs, which normally control apoptosis by targeting BCL-2 [59, 60]. The following years revealed a remarkable number of additional examples, establishing the association of miRNAs and cancer to be the norm, rather than the exception. Currently, hundreds of human miRNAs are associated to the onset and progression of several malignancies, including lymphomas, colorectal carcinoma, breast cancer, lung cancer, thyroid cancer and hepatocellular carcinomas [61].

Several miRNAs may be differentially expressed in cancer patients, when compared to normal samples, acting either as oncogenes or tumor suppressors [62] (**Table 1**). Most often, miRNAs are detected as tumor suppressors, with reduced expression in tumors when compared to normal tissues [63, 64]. These miRNAs have commonly been shown to negatively regulate protein-coding oncogenes. Thus, HER2 and HER3, two oncogenes which are significantly correlated with decreased disease-specific survival in breast cancer patients [65], are suppressed by miR-125a or miR-125b [66]. Additionally, the let-7 family of miRNAs targets several genes associated with cell cycle and cell division, including the RAS oncogene [67]. Inhibition of epidermal growth factor receptor by miR-128b in non-small cell lung cancer (NSCLC) [68] and miR-7 in glioma [69] are additional pertinent examples of miRNAs acting as tumor suppressors. However, several miRNAs have also been found to be overexpressed in cancer, being classified as oncomiRs, often repressing known tumor suppressors. Thus, overexpression of miR-155 and miR-21 is sufficient to induce lymphomagenesis in mice [70, 71].

miRNA	Cancer phenotype	Target mRNA	Cancer association	References
miR-15a	Tumor suppressor	*BCL2*	Chronic lymphocytic leukemia	[59, 60]
miR-16-1	Tumor suppressor	*BCL2*	Chronic lymphocytic leukemia	[59, 60]
miR-125a	Tumor suppressor	*HER2/HER3*	Breast cancer	[66]
miR-125b	Tumor suppressor	*HER2/HER3*	Breast cancer	[66]
let-7	Tumor suppressor	*RAS*	Lung tumor	[67]
miR128-b	Tumor suppressor	*EGFR*	Non-small lung cancer	[68]
miR128-b	Tumor suppressor	*EGFR*	Acute lymphoblastic leukemia	[77]
miR-7	Tumor suppressor	*EGFR*	Glioma	[69]
miR-155	Oncogenic	*BIC*	Lymphoma	[70, 71]
miR-21	Oncogenic	*NA*	Lymphoma	[70, 71]
miR-127	Tumor suppressor	*BCL6*	Prostate cancer	[75, 76]
miR-372/373	Oncogenic	*RAS, p53*	Testicular germ cell tumor	[170]
miR-17	Tumor suppressor	*c-MYC*	Large B-cell lymphoma	[72, 171]
miR-34	Tumor suppressor	*P53*	Ovarian cancer	[73]
miR-210	Tumor suppressor	*DIMT1*	Multiple myeloma	[172]
miR-10b	Tumor suppressor	*TIAM1*	Gastric cancer	[173]
miR-126	Tumor suppressor	ADAM9	Breast cancer	[174]
miR-335	Tumor suppressor	*BRCA1*	Breast cancer	[175]

Table 1. List of miRNAs involved in cancer and their respective mRNA targets.

Mapping efforts have revealed that many miRNAs are located in fragile regions of the genome, which are deleted, amplified or translocated in cancer, directly altering miRNAs genes expression, hence leading to aberrant expression of downstream target mRNAs [59]. In addition to genomic alterations, miRNA expression is also modulated by tumor suppressor or oncogenic factors, which function as transcriptional activators or repressors to control pre-miRNA transcription. One of the first examples of this interaction is the transcriptional upregulation of the miR-17/92 cluster by the c-*myc* oncogene product, counterbalancing the apoptotic activity of E2F1 and allowing c-Myc mediated-proliferation [72]. Likewise, p53 stimulates transcription of the miR-34 family, inducing apoptosis and senescence. Loss of p53 function induces downregulation of the miR-34 family in a very high percentage of ovarian cancer patients with a p53 mutation [73]. The expression of miRNA genes may also be indirectly modulated. Aberrant epigenetic changes, such as DNA hypermethylation of tumor suppressor genes, extensive genomic DNA hypomethylation and alteration of histone modification patterns, are a well-known feature of cancer cells. In fact, epigenetic modifications represent another common mechanism related to the alteration of miRNA expression in cancer. Tumor-suppressing miRNAs are usually found to be hypermethylated in cancer, which, in turn, allows overexpression of their oncogenic targets [74]. Thus, epigenetic repression of the tumor-suppressor miR-127 in primary prostate cancer [75] and bladder tumor causes upregulation of its target transcripts, including that of the proto-oncogene BCL6 [76]. A cancer-driving alteration may arise early in the biogenesis of miRNAs, during transcription of the pri-miRNA. For example, a point mutation in miR-128b gene blocks processing of pri-miR-128b and reduces the levels of mature miR-128b, thus leading to glucocorticoid resistance in acute lymphoblastic leukemia (ALL) [77]. Another mechanism which can lead to an aberrant expression of miRNAs and, thus, to cancer, is the altered expression and/or function of the enzymes involved in the biogenesis of microRNAs, such as DROSHA and DICER. Aberrant expression of these proteins affects the biogenesis of all miRNAs in the cell, influencing the regulation of a multitude of genes. Thus, the first heterozygous germline mutations in DICER1 were identified as causing pleuropulmonary blastoma (PPB), a rare pediatric lung tumor that arises during fetal lung development [78]. Likewise, decreased expression of DROSHA and DICER has been found in 39% of ovarian cancer patients [79]. miRNA biogenesis may also be modulated during nuclear translocation by exportin 5 (XPO5). XPO5 mutations in some tumors generate pre-miRNA accumulation in the nucleus, reducing miRNA maturation and availability in the cytoplasm [80]. miRNA processing is orchestrated by a large number of proteins assisting the basic machinery. Several of these modulatory proteins, such as DDX5 and DDX17, were shown to be either directly mutated or to serve as targets for oncoproteins or tumor suppressors, modulating miRNA biogenesis [81].

The functional outcomes of miRNAs deregulation coincide with the hallmarks of malignant cells, namely: (1) self-sufficiency in growth signals (let-7 family), (2) insensitivity to anti-growth signals (miR-17-92 cluster), (3) apoptosis evasion (miR-34a), (4) limitless replicative potential (miR-372/373 cluster), (5) angiogenesis (miR-210) and (6) invasion and metastases (miR-10b). miRNAs have also been shown to regulate the generation of cancer stem cells (CSCs) [82, 83] and epithelial-mesenchymal transition (EMT), paramount for the metastatic process [84]. Thus, as breast cancer cells metastasize, expression of miR-126 and miR-335 is lost. Overexpressing these miRNAs in cancer cells decreases lung and bone metastasis in vivo [85].

The high number of human miRNAs, regulating a wide range of cancer-related processes, renders these small non-coding RNAs an ideal profiling tool. miRNA expression profiles can distinguish not only between normal and cancerous tissue, but also help to discriminate different subtypes of a particular cancer, or even specific oncogenic abnormalities [86], increasing the accuracy of tumor classification. These expression profiles were able to classify tumors according to their tissue of origin with accuracy higher than 90%. miRNAs regulation of cancer progression also allows these molecules to serve as efficient predictors of prognosis, tumor metastasis and therapy selection. Specific miRNA signatures have recently been shown to correlate to metastatic breast and colon tumors, arising as potent biomarkers to predict metastatic outcome. miRNA profiles may also be applied to select for more personalized and efficient therapies and to adjust the therapeutic scheme during treatment to achieve a better outcome. Noteworthy, in ovarian cancer, miRNA signatures are able to predict chemoresistant tumors, while a polymorphism (SNP34091), which creates a new binding site for miR-191, was suggested as a modulator of tumor chemosensitivity [75].

miRNAs are highly stable molecules present in body fluids including plasma, blood, serum, urine, saliva and milk, being potential cancer biomarkers which may be found in different phases of the tumoral process [87, 88]. Although understanding of how miRNAs are selectively released from cells and how circulating miRNAs are related to disease remains largely unclear, circulating miRNAs may serve as novel diagnostic and prognostic biomarkers for human diseases, including cancer [89].

4. Long non-coding RNAs

Recent studies based on the Encyclopedia of DNA elements (ENCODE) project indicate that more than 80% of the human genome contains functional DNA that includes protein coding genes, non-protein coding regulatory DNA elements and non-coding RNAs (ncRNAs) [90]. Non-coding RNAs is a class of genetic regulators, containing short (<200 nucleotides) and long (>200 nucleotides) transcripts with novel abilities to be used as biomarkers due to their role in disease development and their implications for genomic organization [91, 92]. Short ncRNAs include ribosomal RNAs (rRNAs), transfer RNAs (tRNAs), small nuclear RNAs (snRNAs) and small nucleolar RNAs (snoRNAs). Regulatory long non-coding RNAs (lncRNAs) have been found in a large variety of organisms, ranging from yeasts to mammals, including mice and humans [93]. lncRNAs have emerged as a fundamental molecular class whose members play critical roles in genome regulation and in tissue development and maintenance [92]. Based on their positions relative to the protein coding genes in the genome, lncRNAs can be classified into natural antisense transcripts (NATs), long intronic ncRNAs and long intergenic ncRNAs (lincRNAs) [93].

Recent transcriptional profiling of multiple human tissues, including both normal and tumor samples, has led to the assumption that misregulation of lncRNAs could disrupt these delicate processes and lead to tumorigenesis [94–97]. These studies have validated the tissue-specific expression of lncRNAs in normal tissues, and have identified large sets of lncRNAs which are aberrantly expressed in either a specific cancer or multiple types of cancer, suggesting these RNAs act as master regulators of gene expression [98, 99]. Differential expression of lncRNAs is increasingly recognized as a hallmark feature in cancer [100]. lncRNAs are a novel class of mRNA-like transcripts, which contribute to cancer development and progression, accelerating cancer cells proliferation, apoptosis, invasion and metastasis [101] (**Table 2**).

General mechanisms of lncRNA function implicated in cancer progression are associated with a wide-repertoire of biological processes. Among the main biological pathways, lncRNAs may be involved in epigenetic silencing, splicing regulation, translational control, regulation of apoptosis and cell cycle control [102]. Like protein-coding genes, lncRNAs can function as oncogenes or tumor suppressors. Many lncRNAs shuttle between the nucleus and the cytoplasm, suggesting that they may have dual functions, while others are restricted to the nucleus [103]. In the nucleus, lncRNAs are often part of the nuclear architecture and, in some cases, are critical for maintenance of sub-nuclear structures [104].

LncRNA	Cancer phenotype	Molecular mechanism	Cancer association	References
HOTAIR	Oncogenic, promotes metastasis and invasion	Interacts with PRC2 and LSD1 complex, promotes silencing of HOX genes in *trans* epigenetically	Overexpressed in liver, breast, lung and pancreatic tumors	[109, 176, 177]
GAS5	Tumor suppressor, induces growth arrest and sensitizes cells to apoptosis	Inhibits and binds glucocorticoid receptor (GR) from activating target genes	Downregulated in breast cancer	[178, 179]
H19	Oncogenic, promotes cell proliferation and tumor growth	Unknown	Breast cancer	[180]
MALAT1	Oncogenic, promotes cell proliferation and metastasis	Related to alternative splicing and active transcription, regulation of gene expression	Overexpressed in lung, breast, pancreatic, colon, prostate and hepatocellular carcinomas	[117, 181, 182]
MEG3	Tumor suppressor, inhibits cell proliferation and induces apoptosis	Enhancing p53's transcriptional activity on its target genes. Controls expression of gene loci through recruitment of PRC2	Downregulated in multiple tumor types	[183, 184]
PTENP1	Tumor suppressor; Inhibits cell proliferation, migration, invasion and tumor growth	Binds and inhibits miRNAs from targeting and repressing *PTEN*	Locus lost in prostate cancer, colon cancer and melanoma	[185–187]
ZFas1	Tumor suppressor and inhibits proliferation	Unknown	Breast cancer and dysregulated in many types of tumors	[128, 188]

Table 2. List of lncRNAs involved in cancer with their proposed functions.

lncRNAs bind to and target chromatin regulators allowing connection between RNA and chromatin, acting on the control of gene expression at the transcriptional level [105]. Moreover, several lncRNAs mechanistic themes have emerged, both at the transcriptional and post-transcriptional levels, such as decoys, scaffolds and guides [106]. Examples of the mechanisms of action of some lncRNAs on the control of gene expression and mammalian cells regulation are described below.

HOTAIR (Hox transcript antisense intergenic RNA) is expressed from the HOXC locus and was the first lncRNA shown to be acting in *trans*. *HOTAIR* binds to and targets the PRC2 complex to the HOXD locus [107], functioning as an RNA scaffold containing two main functional domains. The 5′ domain of *HOTAIR* binds PRC2, whereas a 3′ domain binds the LSD1/CoREST/REST H3K4 demethylase complex [108], thus bridging two repressive complexes in order to coordinate their functions in gene silencing. Ectopic *HOTAIR* expression in epithelial cancer cells induces genome-wide retargeting of PRC2, leading to widespread changes in repressive (H3K27me3) and active (H3K4me3) chromatin markers, resembling those found in embryonic fibroblasts. This results in more invasive and metastatic cells and *HOTAIR* expression is predictive of cancer survival [109].

lncRNAs can also participate in global cellular behavior by controlling cell growth. The growth-arrest-specific 5 (*GAS5*) lncRNA sensitizes the cell to apoptosis by regulating the activity of glucocorticoids in response to nutrient starvation [110]. *GAS5* binds to the DNA-binding domain (DBD) of the glucocorticoid receptor (GR), where it acts as a decoy, preventing GR interaction with cognate glucocorticoid response elements (GRE). Under normal conditions, GR target genes are involved in apoptosis suppression, such as cellular inhibitor of apoptosis 2 (cIAP2) and inhibit the cell-death executioners caspases 3, 7 and 9 [111]. However, upon growth arrest, *GAS5* activation compromises GR ability to bind to the cIAP2 GRE, reducing cIAP2 expression levels, thereby removing its suppressive effect on caspases [110]. *GAS5* has also been associated with breast cancer because its transcript levels are significantly reduced, when compared to unaffected normal breast epithelium [110]. Therefore, *GAS5* could act as a tumor suppressor if reduced levels of this lncRNA are unable to maintain sufficient caspase activity to activate an appropriate apoptotic response in disease-compromised cells.

H19 is an imprinted gene expressed exclusively from the maternal allele, which maintains silencing of IGF2. *H19* is highly expressed in a wide variety of solid tumors. The majority of cancers express high levels of *H19* when compared to normal tissues. *H19* is generally overexpressed in stromal cells, rarely in tumor epithelial cells and has been found to be associated with the presence of estrogen receptor (ER) and progesterone receptor (PR) [112]. Data indicating both oncogenic and tumor suppressive roles for *H19* in different cancers are available [113]. In cancer cell lines, *H19* RNA expression is directly regulated by E2F1, promoting cell cycle progression [114].

The lncRNA *MALAT1* (metastasis associated in lung adenocarcinoma transcript) was identified in an attempt to characterize transcripts associated with early stage non-small cell lung cancer (NSCLC) [115]. Some studies found that *MALAT1* regulates alternative splicing through its interaction with the serine/arginine-rich (SR) family of nuclear phosphoproteins, which are involved in the splicing machinery [116, 117]. Because the SR family of proteins affects the alternative splicing patterns of many pre-mRNAs, its activity must be tightly regulated. Small changes in SR protein concentration or phosphorylation status can upset the fragile balance that controls mRNA variability among different cells and tissue types [118]. Therefore, the lncRNA *MALAT1* has been suggested to serve as a fine-tuning mechanism to modulate the activity of SR proteins.

The maternally expressed gene 3 (*MEG3*) is an imprinted lncRNA located on chromosome 14q32 is expressed exclusively from the maternal allele. *MEG3* has been shown to activate p53 and facilitate p53 signaling, including enhancement of p53 binding to target genes [119]. Furthermore, *MEG3* regulates genes of the TGF-β pathway through formation of RNA-DNA triplex structures [120]. *MEG3* overexpression in meningioma, hepatocellular carcinoma and breast cancer cell lines leads to suppression of cell proliferation [121–123].

The *PTEN* (phosphatase and tensin homolog) gene encodes a tumor suppressor that functions by negatively regulating the AKT/PKB signaling pathway [124, 125]. Mutations of this gene constitute a step into the development of many cancers and it is one of the most commonly lost tumor suppressors in human cancer [126]. A highly homologous processed of *PTENP1* (phosphatase and tensin Homolog pseudogene 1) is a pseudogene which is associated with the lncRNA class found on chromosome 9, regulating *PTEN* by both sense and antisense RNAs. This long non-coding RNA acts as a decoy for *PTEN*, targeting microRNAs and exerting a tumor suppressive activity [125, 127].

The lncRNA *Zfas1* (Znfx1 antisense 1) is a transcript antisense to the 5′ end of the protein-coding gene Znfx1, which has functions in epithelial cells and was identified in large-scale studies aimed at isolating differentially expressed genes during mammary development [128]. *Zfas1* intronically hosts three C/D box snoRNAs (*Snord12*, *Snord12b* and *Snord12c*) [128] and recently has been associated with ribosomes cancer cells [129].

The highly specific lncRNA expression signatures render them as attractive markers for accurate disease diagnosis and patients prognosis. In addition, advancement of RNA-based therapeutics opens new avenues for lncRNAs as new targets for cancer therapy.

5. mRNA decay

mRNA degradation is an important mechanism for post-transcriptional control of gene expression, controlling both the quality and the abundance of cellular mRNAs. Deadenylation of the mRNA is the default process, often representing a rate-limiting step in cytoplasmic mRNA decay, in which the poly(A) tail of the transcript is degraded through recruitment of deadenylase complexes [130–132]. In the literature, different deadenylases or poly(A)-specific ribonucleases have been described, namely PARN (poly(A)-specific ribonuclease), Pan2/Pan3 (poly(A) nuclease 2/3) complex and CCR4–NOT (carbon catabolite repression 4) complex [131, 133]. The PARN deadenylase is involved in destabilization of different transcripts related to cell cycle progression and cell proliferation [133, 134], as well as in degradation of oncogenic miRNAs, such as miR-21 [135]. In addition, its expression is altered in different tumors, such as gastric tumors [136] and acute leukemias [137].

Different proteins are able to interact with each other and promote the recruitment of deadenylases to the mRNA poly(A) tail. Members of BTG/Tob family, associated with anti-proliferative activities [138], are able to associate with both Caf1a and Caf1b (enzymatic subunits of the CCR4-NOT complex) [139], and, also, with PABPC1 (cytoplasmic poly(A)-binding protein) [139, 140], promoting mRNA poly(A) tail removal and cytoplasmic mRNA decay. Expression of the BTG/Tob proteins is classically associated with inhibition of cell cycle progression [138]. The Tob/Caf1 complex is also involved in the negative regulation of c-*myc* proto-oncogene expression by accelerating deadenylation and decay of its mRNA [141]. In addition, BTG2 has been characterized as a p53 transcriptional-target, being an essential component for suppression of Ras-induced transformation by p53 [142]. In agreement, reduced expression of BTG2 and TOB proteins are observed in human samples derived from different types of tumor [143–146]. On the other hand, interaction of Tob1 with Caf1a (but not with Caf1b) was recently associated with the metastatic phenotype in mouse mammary carcinoma model and the deadenylase activity of Caf1a was shown to be required for promotion of metastatic disease [147]. Using a human breast cancer model, it has also been shown that high expression of either TOB1 or CNOT1 (the scaffold subunit of the CCR4-NOT complex) correlated with poor survival [147] and was associated with poor distant metastasis free survival in breast cancer patients [148]. Interestingly, PABPC1 has also been described as an oncogenic protein in gastric carcinoma. Zhu and collaborators showed that PABPC1 is upregulated in gastric carcinoma tissues, predicting poor survival and inhibits apoptosis by targeting miR-34c [149]. Following shortening of the poly(A) tail, mRNA can either be degraded through the 3′ pathway, by the eukaryotic exosome complex, or, alternatively, by removal of the cap by Dcp2 and exonuclease decay through the 5′ pathway, promoted by exonuclease Xrn1 [130, 131].

AU-rich elements (ARE) are critical *cis*-acting elements in the 3′-UTRs of a variety of short-lived transcripts. Tristetraprolin (TTP) and human antigen R (HuR) are two important RNA-binding proteins which can bind to AREs in their target mRNAs. TTP promotes deadenylation and degradation of target mRNAs, whereas HuR, as already mentioned, is involved in stabilization of target mRNAs. It has been extensively described that TTP expression is significantly decreased in different types of tumors [150] and that it is involved in cell cycle control, angiogenesis and tumor metastasis [151]. Recently, it has been reported that TTP inhibits the epithelial-mesenchymal transition (EMT) of cancer cells through mRNA degradation of the EMT inducers, specifically, Twist1 and Snail1, and inhibits cell proliferation through down-regulation of c-*fos*, CDC34 and VEGF [152]. Interestingly, TTP appears to bind to AREs and interact with proteins involved in mRNA decay, such as the PM-scl75 exosome component, Xrn1 5′–3′ exonuclease, CCR4deadenylase and Dcp1 decapping enzyme [153], supporting a model in which TTP promotes mRNA decay through the ability to recruit components of the cellular mRNA decay machinery to the target mRNAs. In recent publications, high expression levels of HuR have been correlated with tumor progression and aggressiveness by affecting cell cycle progression, migration, invasion, metastasis and apoptosis in different tumor models [154–157]. HuR enhances the stability of the human epidermal growth factor receptor 2 (ERBB2/HER-2) mRNA, modulating the estrogen receptor-alpha-positive (ER+) breast cancer cells responsiveness to tamoxifen [158].

In addition, deadenylase complexes could be recruited to the mRNA poly(A) tail through the action of miRNAs. GW182 proteins, which participate of the miRNA-induced silencing complex (miRISC), directly interact with PAN3 and NOT1 subunits, leading to recruitment of the PAN2-PAN3 and CCR4-CAF1-NOT deadenylase complexes to the 3′-UTR of target mRNAs [159]. Also, it has been described that PARN deadenylase binds to the 3′ UTR of p53 mRNA through recruitment mediated by miR-125b-loaded miRISC, promoting p53 mRNA decay [134]. Interestingly, this effect can be reverted by HuR proteins, which bind to the p53 AREs and increase p53 mRNA stability [134].

The deadenylation machinery is also an important target for antitumor agents and anticancer therapy. Cantharidin (an inhibitor of protein phosphatase 2A) inhibits the invasive ability of pancreatic cancer cells, with concomitant deadenylation-dependent degradation of MMP2 mRNA [20]. Resveratrol (3,5,4′-trihydroxystilbene), a naturally occurring compound, induces

TPP expression in U87MG human glioma cells and leads to the decay of urokinase plasminogen activator (uPA) and urokinase plasminogen activator receptor (uPAR) mRNAs, promoting suppression of cell growth and inducing apoptosis [160].

Additionally, several mature mRNAs surveillance mechanisms guarantee quality and fidelity to encode a functional protein in a translation-dependent manner. The nonsense-mediated decay (NMD) pathway is the best understood surveillance mechanism; detecting and degrading transcripts which contain premature termination codons (PTCs), avoiding the expression of semi-functional and truncated proteins [161]. The UPF-1 (up-frameshift1) protein, a key component of the NMD mechanism, interacts with both Dcp2 and PARP, linking NMD with the decapping and deadenylation processes [162]. Low expression levels of UPF-1 protein as well as inactivation of UPF-1 function were described in several types of human cancer, suggesting that NMD downregulation is related to tumorigenesis. Decreased levels of UPF-1 were detected in lung adenocarcinoma in comparison to normal tissues, and its downregulation was correlated to poor prognosis and higher histological grade [163]. The pancreatic adenosquamous carcinoma (ASC) is an aggressive tumor which is associated with high metastatic potential and poor prognosis. In these tumors, a mutation that promotes *UPF-1* alternative splicing and results in a non-functional UPF-1 protein, has been observed. Inactivation of the NMD pathway promotes selective accumulation of a p53 isoform, which acts in a dominant-negative manner, contributing to tumorigenesis [164].

NMD can also be inhibited by a wide variety of cellular stresses, some of which are associated to the tumoral context [165]. In response to stress events, phosphorylation of the alpha subunit of the eukaryotic initiation factor 2 (eIF2α) is able to inhibit NMD. It has been described that phospho-eIF2α is necessary for oncogene c-*myc*-mediated NMD inhibition [106]. Inhibition of NMD by cellular stress promotes stabilization of the SLC7A11 mRNA, which encodes a subunit of the cystine/glutamate aminoacid transport system, leading to increased intracellular levels of cysteine, accelerating the production of glutathione. SLC7A11 is upregulated in hypoxic cells, promotes tumorigenesis and chemotherapy resistance, suggesting that it could be an adaptive response that protects tumor cells against oxidative stress [166]. It has recently been described that NMD regulates the epithelial-mesenchymal transition (EMT) in the lung adenocarcinoma model, by targeting the TGF-β signaling pathway [163]. In addition, the NMD mechanism controls the expression of a novel human E-cadherin variant mRNA produced by alternative splicing. Overexpression of this alternatively spliced E-cadherin variant in MCF-7, breast cancer cells was able to induce EMT by promoting higher expression levels of Twist, Snail, Zeb1 and Slug, with a concomitant decrease in the wild type E-cadherin mRNA levels [167].

Several promising NMD targets mRNAs for cancer therapy have been proposed. The MDM4 protein, which is undetectable in normal tissues, is frequently upregulated in cancer cells, acting by inhibiting the p53 tumor-suppressor function [168]. The abundance of the MDM4 protein is controlled, at least in part, by alternative splicing mechanisms and the NMD pathway. In most normal adult tissues, the lack of exon 6 in the Mdm4-spliced variant leads to the production of an unstable transcript (Mdm4-S), which contains a PTC and is targeted to NMD [168]. On the other hand, the oncogenic splicing-factor SRSF3 supports exon 6 inclusion in the Mdm4 mRNA transcript (full-length Mdm4 variant), which is not efficiently degraded by NMD. Therapeutic strategies which lead to antisense oligonucleotide-mediated (ASO-mediated) Mdm4 exon 6 skipping efficiently decreases MDM4 abundance and inhibits tumor cell growth in melanoma and diffuse large B cell lymphoma models, as well as increases sensitivity to MAPK-targeting therapies [169].

6. Final considerations

Different post-transcriptional mechanisms have been associated with gene expression control, leading to complex transcriptional signatures in cancer. The mechanisms presented in this chapter constitute fine regulators of gene expression which influence multiple and highly relevant pathways in cancer development (summarized in **Figure 1**). Several splicing

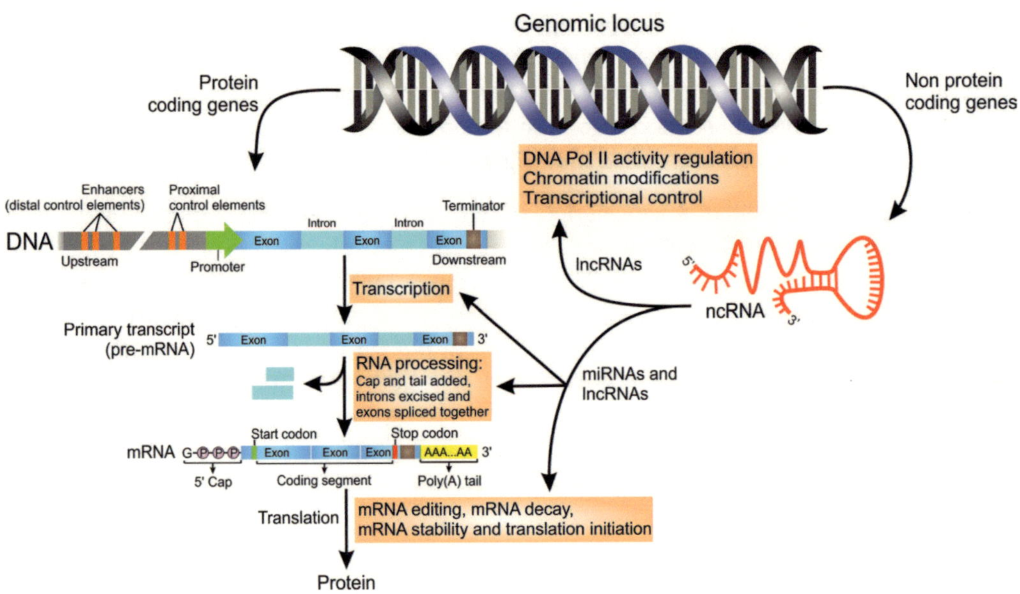

Figure 1. Schematic representation and key roles of different RNA species in the control of gene expression in mammalian cells. This scheme represents a genomic locus and the main molecular mechanisms associated with the control of gene expression pattern. Proximal control elements are located close to the promoter, while distal elements (called enhancers) may be far away from a gene or even located in an intron. Alternative splicing (AS) generates transcriptome diversity. During AS, *cis*-acting regulatory elements, present in the pre-mRNA sequence, determine which exons are retained and which exons are spliced out. For an individual pre-mRNA, several alternative exons show different types of alternative-splicing patterns. Addition of 5′ Cap and Poly(A) tail are controlled events which are extremely important for the stability of the mRNA and its transport from the cytoplasm to the nucleus. Non-coding RNAs (ncRNAs) with regulatory functions can act in multiple pathways during the transcription process by controlling specific events which culminate in synthesis of different proteins. Long non-coding RNAs (lncRNAs) target protein complexes to specific genomic loci affecting transcription patterns (transcriptional interference), leading to chromatin modifications (interplay between epigenetic marks, such as DNA methylation and histone acetylation) and DNA polymerase II activity. Advances in transcriptomics have resulted in the discovery of large numbers of ncRNAs (miRNAs e lncRNAs), many of which display the capacity to regulate gene expression at the levels of transcription (control of AS), post-transcription (mRNA editing, mRNA decay and mRNA stability) and translation (translation initiation).

variants, miRNAs and lncRNAs, have been shown to act as possible oncoRNAs or as tumor suppressors. The functional roles of these RNAs are only beginning to be elucidated providing an uncharted resource for the development of diagnostic methods and novel cancer therapies.

Abbreviations

ADAR	Adenosine deaminases acting on RNA
AGO	Argonaut
Akt/PKB	Protein kinase B
Apaf-1	Apoptotic protease activating factor 1
APOBEC	Apolipoprotein B Mrna editing enzyme, catalytic polypeptide-like
ARE	AU-rich elements
AS	Alternative splicing
ASC	Pancreatic adenosquamous carcinoma
ASO	Antisense oligonucleotide
AZIN1	Antizyme inhibitor 1
BCL	B cell lymphoma gene family
BrdU	Bromodeoxyuridine (5-bromo-2′-deoxyuridine)
BTG	BTG anti-proliferation factor
Caf1	Chromatin assembly factor-1 complex
Casp	Caspase
CCR4	C-C motif chemokine receptor 4
CCR4–NOT	Carbon catabolite repression 4 complex
CD44	CD44 molecule (Indian blood group)
CD6	Cluster of differentiation 6
CDC34	Cell division cycle 34
CDS	Coding DNA sequence
c-fos	Proto-oncogene c-Fos
cIAP2	Cellular inhibitor of apoptosis 2

CLL	Chronic lymphocytic leukemia
c-Myc	Myc proto-oncogene
CNOT1	CCR4-NOT transcription complex subunit 1
CoREST	REST corepressor 1
CSCs	Cancer stem cells
DBD	DNA-binding domain
Dcp1	Decapping protein 1
DDX	DEAD-box helixases
DICER	Dicer 1, ribonuclease III
DROSHA	Drosha ribonuclease III
E2F1	E2F transcription factor 1
eIF2α	Eukaryotic initiation factor 2
EMT	Epithelial-mesenchymal transition
ENCODE	Encyclopedia of DNA elements
ER	Estrogen receptor
ER^+	Estrogen receptor-alpha-positive
ERBB2/HER	Human epidermal growth factor receptor 2
EXP5	Exportin 5
GAS5	Growth-arrest-specific 5
GR	Glucocorticoid receptor
GRE	Glucocorticoid response elements
H19	H19, imprinted maternally expressed transcript
H3K4	Histone H3 lysine 4
hnRNP	Heterologous nuclear ribonuclear particle
HOTAIR	Hox transcript antisense intergenic RNA
HOXC	Homeobox C cluster
HuR	Human antigen R
IGF2	Insulin-like growth factor 2
lincRNAs	Long intergenic ncRNAs

lncRNAs	long non-coding RNAs
LSD1	Lysine-specific histone demethylase 1
MALAT1	Metastasis associated in lung adenocarcinoma transcript
MAPK	mitogen-activated kinase-like protein
MDM4	MDM4, p53 regulator
MEG3	Maternally expressed gene 3
miRISC	miRNA-induced silencing complex
miRNA/miR	microRNA
MMP2	Matrix metalloproteinase 2
NATs	Natural antisense transcripts
ncRNAs	Non-coding RNAs
NMD	Nonsense-mediated decay
NSCLC	Non-small cell lung cancer
ODC	Ornithine decarboxylase
p53	Tumor protein p53
PABPC1	Cytoplasmic poly(A)-binding protein
PABPC1	Poly(A) binding protein cytoplasmic 1
Pan2/Pan3	Poly(A) nuclease 2/3 complex
PARN	Poly(A)-specific ribonuclease
piRNA	PIWI-interacting RNA
Pol II	RNA polymerase II
PPB	Pleuropulmonary blastoma
PR	Progesterone receptor
PRC2	Polycomb repressive complex 2
Pri-miRNA	miRNA primary transcript
PTCs	Premature termination codons
PTEN	Phosphatase and tensin homolog
PTENP1	Phosphatase and tensin homolog pseudogene 1
Ras	HRas proto-oncogene, GTPase

REST	RE1-silencing transcription factor
RISC	RNA-induced silencing complex
rRNAs	Ribosomal RNAs
siRNA	Small interfering RNA
SLC7A11	Solute carrier family 7 member 11
Slug	Snail family transcriptional repressor 2
Snail1	Snail family transcriptional repressor 1
snoRNAs	Small nucleolar RNAs
SNPs	Single-nucleotide polymorphisms
snRNAs	Small nuclear RNAs
snRNP	Small nuclear ribonucleoprotein particles
SRP	Serine-rich protein
SRSF1	Serine and arginine-rich splicing factor 1
TGF-β	Transforming growth factor beta 1
Tob	Transducer of ERBB2
tRNAs	Transfer RNAs
TTP	Tristetraprolin
Twist1	Twist family BHLH transcription factor 1
uPA	Urokinase plasminogen activator
uPAR	Urokinase plasminogen activator receptor
UPF-1	Up-frameshift1 protein
UTR	Untranslated region
VEGF	Vascular endothelial growth factor
XPO5	Exportin 5
Xrn1	5′–3′ exoribonuclease 1
Zeb1	Zinc finger E-box binding homeobox 1
Zfas1	Znfx1 sntisense 1
Znfx1	Zinc finger NFX1-type containing 1

Author details

Carlos DeOcesano-Pereira[1,2], Fernando Janczur Velloso[1], Ana Claudia Oliveira Carreira[1], Carolina Simões Pires Ribeiro[3], Sheila Maria Brochado Winnischofer[3], Mari Cleide Sogayar[1,4] and Marina Trombetta-Lima[1]*

*Address all correspondence to: marinatlima@gmail.com

1 NUCEL-NETCEM, Internal Medicine Department, Medical School, University of São Paulo, São Paulo, SP, Brazil

2 Centre of Excellence in New Target Discovery (CENTD), Butantan Institute, São Paulo, SP, Brazil

3 Biochemistry and Molecular Biology Department, Federal University of Paraná, Curitiba, PR, Brazil

4 Chemistry Institute, Biochemistry Department, University of São Paulo, São Paulo, SP, Brazil

References

[1] Hanahan D, Weinberg RA. Hallmarks of cancer: The next generation. Cell. 2011;**144**(5): 646-674

[2] Zhang L, Zhou W, Velculescu VE, Kern SE, Hruban RH, Hamilton SR, et al. Gene expression profiles in normal and cancer cells. Science. 1997;**276**(5316):1268-1272

[3] Bouska A, Bi C, Lone W, Zhang W, Kedwaii A, Heavican T, et al. Adult high grade B-cell lymphoma with Burkitt lymphoma signature: Genomic features and potential therapeutic targets. Blood. 2017

[4] Kuang M, Cheng J, Zhang C, Feng L, Xu X, Zhang Y, et al. A novel signature for stratifying the molecular heterogeneity of the tissue-infiltrating T-cell receptor repertoire reflects gastric cancer prognosis. Scientific Reports. 2017;**7**(1):7762

[5] Castle JC, Zhang C, Shah JK, Kulkarni AV, Kalsotra A, Cooper TA, et al. Expression of 24,426 human alternative splicing events and predicted cis regulation in 48 tissues and cell lines. Nature Genetics. 2008;**40**(12):1416-1425

[6] Sharp PA. Splicing of messenger RNA precursors. Science. 1987;**235**(4790):766-771

[7] McManus CJ, Graveley BR. RNA structure and the mechanisms of alternative splicing. Current Opinion in Genetics & Development. 2011;**21**(4):373-379

[8] Lander ES, Linton LM, Birren B, Nusbaum C, Zody MC, Baldwin J, et al. Initial sequencing and analysis of the human genome. Nature. 2001;**409**(6822):860-921

[9] Pan Q, Shai O, Lee LJ, Frey BJ, Blencowe BJ. Deep surveying of alternative splicing complexity in the human transcriptome by high-throughput sequencing. Nature Genetics. 2008;**40**(12):1413-1415

[10] Sveen A, Kilpinen S, Ruusulehto A, Lothe RA, Skotheim RI. Aberrant RNA splicing in cancer; expression changes and driver mutations of splicing factor genes. Oncogene. 2016;**35**(19):2413-2427

[11] Venables JP, Klinck R, Koh C, Gervais-Bird J, Bramard A, Inkel L, et al. Cancer-associated regulation of alternative splicing. Nature Structural & Molecular Biology. 2009;**16**(6):670-676

[12] Xi L, Feber A, Gupta V, Wu M, Bergemann AD, Landreneau RJ, et al. Whole genome exon arrays identify differential expression of alternatively spliced, cancer-related genes in lung cancer. Nucleic Acids Research. 2008;**36**(20):6535-6547

[13] Armero VES, Tremblay MP, Allaire A, Boudreault S, Martenon-Brodeur C, Duval C, et al. Transcriptome-wide analysis of alternative RNA splicing events in Epstein-Barr virus-associated gastric carcinomas. PLoS One. 2017;**12**(5):e0176880

[14] Silipo M, Gautrey H, Tyson-Capper A. Deregulation of splicing factors and breast cancer development. Journal of Molecular Cell Biology. 2015;**7**(5):388-401

[15] Srebrow A, Kornblihtt AR. The connection between splicing and cancer. Journal of Cell Science. 2006;**119**(Pt 13):2635-2641

[16] Venables JP, Koh CS, Froehlich U, Lapointe E, Couture S, Inkel L, et al. Multiple and specific mRNA processing targets for the major human hnRNP proteins. Molecular and Cellular Biology. 2008;**28**(19):6033-6043

[17] Oltean S, Bates DO. Hallmarks of alternative splicing in cancer. Oncogene. 2014;**33**(46): 5311-5318

[18] Jiang L, Huang J, Higgs BW, Hu Z, Xiao Z, Yao X, et al. Genomic landscape survey identifies SRSF1 as a key Oncodriver in small cell lung cancer. PLoS Genetics. 2016;**12**(4):e1005895

[19] Anczuków O, Rosenberg AZ, Akerman M, Das S, Zhan L, Karni R, et al. The splicing factor SRSF1 regulates apoptosis and proliferation to promote mammary epithelial cell transformation. Nature Structural & Molecular Biology. 2012;**19**(2):220-228

[20] Anczuków O, Akerman M, Cléry A, Wu J, Shen C, Shirole NH, et al. SRSF1-regulated alternative splicing in breast cancer. Molecular Cell. 2015;**60**(1):105-117

[21] Shultz JC, Goehe RW, Murudkar CS, Wijesinghe DS, Mayton EK, Massiello A, et al. SRSF1 regulates the alternative splicing of caspase 9 via a novel intronic splicing enhancer affecting the chemotherapeutic sensitivity of non-small cell lung cancer cells. Molecular Cancer Research. 2011;**9**(7):889-900

[22] Loh TJ, Moon H, Jang HN, Liu Y, Choi N, Shen S, et al. SR proteins regulate V6 exon splicing of CD44 pre-mRNA. BMB Reports. 2016;**49**(11):612-616

[23] Amin EM, Oltean S, Hua J, Gammons MV, Hamdollah-Zadeh M, Welsh GI, et al. WT1 mutants reveal SRPK1 to be a downstream angiogenesis target by altering VEGF splicing. Cancer Cell. 2011;**20**(6):768-780

[24] Schwerk C, Schulze-Osthoff K. Regulation of apoptosis by alternative pre-mRNA splicing. Molecular Cell. 2005;**19**(1):1-13

[25] Green DR, Reed JC. Mitochondria and apoptosis. Science. 1998;**281**(5381):1309-1312

[26] Seol DW, Billiar TR. A caspase-9 variant missing the catalytic site is an endogenous inhibitor of apoptosis. The Journal of Biological Chemistry. 1999;**274**(4):2072-2076

[27] Srinivasula SM, Ahmad M, Guo Y, Zhan Y, Lazebnik Y, Fernandes-Alnemri T, et al. Identification of an endogenous dominant-negative short isoform of caspase-9 that can regulate apoptosis. Cancer Research. 1999;**59**(5):999-1002

[28] Shultz JC, Goehe RW, Wijesinghe DS, Murudkar C, Hawkins AJ, Shay JW, et al. Alternative splicing of caspase 9 is modulated by the phosphoinositide 3-kinase/Akt pathway via phosphorylation of SRp30a. Cancer Research. 2010;**70**(22):9185-9196

[29] Lin Y, Li Z, Ozsolak F, Kim SW, Arango-Argoty G, Liu TT, et al. An in-depth map of polyadenylation sites in cancer. Nucleic Acids Research. 2012;**40**(17):8460-8471

[30] Erson-Bensan AE, Can T. Alternative polyadenylation: Another foe in cancer. Molecular Cancer Research. 2016;**14**(6):507-517

[31] Elkon R, Ugalde AP, Agami R. Alternative cleavage and polyadenylation: Extent, regulation and function. Nature Reviews. Genetics. 2013;**14**(7):496-506

[32] Sandberg R, Neilson JR, Sarma A, Sharp PA, Burge CB. Proliferating cells express mRNAs with shortened 3′ untranslated regions and fewer microRNA target sites. Science. 2008;**320**(5883):1643-1647

[33] Morris AR, Bos A, Diosdado B, Rooijers K, Elkon R, Bolijn AS, et al. Alternative cleavage and polyadenylation during colorectal cancer development. Clinical Cancer Research. 2012;**18**(19):5256-5266

[34] Akman BH, Can T, Erson-Bensan AE. Estrogen-induced upregulation and 3′-UTR shortening of CDC6. Nucleic Acids Research. 2012;**40**(21):10679-10688

[35] Baysal BE, Sharma S, Hashemikhabir S, Janga SC. RNA editing in pathogenesis of cancer. Cancer Research. 2017;**77**(14):3733-3739

[36] Menendez D, Nguyen TA, Snipe J, Resnick MA. The cytidine deaminase APOBEC3 family is subject to transcriptional regulation by p53. Molecular Cancer Research. 2017;**15**(6):735-743

[37] Tomaselli S, Galeano F, Alon S, Raho S, Galardi S, Polito VA, et al. Modulation of microRNA editing, expression and processing by ADAR2 deaminase in glioblastoma. Genome Biology. 2015;**16**:5

[38] Anantharaman A, Gholamalamdari O, Khan A, Yoon JH, Jantsch MF, Hartner JC, et al. RNA-editing enzymes ADAR1 and ADAR2 coordinately regulate the editing and expression of Ctn RNA. FEBS Letters. 2017

[39] Chan TH, Qamra A, Tan KT, Guo J, Yang H, Qi L, et al. ADAR-mediated RNA editing predicts progression and prognosis of gastric cancer. Gastroenterology. 2016;**151**(4):637-650.e10

[40] Zhang L, Yang CS, Varelas X, Monti S. Altered RNA editing in 3′ UTR perturbs microRNA-mediated regulation of oncogenes and tumor-suppressors. Scientific Reports. 2016;**6**:23226

[41] Chen L, Li Y, Lin CH, Chan TH, Chow RK, Song Y, et al. Recoding RNA editing of AZIN1 predisposes to hepatocellular carcinoma. Nature Medicine. 2013;**19**(2):209-216

[42] Qiu S, Liu J, Xing F. Antizyme inhibitor 1: A potential carcinogenic molecule. Cancer Science. 2017;**108**(2):163-169

[43] Solomon O, Oren S, Safran M, Deshet-Unger N, Akiva P, Jacob-Hirsch J, et al. Global regulation of alternative splicing by adenosine deaminase acting on RNA (ADAR). RNA. 2013;**19**(5):591-604

[44] Goldberg L, Abutbul-Amitai M, Paret G, Nevo-Caspi Y. Alternative splicing of STAT3 is affected by RNA editing. DNA and Cell Biology. 2017;**36**(5):367-376

[45] Ishizu H, Siomi H, Siomi MC. Biology of PIWI-interacting RNAs: New insights into biogenesis and function inside and outside of germlines. Genes & Development. 2012;**26**(21):2361-2373

[46] Axtell MJ, Westholm JO, Lai EC. Vive la différence: Biogenesis and evolution of microRNAs in plants and animals. Genome Biology. 2011;**12**(4):221

[47] Ghildiyal M, Zamore PD. Small silencing RNAs: An expanding universe. Nature Reviews. Genetics. 2009;**10**(2):94-108

[48] Fire A, Xu S, Montgomery MK, Kostas SA, Driver SE, Mello CC. Potent and specific genetic interference by double-stranded RNA in *Caenorhabditis elegans*. Nature. 1998;**391**(6669):806-811

[49] Bartel DP. MicroRNAs: Genomics, biogenesis, mechanism, and function. Cell. 2004;**116**(2):281-297

[50] Iorio MV, Croce CM. MicroRNAs in cancer: Small molecules with a huge impact. Journal of Clinical Oncology. 2009;**27**(34):5848-5856

[51] Kozomara A, Griffiths-Jones S. miRBase: Annotating high confidence microRNAs using deep sequencing data. Nucleic Acids Research. 2014;**42**(Database issue):D68-D73

[52] Lee Y, Jeon K, Lee JT, Kim S, Kim VN. MicroRNA maturation: Stepwise processing and subcellular localization. The EMBO Journal. 2002;**21**(17):4663-4670

[53] Huntzinger E, Izaurralde E. Gene silencing by microRNAs: Contributions of translational repression and mRNA decay. Nature Reviews. Genetics. 2011;**12**(2):99-110

[54] Ketting RF, Fischer SE, Bernstein E, Sijen T, Hannon GJ, Plasterk RH. Dicer functions in RNA interference and in synthesis of small RNA involved in developmental timing in *C. elegans*. Genes & Development. 2001;**15**(20):2654-2659

[55] Kawamata T, Tomari Y. Making RISC. Trends in Biochemical Sciences. 2010;**35**(7):368-376

[56] Bartel DP. MicroRNAs: Target recognition and regulatory functions. Cell. 2009;**136**(2): 215-233

[57] Friedman RC, Farh KK, Burge CB, Bartel DP. Most mammalian mRNAs are conserved targets of microRNAs. Genome Research. 2009;**19**(1):92-105

[58] Ha M, Kim VN. Regulation of microRNA biogenesis. Nature Reviews. Molecular Cell Biology. 2014;**15**(8):509-524

[59] Calin GA, Sevignani C, Dumitru CD, Hyslop T, Noch E, Yendamuri S, et al. Human microRNA genes are frequently located at fragile sites and genomic regions involved in cancers. Proceedings of the National Academy of Sciences of the United States of America. 2004;**101**(9):2999-3004

[60] Cimmino A, Calin GA, Fabbri M, Iorio MV, Ferracin M, Shimizu M, et al. miR-15 and miR-16 induce apoptosis by targeting BCL2. Proceedings of the National Academy of Sciences of the United States of America. 2005;**102**(39):13944-13949

[61] Di Leva G, Calin GA, Croce CM. MicroRNAs: Fundamental facts and involvement in human diseases. Birth Defects Research. Part C, Embryo Today. 2006;**78**(2):180-189

[62] Malumbres M. miRNAs versus oncogenes: The power of social networking. Molecular Systems Biology. 2012;**8**:569

[63] Bucay N, Sekhon K, Yang T, Majid S, Shahryari V, Hsieh C, et al. MicroRNA-383 located in frequently deleted chromosomal locus 8p22 regulates CD44 in prostate cancer. Oncogene. 2017;**36**(19):2667-2679

[64] Volinia S, Galasso M, Costinean S, Tagliavini L, Gamberoni G, Drusco A, et al. Reprogramming of miRNA networks in cancer and leukemia. Genome Research. 2010;**20**(5):589-599

[65] Wiseman SM, Makretsov N, TO N, Gilks B, Yorida E, Cheang M, et al. Coexpression of the type 1 growth factor receptor family members HER-1, HER-2, and HER-3 has a synergistic negative prognostic effect on breast carcinoma survival. Cancer. 2005;**103**(9):1770-1777

[66] Scott GK, Goga A, Bhaumik D, Berger CE, Sullivan CS, Benz CC. Coordinate suppression of ERBB2 and ERBB3 by enforced expression of micro-RNA miR-125a or miR-125b. The Journal of Biological Chemistry. 2007;**282**(2):1479-1486

[67] Johnson SM, Grosshans H, Shingara J, Byrom M, Jarvis R, Cheng A, et al. RAS is regulated by the let-7 microRNA family. Cell. 2005;**120**(5):635-647

[68] Weiss GJ, Bemis LT, Nakajima E, Sugita M, Birks DK, Robinson WA, et al. EGFR regulation by microRNA in lung cancer: Correlation with clinical response and survival to gefitinib and EGFR expression in cell lines. Annals of Oncology. 2008;**19**(6):1053-1059

[69] Kefas B, Godlewski J, Comeau L, Li Y, Abounader R, Hawkinson M, et al. microRNA-7 inhibits the epidermal growth factor receptor and the Akt pathway and is down-regulated in glioblastoma. Cancer Research. 2008;**68**(10):3566-3572

[70] Costinean S, Zanesi N, Pekarsky Y, Tili E, Volinia S, Heerema N, et al. Pre-B cell proliferation and lymphoblastic leukemia/high-grade lymphoma in E(mu)-miR155 transgenic mice. Proceedings of the National Academy of Sciences of the United States of America. 2006;**103**(18):7024-7029

[71] Medina PP, Nolde M, Slack FJ. OncomiR addiction in an in vivo model of microRNA-21-induced pre-B-cell lymphoma. Nature. 2010;**467**(7311):86-90

[72] O'Donnell KA, Wentzel EA, Zeller KI, Dang CV, Mendell JT. c-Myc-regulated microRNAs modulate E2F1 expression. Nature. 2005;**435**(7043):839-843

[73] Corney DC, Flesken-Nikitin A, Godwin AK, Wang W, Nikitin AY. MicroRNA-34b and MicroRNA-34c are targets of p53 and cooperate in control of cell proliferation and adhesion-independent growth. Cancer Research. 2007;**67**(18):8433-8438

[74] Di Leva G, Garofalo M, Croce CM. MicroRNAs in cancer. Annual Review of Pathology. 2014;**9**:287-314

[75] Acunzo M, Romano G, Wernicke D, Croce CM. MicroRNA and cancer—A brief overview. Advances in Biological Regulation. 2015;**57**:1-9

[76] Saito Y, Liang G, Egger G, Friedman JM, Chuang JC, Coetzee GA, et al. Specific activation of microRNA-127 with downregulation of the proto-oncogene BCL6 by chromatin-modifying drugs in human cancer cells. Cancer Cell. 2006;**9**(6):435-443

[77] Kotani A, Ha D, Schotte D, den Boer ML, Armstrong SA, Lodish HF. A novel mutation in the miR-128b gene reduces miRNA processing and leads to glucocorticoid resistance of MLL-AF4 acute lymphocytic leukemia cells. Cell Cycle. 2010;**9**(6):1037-1042

[78] Hill DA, Ivanovich J, Priest JR, Gurnett CA, Dehner LP, Desruisseau D, et al. DICER1 mutations in familial pleuropulmonary blastoma. Science. 2009;**325**(5943):965

[79] Merritt WM, Lin YG, Han LY, Kamat AA, Spannuth WA, Schmandt R, et al. Dicer, Drosha, and outcomes in patients with ovarian cancer. The New England Journal of Medicine. 2008;**359**(25):2641-2650

[80] Melo SA, Moutinho C, Ropero S, Calin GA, Rossi S, Spizzo R, et al. A genetic defect in exportin-5 traps precursor microRNAs in the nucleus of cancer cells. Cancer Cell. 2010;**18**(4):303-315

[81] Lin S, Gregory RI. MicroRNA biogenesis pathways in cancer. Nature Reviews. Cancer. 2015;**15**(6):321-333

[82] Peter ME. Regulating cancer stem cells the miR way. Cell Stem Cell. 2010;**6**(1):4-6

[83] Shimono Y, Zabala M, Cho RW, Lobo N, Dalerba P, Qian D, et al. Downregulation of miRNA-200c links breast cancer stem cells with normal stem cells. Cell. 2009;**138**(3):592-603

[84] Adam L, Zhong M, Choi W, Qi W, Nicoloso M, Arora A, et al. miR-200 expression regulates epithelial-to-mesenchymal transition in bladder cancer cells and reverses resistance to epidermal growth factor receptor therapy. Clinical Cancer Research. 2009;**15**(16):5060-5072

[85] Tavazoie SF, Alarcón C, Oskarsson T, Padua D, Wang Q, Bos PD, et al. Endogenous human microRNAs that suppress breast cancer metastasis. Nature. 2008;**451**(7175):147-152

[86] Iorio MV, Croce CM. microRNA involvement in human cancer. Carcinogenesis. 2012;**33**(6):1126-1133

[87] Cheng L, Sun X, Scicluna BJ, Coleman BM, Hill AF. Characterization and deep sequencing analysis of exosomal and non-exosomal miRNA in human urine. Kidney International. 2014;**86**(2):433-444

[88] Huang X, Yuan T, Tschannen M, Sun Z, Jacob H, Du M, et al. Characterization of human plasma-derived exosomal RNAs by deep sequencing. BMC Genomics. 2013;**14**:319

[89] Kosaka N, Iguchi H, Ochiya T. Circulating microRNA in body fluid: A new potential biomarker for cancer diagnosis and prognosis. Cancer Science. 2010;**101**(10):2087-2092

[90] Thomas DJ, Rosenbloom KR, Clawson H, Hinrichs AS, Trumbower H, Raney BJ, et al. The ENCODE Project at UC Santa Cruz. Nucleic Acids Research. 2007;**35**(Database):D663-D667

[91] Kapranov P, Willingham AT, Gingeras TR. Genome-wide transcription and the implications for genomic organization. Nature Reviews. Genetics. 2007;**8**(6):413-423

[92] Morris KV, Mattick JS. The rise of regulatory RNA. Nature Reviews. Genetics. 2014;**15**(6):423-437

[93] Shao J, Chen H, Yang D, Jiang M, Zhang H, Wu B, et al. Genome-wide identification and characterization of natural antisense transcripts by strand-specific RNA sequencing in Ganoderma lucidum. Scientific Reports. 2017;**7**(1):5711

[94] Hung T, Chang HY. Long noncoding RNA in genome regulation: Prospects and mechanisms. RNA Biology. 2010;**7**(5):582-585

[95] Hansji H, Leung EY, Baguley BC, Finlay GJ, Askarian-Amiri ME. Keeping abreast with long non-coding RNAs in mammary gland development and breast cancer. Frontiers in Genetics. 2014;**5**:379

[96] Malek E, Jagannathan S, Driscoll JJ. Correlation of long non-coding RNA expression with metastasis, drug resistance and clinical outcome in cancer. Oncotarget. 2014;**5**(18): 8027-8038

[97] Necsulea A, Soumillon M, Warnefors M, Liechti A, Daish T, Zeller U, et al. The evolution of lncRNA repertoires and expression patterns in tetrapods. Nature. 2014;**505**(7485): 635-640

[98] Brunner AL, Beck AH, Edris B, Sweeney RT, Zhu SX, Li R, et al. Transcriptional profiling of long non-coding RNAs and novel transcribed regions across a diverse panel of archived human cancers. Genome Biology. 2012;**13**(8):R75

[99] Rinn JL, Chang HY. Genome regulation by long noncoding RNAs. Annual Review of Biochemistry. 2012;**81**:145-166

[100] Gutschner T, Diederichs S. The hallmarks of cancer: A long non-coding RNA point of view. RNA Biology. 2012;**9**(6):703-719

[101] Wapinski O, Chang HY. Long noncoding RNAs and human disease. Trends in Cell Biology. 2011;**21**(6):354-361

[102] Schmitt AM, Chang HY. Long noncoding RNAs in cancer pathways. Cancer Cell. 2016;**29**(4):452-463

[103] Engreitz JM, Ollikainen N, Guttman M. Long non-coding RNAs: Spatial amplifiers that control nuclear structure and gene expression. Nature Reviews. Molecular Cell Biology. 2016;**17**(12):756-770

[104] Geisler S, Coller J. RNA in unexpected places: Long non-coding RNA functions in diverse cellular contexts. Nature Reviews. Molecular Cell Biology. 2013;**14**(11):699-712

[105] Holoch D, Moazed D. RNA-mediated epigenetic regulation of gene expression. Nature Reviews. Genetics. 2015;**16**(2):71-84

[106] Villares GJ, Zigler M, Dobroff AS, Wang H, Song R, Melnikova VO, et al. Protease activated receptor-1 inhibits the Maspin tumor-suppressor gene to determine the melanoma metastatic phenotype. Proceedings of the National Academy of Sciences of the United States of America. 2011;**108**(2):626-631

[107] Rinn JL, Kertesz M, Wang JK, Squazzo SL, Xu X, Brugmann SA, et al. Functional demarcation of active and silent chromatin domains in human HOX loci by noncoding RNAs. Cell. 2007;**129**(7):1311-1323

[108] Tsai MC, Manor O, Wan Y, Mosammaparast N, Wang JK, Lan F, et al. Long non-coding RNA as modular scaffold of histone modification complexes. Science. 2010;**329**(5992):689-693

[109] Gupta RA, Shah N, Wang KC, Kim J, Horlings HM, Wong DJ, et al. Long non-coding RNA HOTAIR reprograms chromatin state to promote cancer metastasis. Nature. 2010;**464**(7291):1071-1076

[110] Kino T, Hurt DE, Ichijo T, Nader N, Chrousos GP. Noncoding RNA gas5 is a growth arrest- and starvation-associated repressor of the glucocorticoid receptor. Science Signaling. 2010;**3**(107):ra8

[111] Webster JC, Huber RM, Hanson RL, Collier PM, Haws TF, Mills JK, et al. Dexamethasone and tumor necrosis factor-alpha act together to induce the cellular inhibitor of apoptosis-2 gene and prevent apoptosis in a variety of cell types. Endocrinology. 2002;**143**(10):3866-3874

[112] Adriaenssens E, Dumont L, Lottin S, Bolle D, Lepretre A, Delobelle A, et al. H19 over-expression in breast adenocarcinoma stromal cells is associated with tumor values and steroid receptor status but independent of p53 and Ki-67 expression. The American Journal of Pathology. 1998;**153**(5):1597-1607

[113] Gabory A, Jammes H, Dandolo L. The H19 locus: Role of an imprinted non-coding RNA in growth and development. BioEssays. 2010;**32**(6):473-480

[114] Berteaux N, Lottin S, Monte D, Pinte S, Quatannens B, Coll J, et al. H19 mRNA-like noncoding RNA promotes breast cancer cell proliferation through positive control by E2F1. The Journal of Biological Chemistry. 2005;**280**(33):29625-29636

[115] Ji P, Diederichs S, Wang W, Böing S, Metzger R, Schneider PM, et al. MALAT-1, a novel noncoding RNA, and thymosin beta4 predict metastasis and survival in early-stage non-small cell lung cancer. Oncogene. 2003;**22**(39):8031-8041

[116] Bernard D, Prasanth KV, Tripathi V, Colasse S, Nakamura T, Xuan Z, et al. A long nuclear-retained non-coding RNA regulates synaptogenesis by modulating gene expression. The EMBO Journal. 2010;**29**(18):3082-3093

[117] Tripathi V, Ellis JD, Shen Z, Song DY, Pan Q, Watt AT, et al. The nuclear-retained non-coding RNA MALAT1 regulates alternative splicing by modulating SR splicing factor phosphorylation. Molecular Cell. 2010;**39**(6):925-938

[118] Long JC, Caceres JF. The SR protein family of splicing factors: Master regulators of gene expression. The Biochemical Journal. 2009;**417**(1):15-27

[119] Zhou Y, Zhong Y, Wang Y, Zhang X, Batista DL, Gejman R, et al. Activation of p53 by MEG3 non-coding RNA. The Journal of Biological Chemistry. 2007;**282**(34):24731-24742

[120] Mondal T, Subhash S, Vaid R, Enroth S, Uday S, Reinius B, et al. MEG3 long noncoding RNA regulates the TGF-β pathway genes through formation of RNA-DNA triplex structures. Nature Communications. 2015;**6**:7743

[121] Zhang X, Zhou Y, Mehta KR, Danila DC, Scolavino S, Johnson SR, et al. A pituitary-derived MEG3 isoform functions as a growth suppressor in tumor cells. The Journal of Clinical Endocrinology and Metabolism. 2003;**88**(11):5119-5126

[122] Zhang X, Gejman R, Mahta A, Zhong Y, Rice KA, Zhou Y, et al. Maternally expressed gene 3, an imprinted noncoding RNA gene, is associated with meningioma pathogenesis and progression. Cancer Research. 2010;**70**(6):2350-2358

[123] Braconi C, Kogure T, Valeri N, Huang N, Nuovo G, Costinean S, et al. microRNA-29 can regulate expression of the long non-coding RNA gene MEG3 in hepatocellular cancer. Oncogene. 2011;**30**(47):4750-4756

[124] Chen CL, Tseng YW, JC W, Chen GY, Lin KC, Hwang SM, et al. Suppression of hepatocellular carcinoma by baculovirus-mediated expression of long non-coding RNA PTENP1 and MicroRNA regulation. Biomaterials. 2015;**44**:71-81

[125] Tang J, Ning R, Zeng B, Li Y. Molecular evolution of PTEN Pseudogenes in mammals. PLoS One. 2016;**11**(12):e0167851

[126] Chen TH, Yen AM, GH W, Chen LS, Chiu YH. Multiple detection modalities and disease natural history of breast cancer. Studies in Health Technology and Informatics. 2007;**129**(Pt 1):78-81

[127] Welch JD, Baran-Gale J, Perou CM, Sethupathy P, Prins JF. Pseudogenes transcribed in breast invasive carcinoma show subtype-specific expression and ceRNA potential. BMC Genomics. 2015;**16**:113

[128] Askarian-Amiri ME, Crawford J, French JD, Smart CE, Smith MA, Clark MB, et al. SNORD-host RNA Zfas1 is a regulator of mammary development and a potential marker for breast cancer. RNA. 2011;**17**(5):878-891

[129] Hansji H, Leung EY, Baguley BC, Finlay GJ, Cameron-Smith D, Figueiredo VC, et al. ZFAS1: A long noncoding RNA associated with ribosomes in breast cancer cells. Biology Direct. 2016;**11**(1):62

[130] Schoenberg DR, Maquat LE. Regulation of cytoplasmic mRNA decay. Nature Reviews. Genetics. 2012;**13**(4):246-259

[131] Wahle E, Winkler GS. RNA decay machines: Deadenylation by the Ccr4-not and Pan2-Pan3 complexes. Biochimica et Biophysica Acta. 2013;**1829**(6-7):561-570

[132] Rambout X, Detiffe C, Bruyr J, Mariavelle E, Cherkaoui M, Brohée S, et al. The transcription factor ERG recruits CCR4-NOT to control mRNA decay and mitotic progression. Nature Structural & Molecular Biology. 2016;**23**(7):663-672

[133] Balatsos NA, Maragozidis P, Anastasakis D, Stathopoulos C. Modulation of poly(A)-specific ribonuclease (PARN): Current knowledge and perspectives. Current Medicinal Chemistry. 2012;**19**(28):4838-4849

[134] Zhang X, Devany E, Murphy MR, Glazman G, Persaud M, Kleiman FE. PARN deadenylase is involved in miRNA-dependent degradation of TP53 mRNA in mammalian cells. Nucleic Acids Research. 2015;**43**(22):10925-10938

[135] Boele J, Persson H, Shin JW, Ishizu Y, Newie IS, Søkilde R, et al. PAPD5-mediated 3′adenylation and subsequent degradation of miR-21 is disrupted in proliferative disease. Proceedings of the National Academy of Sciences of the United States of America. 2014;**111**(31):11467-11472

[136] Zhang LN, Yan YB. Depletion of poly(A)-specific ribonuclease (PARN) inhibits proliferation of human gastric cancer cells by blocking cell cycle progression. Biochimica et Biophysica Acta. 2015;**1853**(2):522-534

[137] Maragozidis P, Karangeli M, Labrou M, Dimoulou G, Papaspyrou K, Salataj E, et al. Alterations of deadenylase expression in acute leukemias: Evidence for poly(a)-specific ribonuclease as a potential biomarker. Acta Haematologica. 2012;**128**(1):39-46

[138] Winkler GS. The mammalian anti-proliferative BTG/Tob protein family. Journal of Cellular Physiology. 2010;**222**(1):66-72

[139] Ezzeddine N, Chang TC, Zhu W, Yamashita A, Chen CY, Zhong Z, et al. Human TOB, an antiproliferative transcription factor, is a poly(A)-binding protein-dependent positive regulator of cytoplasmic mRNA deadenylation. Molecular and Cellular Biology. 2007;**27**(22):7791-7801

[140] Stupfler B, Birck C, Séraphin B, Mauxion F. BTG2 bridges PABPC1 RNA-binding domains and CAF1 deadenylase to control cell proliferation. Nature Communications. 2016;**7**:10811

[141] Ogami K, Hosoda N, Funakoshi Y, Hoshino S. Antiproliferative protein Tob directly regulates c-myc proto-oncogene expression through cytoplasmic polyadenylation element-binding protein CPEB. Oncogene. 2014;**33**(1):55-64

[142] Boiko AD, Porteous S, Razorenova OV, Krivokrysenko VI, Williams BR, Gudkov AV. A systematic search for downstream mediators of tumor suppressor function of p53 reveals a major role of BTG2 in suppression of Ras-induced transformation. Genes & Development. 2006;**20**(2):236-252

[143] Kawakubo H, Carey JL, Brachtel E, Gupta V, Green JE, Walden PD, et al. Expression of the NF-kappaB-responsive gene BTG2 is aberrantly regulated in breast cancer. Oncogene. 2004;**23**(50):8310-8319

[144] Struckmann K, Schraml P, Simon R, Elmenhorst K, Mirlacher M, Kononen J, et al. Impaired expression of the cell cycle regulator BTG2 is common in clear cell renal cell carcinoma. Cancer Research. 2004;**64**(5):1632-1638

[145] Kawakubo H, Brachtel E, Hayashida T, Yeo G, Kish J, Muzikansky A, et al. Loss of B-cell translocation gene-2 in estrogen receptor-positive breast carcinoma is associated with tumor grade and overexpression of cyclin d1 protein. Cancer Research. 2006;**66**(14):7075-7082

[146] Möllerström E, Kovács A, Lövgren K, Nemes S, Delle U, Danielsson A, et al. Up-regulation of cell cycle arrest protein BTG2 correlates with increased overall survival in breast cancer, as detected by immunohistochemistry using tissue microarray. BMC Cancer. 2010;**10**:296

[147] Faraji F, Hu Y, Yang HH, Lee MP, Winkler GS, Hafner M, et al. Post-transcriptional control of tumor cell autonomous metastatic potential by CCR4-NOT Deadenylase CNOT7. PLoS Genetics. 2016;**12**(1):e1005820

[148] Helms MW, Kemming D, Contag CH, Pospisil H, Bartkowiak K, Wang A, et al. TOB1 is regulated by EGF-dependent HER2 and EGFR signaling, is highly phosphorylated, and indicates poor prognosis in node-negative breast cancer. Cancer Research. 2009;**69**(12):5049-5056

[149] Zhu J, Ding H, Wang X, Lu Q. PABPC1 exerts carcinogenesis in gastric carcinoma by targeting miR-34c. International Journal of Clinical and Experimental Pathology. 2015;**8**(4):3794-3802

[150] Brennan SE, Kuwano Y, Alkharouf N, Blackshear PJ, Gorospe M, Wilson GM. The mRNA-destabilizing protein tristetraprolin is suppressed in many cancers, altering tumorigenic phenotypes and patient prognosis. Cancer Research. 2009;**69**(12):5168-5176

[151] Wang H, Ding N, Guo J, Xia J, Ruan Y. Dysregulation of TTP and HuR plays an important role in cancers. Tumour Biology. 2016;**37**(11):14451-14461

[152] Yoon NA, Jo HG, Lee UH, Park JH, Yoon JE, Ryu J, et al. Tristetraprolin suppresses the EMT through the down-regulation of Twist1 and Snail1 in cancer cells. Oncotarget. 2016;**7**(8):8931-8943

[153] Lykke-Andersen J, Wagner E. Recruitment and activation of mRNA decay enzymes by two ARE-mediated decay activation domains in the proteins TTP and BRF-1. Genes & Development. 2005;**19**(3):351-361

[154] Filippova N, Yang X, Ananthan S, Sorochinsky A, Hackney JR, Gentry Z, et al. Hu antigen R (HuR) multimerization contributes to glioma disease progression. The Journal of Biological Chemistry. 2017

[155] Gauchotte G, Hergalant S, Vigouroux C, Casse JM, Houlgatte R, Kaoma T, et al. Cytoplasmic overexpression of RNA-binding protein HuR is a marker of poor prognosis in meningioma, and HuR knockdown decreases meningioma cell growth and resistance to hypoxia. The Journal of Pathology. 2017;**242**(4):421-434

[156] Lang M, Berry D, Passecker K, Mesteri I, Bhuju S, Ebner F, et al. HuR small-molecule inhibitor elicits differential effects in adenomatosis polyposis and colorectal carcinogenesis. Cancer Research. 2017;**77**(9):2424-2438

[157] Xu X, Song C, Chen Z, Yu C, Wang Y, Tang Y, et al. Downregulation of HuR inhibits the progression of esophageal cancer through Interleukin-18. Cancer Research and Treatment. 2017

[158] Tan S, Ding K, Chong QY, Zhao J, Liu Y, Shao Y, et al. Post-transcriptional regulation of ERBB2 by miR26a/b and HuR confers resistance to tamoxifen in estrogen receptor-positive breast cancer cells. The Journal of Biological Chemistry. 2017;**292**(33): 13551-13564

[159] Braun JE, Huntzinger E, Fauser M, Izaurralde E. GW182 proteins directly recruit cytoplasmic deadenylase complexes to miRNA targets. Molecular Cell. 2011;**44**(1):120-133

[160] Ryu J, Yoon NA, Seong H, Jeong JY, Kang S, Park N, et al. Resveratrol induces glioma cell apoptosis through activation of tristetraprolin. Molecules and Cells. 2015;**38**(11):991-997

[161] Lykke-Andersen S, Jensen TH. Nonsense-mediated mRNA decay: An intricate machinery that shapes transcriptomes. Nature Reviews. Molecular Cell Biology. 2015;**16**(11): 665-677

[162] Lejeune F, Li X, Maquat LE. Nonsense-mediated mRNA decay in mammalian cells involves decapping, deadenylating, and exonucleolytic activities. Molecular Cell. 2003;**12**(3):675-687

[163] Cao L, Qi L, Zhang L, Song W, Yu Y, Xu C, et al. Human nonsense-mediated RNA decay regulates EMT by targeting the TGF-ß signaling pathway in lung adenocarcinoma. Cancer Letters. 2017;**403**:246-259

[164] Liu C, Karam R, Zhou Y, Su F, Ji Y, Li G, et al. The UPF1 RNA surveillance gene is commonly mutated in pancreatic adenosquamous carcinoma. Nature Medicine. 2014; **20**(6):596-598

[165] Gardner LB. Nonsense-mediated RNA decay regulation by cellular stress: Implications for tumorigenesis. Molecular Cancer Research. 2010;**8**(3):295-308

[166] Martin L, Gardner LB. Stress-induced inhibition of nonsense-mediated RNA decay regulates intracellular cystine transport and intracellular glutathione through regulation of the cystine/glutamate exchanger SLC7A11. Oncogene. 2015;**34**(32):4211-4218

[167] Matos ML, Lapyckyj L, Rosso M, Besso MJ, Mencucci MV, Briggiler CI, et al. Identification of a novel human E-cadherin splice variant and assessment of its effects upon EMT-related events. Journal of Cellular Physiology. 2017;**232**(6):1368-1386

[168] Bezzi M, Teo SX, Muller J, Mok WC, Sahu SK, Vardy LA, et al. Regulation of constitutive and alternative splicing by PRMT5 reveals a role for Mdm4 pre-mRNA in sensing defects in the spliceosomal machinery. Genes & Development. 2013;**27**(17):1903-1916

[169] Dewaele M, Tabaglio T, Willekens K, Bezzi M, Teo SX, Low DH, et al. Antisense oligonucleotide-mediated MDM4 exon 6 skipping impairs tumor growth. The Journal of Clinical Investigation. 2016;**126**(1):68-84

[170] Voorhoeve PM, le Sage C, Schrier M, Gillis AJ, Stoop H, Nagel R, et al. A genetic screen implicates miRNA-372 and miRNA-373 as oncogenes in testicular germ cell tumors. Cell. 2006;**124**(6):1169-1181

[171] Ota A, Tagawa H, Karnan S, Tsuzuki S, Karpas A, Kira S, et al. Identification and characterization of a novel gene, C13orf25, as a target for 13q31-q32 amplification in malignant lymphoma. Cancer Research. 2004;**64**(9):3087-3095

[172] Ikeda S, Kitadate A, Abe F, Saitoh H, Michishita Y, Hatano Y, et al. Hypoxia-inducible microRNA-210 regulates the DIMT1-IRF4 oncogenic axis in multiple myeloma. Cancer Science. 2017;**108**(4):641-652

[173] Li Z, Lei H, Luo M, Wang Y, Dong L, Ma Y, et al. DNA methylation downregulated mir-10b acts as a tumor suppressor in gastric cancer. Gastric Cancer. 2015;**18**(1):43-54

[174] Wang CZ, Yuan P, Li Y. MiR-126 regulated breast cancer cell invasion by targeting ADAM9. International Journal of Clinical and Experimental Pathology. 2015;**8**(6):6547-6553

[175] Heyn H, Engelmann M, Schreek S, Ahrens P, Lehmann U, Kreipe H, et al. MicroRNA miR-335 is crucial for the BRCA1 regulatory cascade in breast cancer development. International Journal of Cancer. 2011;**129**(12):2797-2806

[176] Bhan A, Mandal SS. LncRNA HOTAIR: A master regulator of chromatin dynamics and cancer. Biochimica et Biophysica Acta. 2015;**1856**(1):151-164

[177] Zhang J, Zhang P, Wang L, Piao HL, Ma L. Long non-coding RNA HOTAIR in carcinogenesis and metastasis. Acta Biochimica et Biophysica Sinica. 2014;**46**(1):1-5

[178] Pickard MR, Williams GT. The hormone response element mimic sequence of GAS5 lncRNA is sufficient to induce apoptosis in breast cancer cells. Oncotarget. 2016;**7**(9):10104-10116

[179] Mourtada-Maarabouni M, Pickard MR, Hedge VL, Farzaneh F, Williams GT. GAS5, a non-protein-coding RNA, controls apoptosis and is downregulated in breast cancer. Oncogene. 2009;**28**(2):195-208

[180] Berteaux N, Aptel N, Cathala G, Genton C, Coll J, Daccache A, et al. A novel H19 antisense RNA overexpressed in breast cancer contributes to paternal IGF2 expression. Molecular and Cellular Biology. 2008;**28**(22):6731-6745

[181] Jadaliha M, Zong X, Malakar P, Ray T, Singh DK, Freier SM, et al. Functional and prognostic significance of long non-coding RNA MALAT1 as a metastasis driver in ER negative lymph node negative breast cancer. Oncotarget. 2016

[182] Gutschner T, Hammerle M, Diederichs S. MALAT1—A paradigm for long noncoding RNA function in cancer. Journal of Molecular Medicine. 2013;**91**(7):791-801

[183] Sun L, Li Y, Yang B. Downregulated long non-coding RNA MEG3 in breast cancer regulates proliferation, migration and invasion by depending on p53's transcriptional activity. Biochemical and Biophysical Research Communications. 2016

[184] Zhou Y, Zhang X, Klibanski A. MEG3 noncoding RNA: A tumor suppressor. Journal of Molecular Endocrinology. 2012;**48**(3):R45-R53

[185] Poliseno L, Marranci A, Pandolfi PP. Pseudogenes in human cancer. Frontiers in Medicine. 2015;**2**:68

[186] Poliseno L, Salmena L, Zhang J, Carver B, Haveman WJ, Pandolfi PP. A coding-independent function of gene and pseudogene mRNAs regulates tumour biology. Nature. 2010;**465**(7301):1033-1038

[187] Poliseno L, Haimovic A, Christos PJ, Vega YSMEC, Shapiro R, Pavlick A, et al. Deletion of PTENP1 pseudogene in human melanoma. The Journal of Investigative Dermatology. 2011;**131**(12):2497-2500

[188] Liu F, Gao H, Li S, Ni X, Zhu Z. Long non-coding RNA ZFAS1 correlates with clinical progression and prognosis in cancer patients. Oncotarget. 2017;**8**(37):61561-61569

Chapter 8

Current Status for Application of RNA Interference Technology as Nucleic Acid Drug

Tomoko Takahashi, Yuko Nakano and
Kumiko Ui-Tei

Additional information is available at the end of the chapter

http://dx.doi.org/10.5772/intechopen.71965

Abstract

RNA interference (RNAi) is a convenient and useful gene suppression technology induced by small interfering RNA (siRNA) composed of 21-nucleotide long double-stranded RNA. The successful application of RNAi for clinical use is expected for a long time. Although siRNA drug is categorized into a nucleic acid drug, it has a prominent advantage that genetic function can be suppressed by destroying mRNA at the posttranscriptional level without wounding genomic DNA. Nevertheless, unfortunately there are no siRNA certified as pharmaceuticals passing through clinical trials, since there are several problems, such as gene suppression efficiency, stability in blood stream, or other undesirable effects. Here, we describe the current status and future prospects for clinical application of the siRNA nucleic acid drug.

Keywords: RNA interference, siRNA, off-target effect, thermodynamic property, chemical modification

1. Introduction

In recent years, nucleic acid drugs have attracted attention as a next-generation medicine following low molecular weight drugs and antibody drugs. Research and development of these drugs for clinical application is advanced in major pharmaceutical companies, bio-ventures, or research institutions including universities. Nucleic acid drugs, such as DNA/RNA or their modified molecules, act directly on molecules causing diseases and regulate their functions by administering chemically synthesized nucleic acid to the body by local administration or subcutaneous injection. Unlike the hitherto known gene therapy, the nucleic acid drugs directly act on the target molecules and relieve symptoms of the diseases without manipulating the genomes. Although the effects of various nucleic acid drugs, including antisense RNA, small interfering RNA (siRNA), aptamer, or decoy, are investigated in the clinical trials, only five examples including four antisense oligos and an aptamer are already approved. However, no siRNA drug is certified so far. In this manuscript, we outline the advantages, current status, and problems to be solved in the development of nucleic acid drugs, in particular, focusing on the development of siRNA drug.

2. RNA interference

RNA interference (RNAi) is a highly regulated, evolutionarily conserved mechanism of post-transcriptional gene regulation. siRNA, consists of double-stranded RNA with 19 nucleotides in length with 2 nucleotides overhangs, is the intermediate utilized in this mechanism [1].

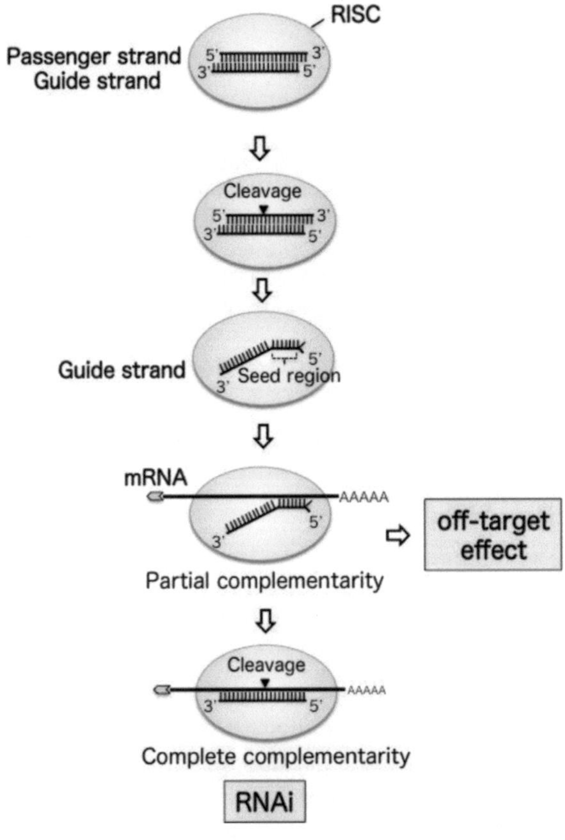

Figure 1. Mechanism of RNA interference. siRNA is the approximately 21-nt double-stranded RNA composed of the guide strand RNA and the passenger strand RNA. siRNA is incorporated into a protein complex called RISC and unwound into single-stranded RNAs. After unwinding, the guide strand is remained on the AGO protein, while the passenger strand is degraded. The mRNAs only with partial complementarities with the seed region of siRNA guide strand are off-target genes and are repressed by siRNA as a mechanism known to be "off-target effect." the mRNA, which has a complete complementary sequence with the guide strand RNA, is cleaved by "RNAi" as an actual target.

When siRNA is introduced into the cells, it is loaded onto the Argonaute (AGO) protein, which is a component of a protein complex called RNA-induced silencing complex (RISC) [2, 3]. In the RISC, siRNA is unwound into single-stranded RNAs, and a functional RNA strand called the guide strand is remained in the RISC and the opposite passenger strand is degraded [4–8]. The activated guide strand RNA-containing RISC binds to the target transcript in a sequence-specific manner. The perfectly complementary target transcript is then cleaved between the 10th and 11th nucleotide relative to the 5′ end of the guide strand [2]. Thus, gene functions of mRNAs which have the complementary nucleotide sequences of the guide strand are suppressed (**Figure 1**) [9]. This elegant, endogenous process has been extensively utilized in functional genomics studies and shows potential as a therapeutic platform [10]. However, although the clinical application of siRNA is expected for a long time, it has not been put into practical use due to some essential problems. For example, the difficult delivery system of siRNA to the target tissues: siRNA is easily degraded by RNA degradation enzymes when it is introduced into the blood, and it is extremely difficult to deliver siRNA to specific tissues. The other severe problem is off-target effects on messenger RNAs (mRNAs) other than the target gene (**Figure 1**). The siRNA often suppresses unintended mRNAs with partial complementarities in nucleotide sequences of the guide strand. The procedures to overcome such problems have been really expected. There is a new candidate method that has overcome the readily degradable property of RNA by enclosing them in lipid nanoparticles (LNP). Although its clinical trial has reached to phase III, there is no example approved as a formal pharmaceutical so far.

3. Advantages for using RNAi technology for nucleic acid medicine

siRNA with complementary nucleotide sequence to the mRNA of target gene can be designed conveniently, if the nucleotide sequence of the target gene is known. In addition, since siRNA can be chemically synthesized, it is not necessary to undergo complicated manufacturing processes, such as immunization of animals or cell culture like synthesis of antibody drugs. Furthermore, due to the complementary binding of siRNA to the target mRNA, its specificity has been considered to be very high, and siRNA can target molecules, such as mRNAs or other noncoding RNAs at the posttranscriptional level that could not be regulated by traditional drugs. These excellent characteristics are reasons to be expected as the future medicine.

4. Problems to be solved for application of siRNA to nucleic acid medicine

Although clinical trials of siRNA application are performed for a long time, there are no authorized siRNA as a clinical drug until now. The current status of the development in RNAi technology and the major problems for its clinical application are discussed in the following section.

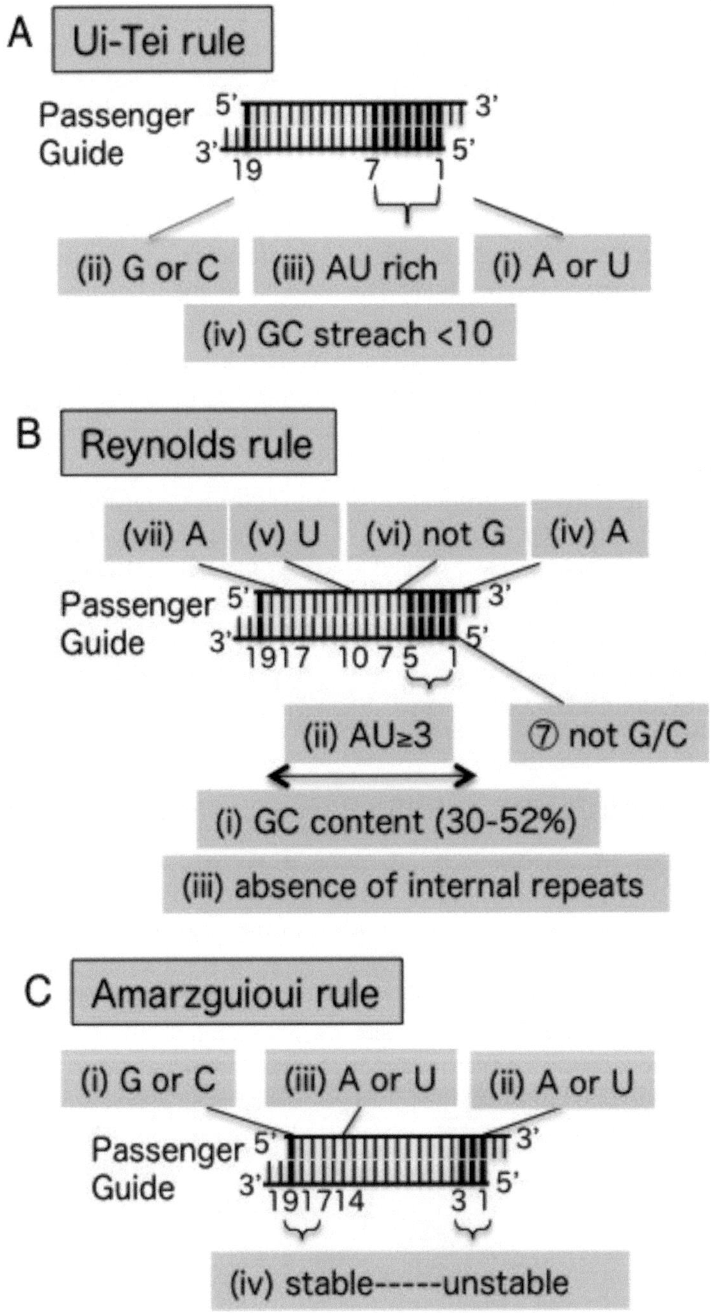

Figure 2. Sequence design algorithms for siRNAs with high RNAi effects. Three widely used siRNA sequence design rules; the Ui-Tei method (A), the Reynolds method (B), and the Amarzguioui method (C). Upper RNA strand indicates the passenger strand, and lower strand indicates the guide strand. The number under the guide strand indicates the nucleotide position measured from the 5′ end of the guide strand. Detailed algorithms are shown in main text.

4.1. Sequence design of highly functional siRNA

The siRNA design is known to define the RNAi efficiency essentially because its effectiveness is dependent on the base-pairing between siRNA and target mRNA. Basic studies so far revealed that the highly efficient RNAi can be induced by almost all siRNAs with any sequences in flies or nematodes, whereas RNAi efficiencies varied greatly depending on the sequences of siRNAs in mammals including human [11]. Among nucleic acid medicines, the nucleotide sequence of aptamer, which specifically acts on a target molecule successfully, is selected by an enormous screening experiment using an artificial nucleic acid library called systematic evolution of ligands by the exponential enrichment (SELEX) method. Such screening requires a great deal of labor and cost. However, the nucleotide sequences of functional siRNAs are designed systematically according to a few reliable algorithms, such as the Ui-Tei rule [11], Reynolds rule [12], or Amarzguioui rule [13] (**Figure 2**). The relationship between siRNA sequence and RNAi was determined by experimental analyses using 62 targets for 4 exogenous and 2 endogenous genes in mammalian cells [11], or 180 siRNAs targeting mRNAs of 2 genes [12], or by the statistical analysis of 49 siRNAs verified by 34 siRNAs [13]. The algorithm of each strategy for the selection of functional siRNA is as follows:

1. Ui-Tei rule
   - i. Nucleotide at the 5′ end of the guide strand is A or U.
   - ii. Nucleotide at the 5′ end of the passenger strand is preferably G or C.
   - iii. A and U are abundant in the region corresponding to the 5′ terminal one-third of the guide strand.
   - iv. It is better not to include a long GC stretch over the entire region.
2. Reynolds rule
   - i. The content of G and C is 30–5% over the entire region.
   - ii. At least three out of five nucleotides at the 3′ end of the passenger strand are preferably A or U.
   - iii. Possible inverted repeats that form hairpin structures are absent.
   - iv. The third nucleotide from the 5′ end of the passenger strand is A.
   - v. The 10th nucleotide from the 5′end of the passenger strand is U.
   - vi. The 13th nucleotide from the 5′end of the passenger strand is other than G.
   - vii. The 19th nucleotide from the 5′end of the passenger strand is preferably A (other than G or C).
3. Amarzguioui rule
   - i. The nucleotide at the 5′ end of the passenger strand is G or C (other than U).
   - ii. A or U is preferable at the 5′ end of the guide strand.

iii. The sixth nucleotide from the 5′ end of the passenger strand is A.

iv. The AU content of three nucleotides at the 5′ end of the passenger strand is relatively lower than that of the passenger strand.

The siRNAs with high RNAi effects can be conveniently designed using these three siRNA design algorithms. The application of these algorithms incorporating each of all criteria is shown to improve potent siRNA selection. However, among them, siRNAs designed by the Ui-Tei rule can suppress the target genes with the highest probability of 95% or more. About 15% of all siRNAs complementary for human transcripts satisfy this algorithm, and such siRNA can be designed using siDirect 2.0 (**Figure 3**), which is an open access website [14, 15].

4.2. Avoid the adverse suppression effects on genes other than the target

The siRNA exerts its RNAi effect by binding to the target mRNA via complete complementarity of nucleotide sequence (**Figure 1**). However, its suppression effects are often observed on the genes, other than the target gene, with nucleotide sequences partially complementary to the siRNA. Such phenomenon is known to be "off-target effects," which is an unintended adverse effect of RNAi [16–19]. Especially, the region called "seed" positioned at nucleotides 2–8 from the 5′ terminus of the guide strand contributed to the off-target effects [18, 19] (**Figure 4**), since the seed region loaded on the Argonaute protein in quasi-helical structure and stably form base-pairings with the off-target mRNAs. To avoid such adverse effects, it is desirable to design siRNAs that do not interact with off-target mRNAs other than the target mRNA as much as possible. However, since the off-target effect by siRNA is induced by sequence complementarity of only seven nucleotides sequence in the seed region, it is impossible to select siRNA sequence with no seven nucleotides complementarities with off-target genes. However, such off-target effect was not always observed. It was revealed that the seed-dependent off-target effect is induced only when the base-pairing stability between the guide strand seed region and the off-target mRNA is strong (**Figure 5**). It means that the off-target effect is avoidable when the stability in the seed-target duplex is weak [19, 20]. The melting temperature of RNA–RNA duplex calculated by the nearest-neighbor procedure may be a useful parameter for evaluating the RNA–RNA duplex stability (**Figure 5**).

Thus, the sequence design of siRNA with high specificity for a target gene without off-target effect on the untargeted genes comes to be possible. First, such siRNA satisfies the functional siRNA selection rules, such as Ui-Tei rules. Second, it is preferable to have a lower thermodynamic stability of base-pairing between the siRNA seed region and the target mRNA. The siRNAs simultaneously satisfying these two conditions are considered to show high RNAi effect and reduced off-target effect. However, only 3% of siRNAs, satisfying both conditions simultaneously, is selectable in human. This is relevant to the fact that it is impossible to select any siRNA sequences for about 5000 genes, one quarter of all human genes. Thus, this limitation is inevitable for sequence design of human siRNA [15].

4.3. Reduction of off-target effects using chemical modifications

The off-target effect has been found to depend on the thermodynamic stability of the seed-target duplex, and such thermodynamic property is basically determined according to the nucleotide

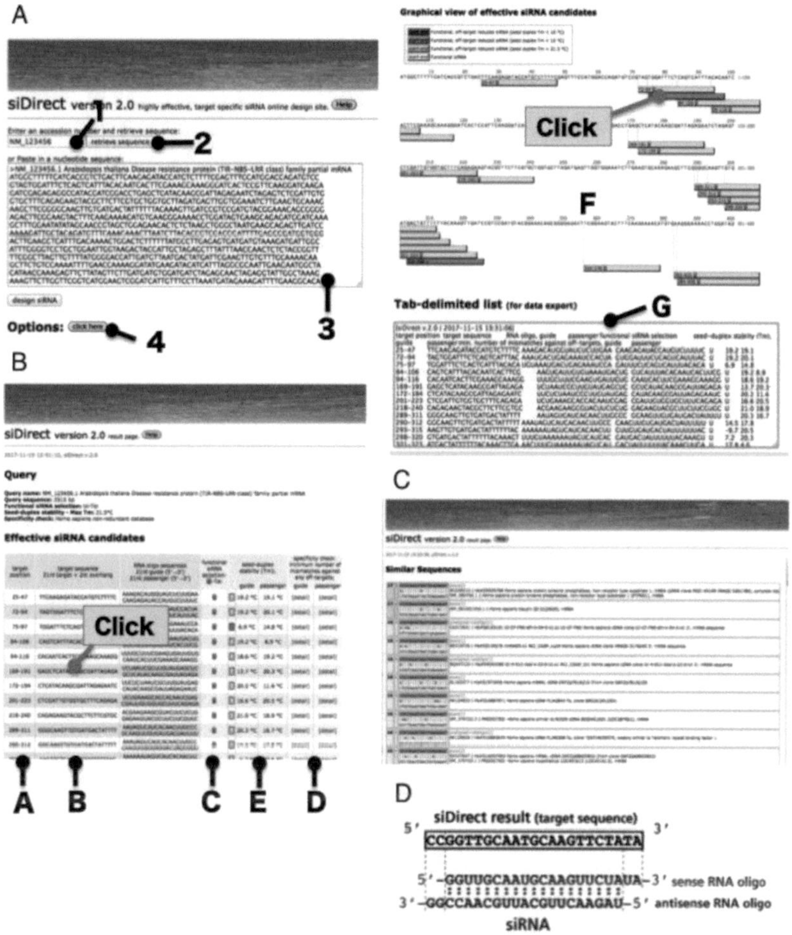

Figure 3. Highly efficient and target-specific siRNA design website: siDirect. (A) the first screen shot. “1” indicates the box to enter the accession number of target gene. When click “2,” you can get nucleotide sequence from GenBank. However, you can directly paste the nucleotide sequence (<10 kbp) in “3.” for design siRNA, click “4.” (B) the second screen “a” indicates the target positions. “B” indicates siRNA target sequences with links to the off-target lists. “C” indicates the functional siRNA design algorithms used for selection of the indicated siRNA. “D” shows homology search results against mRNAs. Numbers of hits with complete match (0), one mismatch, two mismatches, or three mismatches are shown. The number 1 in the 0(+) column usually indicates a complete match against intended target mRNA. “E” shows calculated tm to the siRNA seed region. An siRNA with lower seed tm value reduces off-target effects. “F” is a graphical view of designed siRNA. Off-target lists can be seen by click each siRNA. “G” indicates tab-delimited siRNA list. You can copy and paste the result into excel or text editors, etc. (C) List of off-target candidates for individual siRNA. “6” is siRNA information. “7” shows the alignment between each off-target candidate and each siRNA sequence, clarifying the mismatch positions. (D) Design strategy of guide and passenger strand RNA oligonucleotides based on siDirect result.

sequence. However, the base-pairing stability can be modified by introducing chemical modifications into siRNA. The chemical modifications, including DNA and unlocked nucleic acid (UNA), are known to decrease thermodynamic stabilities. In fact, introduction of DNA molecules into siRNA seed region successfully reduced off-target effects [21, 22], since the DNA-RNA duplex in the seed region shows weak base-pairing stability compared to RNA-RNA duplex.

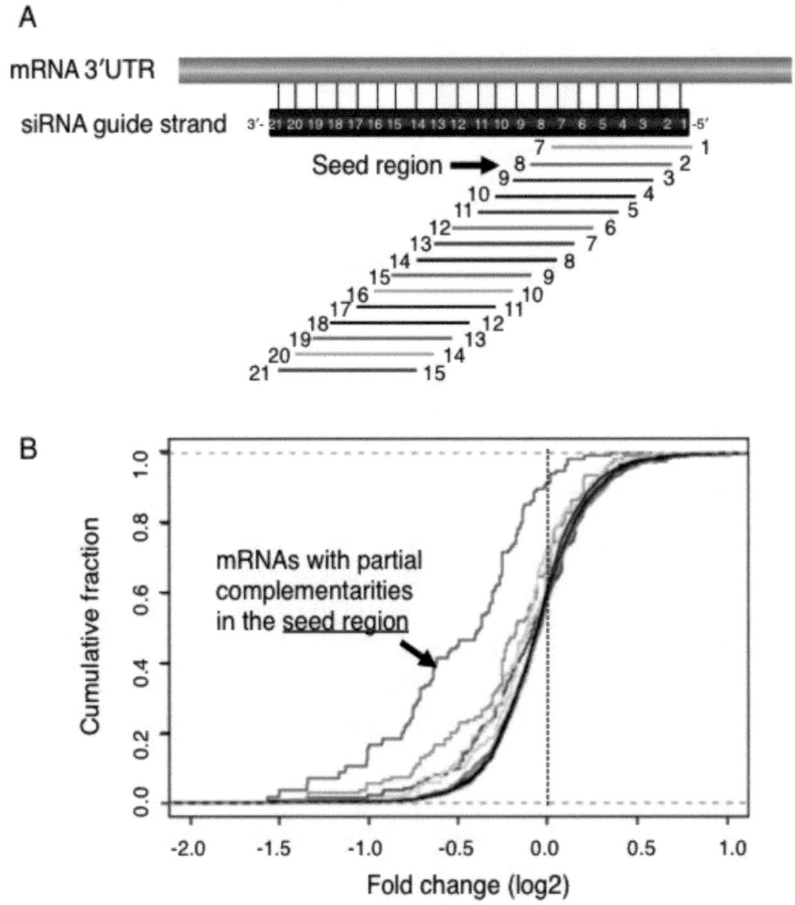

Figure 4. Quantitative analysis of off-target mRNAs by microarray. (A) all of the expressed mRNAs were divided into 15 groups by the region of complementarities with siRNA. (B) Cumulative frequency curve of changes in the expression level of each gene group. When curve shifts to the left, the expression levels of these genes are suppressed. A gene group having a sequence complementary to the siRNA seed region (positions 2–8) in their 3′ UTRs was suppressed.

In contract, the thermodynamic stability of RNA duplex with 2′-O-methyl (2′-OMe) or LNA is known to increase in the protein-free condition. However, we showed that these modifications also reduced the off-target effects [23]. The chemical modification often changes the nucleotide conformation in addition to thermodynamic stability. In RNAi, the guide strand RNA is preloaded on the AGO protein via seed region and form duplex with target mRNA. The 2′-OMe modification in all of the seven nucleotides of siRNA seed region does not disturb the preloading on the AGO protein, but the base-pairing formation with complementary RNA on the AGO protein is apparently disturbed by steric hindrance. As a result, siRNA with 2′-OMe in the guide strand seed region shows weak off-target effect without reduction of RNAi effect [23]. LNA showed more strong effect in the interaction between siRNA and AGO protein or off-target mRNAs. The siRNA modified with LNAs in all of the seven nucleotides in the seed region cannot preload on AGO protein and it cannot base-pair with the complementary RNA. However, siRNA with LNA modifications in three nucleotides among seven

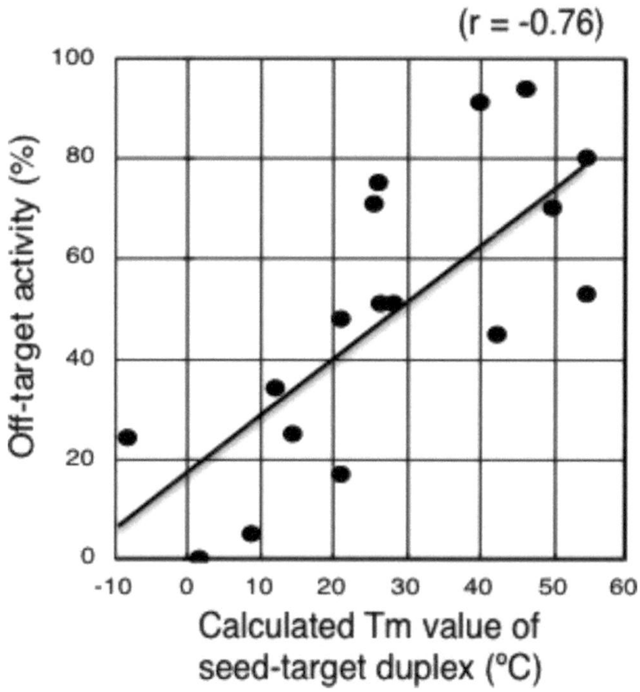

Figure 5. Correlation between thermodynamic stability (Tm value) in the seed-target duplex and off-target effect. siRNAs with low seed tm values in the seed region show low off-target effects, while siRNAs with high seed tm values showed high off-target effects.

can preload on the AGO protein, but it cannot base-pair with the complementary RNA. Thus, siRNA with seven LNA modifications in the seed region has neither RNAi effect nor off-target effect, but siRNA with three LNA modifications shows weak off-target effect without reduction of RNAi effect [23]. Thus, since the chemical modifications can regulate the binding capability of siRNA to the target mRNA depending on the thermodynamic and structural characteristics, the proper application of chemical modifications may be a useful strategy for selection of highly effective and off-target effect-reduced RNAi.

4.4. Increasing stability in blood and efficient transport to the target tissues or cells of siRNA

Nucleic acids are degraded by nucleolytic enzymes when they are released into blood. Fomivirsen is an oligonucleotide used as an antisense antiviral drug that was applied to the treatment of cytomegalovirus retinitis in patients with acquired immunodeficiency syndrome (AIDS). Pegaptanib is a pegylated antivascular endothelial growth factor (VEGF) aptamer and used as an antiangiogenic medicine for the treatment of neovascular age-related macular degeneration (AMD). These nucleic acid drugs are treated by local administration into vitreous bodies. Mipomersen is the second antisense drug used for the treatment of homozygous familial hypercholesterolemia and is administered through subcutaneous injection. The various chemical modifications were introduced into these nucleic acid drugs to increase the stability in the blood. Fomivirsen is involved in the first generation of antisense therapeutics containing phosphorothioate linkages between bases to prevent nuclease digestion. Five 2′-OMe modifications were introduced into mipomersen to allow the resistance to degradation by endonucleases and exonucleases maintaining high affinity and specificity to the target mRNA. Pegaptanib has both modifications of phosphorothioate and 2′-OMe. Incorporation of them greatly improved the aptamer half-life in urine and also improved binding affinity for VEGF. Since it has also reported that siRNAs with chemical modifications, such as 2′-OMe and 2′-fluoro (2′-F), are resistant to degradation by RNA degrading enzymes [24, 25], it is possible to use proper chemical modifications for each siRNA to enhance its stability in blood.

Furthermore, since the nucleic acid has anionic charge, the permeability of the cell membrane is low. Then, the development of drug delivery system (DDS) to transport nucleic acid drugs to target tissues or cells stably using lipid or collagen are also on going. Many trials are performed using lipid nanoparticle (LNP) technology in which pharmacokinetics are indicated to be much better than a naked RNAi approach. Several types of nanoparticles, including LNP, *N*-acetylgalactosamine (GalNAc) conjugates and dynamic polyconjugated (DPCs), are used clinically. The most successful DDS so far is lipid nanoparticle (LNP) developed by Tekmira. LNP, which forms a lipid bilayer membrane similar to the cell membrane, protects siRNA by encapsulation and assists the transport of siRNA to the target tissues. Alnylam has developed a therapeutic agent (ALN-TTR 02) for familial amyloid polyneuropathy by using this LNP, which is currently conducting phase III of clinical trials. In addition, the method for conjugation of atelocollagen and siRNA has also been developed. Atelocollagen makes siRNA less susceptible to degradation by RNase enzymes, which results in a long-lasting RNA silencing effect.

4.5. Suppression of excessive immune response induced by introduction of exogenous nucleic acid

In general, nucleic acid medicine introduces a large amount of artificially synthesized nucleic acids into the body. However, the excessive autoimmune response is often induced by the exogenous introduction of nucleic acids. In mammals, it is well-known that the activation of virus sensor proteins, like Toll-like receptors (TLRs) [26, 27] and RIG-I-like receptors (RLRs) [28], or Protein kinase R (PKR) [29] induces interferon response. Interferon response may upregulate the production of inflammatory cytokines and can possibly cause systemic inflammation. It has been reported that LNA- or 2′-OMe-modified siRNA suppresses the activation of TLR 7/8 and does not induce the excessive immune response without reducing RNAi activity [30, 31]. It was also reported that induction of interferon response was not observed even when a complex of atelocollagen and siRNA was introduced into the cells [32]. By revealing the detailed molecular mechanism of the immune response by introduction of the exogenous nucleic acids, more appropriate chemical modifications to avoid such immune response should be developed.

5. Conclusion

RNAi is a field in which its clinical application is strongly expected, but its first wave for clinical application failed due to the difficulties in the initial stage. However, due to the improvement of its delivery system and the sequence selection method, the new wave has come in 2012. Current clinical trials are applied to targets, including the eye, liver, cancer, blood, gastrointestinal tract, dermis, and others, since it is relatively easy to deliver siRNA to these tissues with currently available nanoparticles [33].

Antibody drugs and low molecular weight drugs were widely used so far. They were synthesized through complicated manufacturing processes, so that mass production at low cost was impossible. However, the nucleic acid drugs can be artificially synthesized by a simple manufacturing process. Then, once a production line is established, it can be synthesized inexpensively in large quantities. In addition, for antibody drugs and low molecular weight drugs, basic data from scratch are required every time when the target changes, but nucleic acid drugs such as siRNA drugs can be designed relatively easily by identifying the nucleotide sequences of target genes. Thus, it is expected that the siRNA is a powerful candidate for nucleic acid therapeutics.

Genome editing techniques such as clustered regularly interspaced short palindromic repeats (CRISPR)/CRISPR-associated proteins 9 (Cas9) system [34] and transcription activator-like effector nucleases (TALEN) [35] can directly modify the genomic DNA that causes disease. Although it is extremely attractive as a potential drug candidate in the future, there are many ethical issues to overcome when the edited genome is transmitted to the next generation. On the other hand, siRNA does not introduce the permanent modification in the genomic DNA and its action is transient, since siRNA knockdown the target mRNA. Then, CRISPR interfering (CRISPRi) system modified from the CRISPR/Cas9 system is developed. CRISPRi inhibit the gene expression without cleavage of genomic DNA by introducing mutations into DNA cleavage domains in Cas9 [36]. Such system may also promote the nucleic acid medicine.

Acknowledgements

We thank Saigo K., Naito Y., Nishi K., Zenno S., Takahashi F., Haraguchi T., Yamato K., Morishita S., Yamada T., Yoshimura J., Juni A., Iribe H., Miyamoto K., Kobayashi Y. and Aida M. to perform the basic studies which serve as foundations of this chapter. This work was mainly supported by grants from the Ministry of Education, Culture, Sports, Science and Technology of Japan (MEXT).

Author details

Tomoko Takahashi, Yuko Nakano and Kumiko Ui-Tei*

*Address all correspondence to: ktei@bs.s.u-tokyo.ac.jp

Department of Biological Sciences, Graduate School of Science, The University of Tokyo, Tokyo, Japan

References

[1] Elbashir SM, Harborth J, Lendeckel W, Yalcin A, Weber K, Tuschl T. Duplexes of 21-nucleotide RNAs mediate RNA interference in cultured mammalian cells. Nature. 2001;**411**:494-498

[2] Hutvagner G, Simard MJ. Argonaute proteins: Key players in RNA silencing. Nature Reviews. Molecular Cell Biology. 2008;**9**:22-32

[3] Doi N, Zenno S, Ueda R, Ohki-Hamazaki H, Ui-Tei K, Saigo K. Short-interfering-RNA-mediated gene silencing in mammalian cells requires dicer and eIF2C translation initiation factors. Current Biology. 2003;**13**:41-46

[4] Matranga C, Tomori Y, Shin C, Bartel DP, Zamore PS. Passenger-strand cleavage facilitates assembly of siRNA into Ago2-containing RNAi enzyme complexes. Cell. 2005;**123**: 607-620

[5] Miyoshi K, Tsukumo H, Nagami T, Siomi H, Siomi MC. Slicer function of *Drosophila* Argonautes and its involvement in RISC formation. Genes & Development. 2005;**19**: 2837-2848

[6] Leuschner PJ, Ameres SL, Kueng S, Martinez J. Cleavage of the siRNA passenger strand during RISC assembly in human cells. EMBO Reports. 2006;**7**:314-320

[7] Kawamata T, Seitz H, Tomari Y. Structural determinants of miRNAs for RISC loading and slicer-independent unwinding. Nature Structural & Molecular Biology. 2009;**16**:953-960

[8] Yoda M, Kawamata T, Paroo Z, Ye X, Iwasaki S, Liu Q, Tomari Y. ATP-dependent human RISC assembly pathways. Nature Structural & Molecular Biology 2009;**17**:117-123

[9] Fire A, Xu S, Montgomery MK, Kostas SA, Driver SE, Mello CC. Potent and specific genetic interference by double-stranded RNA in *Caenorhabditis elegans*. Nature. 1998;**391**: 806-811

[10] Ryther RCC, Flynt AS, Phillips JA, Patton JG. siRNA therapeutics: Big potential from small RNAs. Gene Therapy. 2004;**12**:5-11

[11] Ui-Tei K, Naito Y, Takahashi F, Haraguchi T, Ohki-Hamazaki H, Juni A, Ueda R, Saigo K. Guidelines for the selection of highly effective siRNA sequences for mammalian and chick RNA interference. Nucleic Acids Research. 2004;**32**:936-948

[12] Reynolds A, Leake D, Boese Q, Scringe S, Marchall WS, Khvorova A. Rational siRNA design for RNA interference. Nature Biotechnology. 2004;**22**:326-330

[13] Amarzguioui M, Prydz H. An algorithm for selection of functional siRNA sequences. Biochemical and Biophysical Research Communications. 2004;**316**:1050-1058

[14] Naito Y, Yamada T, Ui-Tei K, Morishita S, Saigo K. siDirect: Highly effective, target-specific siRNA design software for mammalian RNA interference. Nucleic Acids Research. 2004;**32**:W124-W129

[15] Naito Y, Yoshimura J, Morishita S, Ui-Tei K. siDirect 2.0: Updatead software for designing functional siRNA with reduced seed-dependent off-target effect. BMC Bioinformatics. 2009;**10**:392. DOI: 10.1186/1471-2105-10-392

[16] Lin X, Ruan X, Anderson MG, McDowell JA, Kroeger PE, Fesik SW, Shen Y. siRNA-mediated off-target gene silencing triggered by a 7 nt complementation. Nucleic Acids Research. 2005;**33**:4527-4535

[17] Birmingham A, Selfors LM, Forster T, Wrobel D, Kennedy CJ, Shanks E, Santoyo-Lopez J, Dunican DJ, Long A, Kelleher D, Smith Q, Beijersbergen RL, Ghazal P, Sharmu CE. 3'UTR seed matches, but not overall identity, are associated with RNAi off-targets. Nature Methods. 2006;**3**:199-204

[18] Jackson AL, Burchard J, Schelter J, Chau BN, Cleary M, Lim L, Linsley PS. Widespread siRNA "off-target" transcript silencing by seed region sequence complementarity. RNA. 2006;**12**:1179-1187

[19] Ui-Tei K, Naito Y, Nishi K, Juni A, Saigo K. Thermodynamic stability and Watson-crick base pairing in the seed duplex are major determinants of the efficiency of the siRNA-based off-target effects. Nucleic Acids Research. 2008;**36**:7100-7109. DOI: 10.1093/nar/gkn902

[20] Ui-Tei K, Nishi K, Takahashi T, Nagasawa T. Thermodynamic control of small RNA-mediated gene silencing. Frontiers in Genetics. 2012;**3**:101. DOI: 10.3389/fgene.2012.00101

[21] Ui-Tei K, Naito Y, Zenno S, Nishi K, Yamato K, Takahashi F, Juni A, Saigo K. Functional dissection of siRNA sequence by systematic DNA substitution: Modified siRNA with a DNA seed arm is a powerful tool for mammalian gene silencing with significantly reduced off-target effect. Nucleic Acids Research. 2008;**36**:2136-2151. DOI: 10.1093/nar/gkn042

[22] Takahashi T, Zenno S, Ishibashi O, Takizawa T, Saigo K, Ui-Tei K. Interaction between the non-seed region of siRNA and RNA-binding RLC/RISC proteins, ago and TRBP, in mammalian cells. Nucleic Acids Research. 2014;**42**:5256-5269. DOI: 10.1093/nar/gku153

[23] Iribe H, Miyamoto K, Takahashi T, Kobayashi Y, Leo J, Aida M, Ui-Tei K. Chemical modification of the siRNA seed region suppresses off-target effects by steric hindrance to base-pairing with targets. ACS Omega. 2017;**2**:2055-2064. DOI: 10.1021/acsomega.7b00291

[24] Sproat BS, Lamond AI, Beijer B, NEuner P, Ryder U. Highly efficient chemical synthesis of 2′-O-methyloligoribonucleotides and tetrabiotinylated derivatives: Novel probes that are resistant to degradation by RNA or DNA specific nucleases. Nucleic Acids Research. 1989;**17**:3373-3386

[25] Peiken WA, Olsen DB, BEnseler F, Aurup H, Eckstein F. Kinetic characterization of ribonuclease-resistant 2′-modified hammerhead ribozymes. Science. 1991;**253**:314-317

[26] Lemaitre B, Nicolas E, Michaut L, Reichhart JM, Hoffmann JA. The dorsoventral regulatory gene cassette spätzle/toll/cactus controls the potent antifungal response in drosophila adults. Cell. 1996;**86**:973

[27] Medzhitov R, Preston-Hurlburt P, Janeway CA Jr. A human homologue of the drosophila toll protein signals activation of adaptive immunity. Nature 1997;**388**:394-197

[28] Yoneyama M, Kikuchi M, Natsukawa T, Shinobu N, Imaizumi T, Miyagishi M, Taira K, Akira S, Fujita T. The RNA helicase RIG-I has an essential function in double-stranded RNA-induced innate antiviral responses. Nature Immunology. 2004;**5**:730-737

[29] Meurs E, Chong K, Galabru J, Thomas NS, Kerr IM, Williams BR, Hovanessian AG. Molecular cloning and characterization of the human double-stranded RNA-activated protein kinase induced by interferon. Cell. 1990;**62**:379-390

[30] Dahlgren C, Wahlestedt C, Thonberg H. No induction of anti-viral responses in human cell lines HeLa and MCF-7 when transfecting with siRNA or siLNA. Biochemical and Biophysical Research Communications. 2006;**341**:1211-1217

[31] Judge AD, Bola G, Lee AC, MacLachlan I. Design of noninflammatory synthetic siRNA mediating potent gene silencing in vito. Molecular Therapy. 2006;**13**:494-505

[32] Takeshita F, Minakuchi Y, Nagahara S, Honma K, Sasaki H, Hirai K, Teratani T, Namatame N, Yamamoto Y, Hanai K, Kato T, Sano A, Ochiya T. Efficient delivery of small interfering RNA to bone-metastatic tumors by using atelocollagen in vivo. Proceedings of the National Academy of Sciences of the United States of America. 2005;**102**:12177-12182

[33] Bobbin ML, Rossi JJ. RNA interference (RNAi)-based therapeutics: Delivering on the promise ? Annual Review of Pharmacology and Toxicology. 2016;**56**:103-122

[34] Jinek M, Chylinski K, Fonfara I, Hauer M, Doudna JA, Charpentier E. A programmable dual-RNA-guided DNA endonuclease in adaptive bacterial immunity. Science. 2012;**337**:816-821. DOI: 10.1126/science.1225829

[35] Christian M, Cermak T, Doyle EL, Schmidt C, Zhang F, Hummel A, Bogdanove AJ, Voytas DF. Targeting DNA double-strand breads with TAL effector nucleases. Genetics. 2010;**186**:757-761. DOI: 10.1534/genetics.110.120717

[36] Cilbert LA, Larson MH, Morsut L, Liu Z, Brar GA, Torres SE, Stem-Ginossar N, Brandman O, Whitehead EH, Doudna JA, Lim WA, Weissman JS, Qi LS. CRISPR-mediated modular RNA-guided regulation of transcription in eukryotes. Cell. 2013;**154**:442-451. DOI: 10.1016/j.cell.2013.06.044

Section 4

Transcription of Genes that Encode Immune System Regulators

Chapter 9

Gene Expression during the Activation of Human B Cells

Youming Zhang

Additional information is available at the end of the chapter

http://dx.doi.org/10.5772/intechopen.71863

Abstract

Human B lymphocytes not only play a critical role in the humoral immunity to generate antibodies, but also are equally important to cellular immunity as B lymphocytes can present antigens to T lymphocytes and can release a range of potential immune-regulating cytokines after stimulations. Human immunoglobulin class switch recombination (CSR) in activated B cells is an essential process in the humoral immunity and the process is complicated and tightly controlled by many regulators. The recent genomic and genetic approaches in CSR identified novel genes that were actively involved in the process. Understanding the roles of the novel genes in CSR will bring new insights into the mechanisms of the process and new potential therapeutic targets for immunoglobulin-related disorders such as allergic asthma and autoimmune diseases.

Keywords: B cells, immunoglobulin class switch recombination, gene expression, regulation

1. Introduction

Human lymphocytes include T lymphocytes, B lymphocytes and natural killer cells. T lymphocytes are majorly responsible for cell-mediated immunity. B lymphocytes (cells) play the critical roles in the humoral immunity to activate immune system by secreting antibodies. B lymphocytes are also equally critical to cellular immunity as they can also present antigens to T lymphocytes and can also release a range of potential immune-regulating cytokines [1, 2].

The "B" from B cells came from the name of the bursa of Fabricius, a lymphoid organ in birds, where B cells mature. It was first discovered by Chang and Glick [3]. B cells mature in the bone marrow in mammals. B cells express B cell receptors (BCRs) on their cell membrane and BCRs allow the cell to bind to a specific antigen and initiate an antibody response. Each B cell carries a unique receptor for antigen that is composed of the membrane-band form of its antibody. After antigen recognition by the membrane-bound receptor, the B cells can proliferate to increase their numbers and differentiate to secrete their antigen-specific antibodies.

There are three principle classes of B cells in humans according to their ontogeny and anatomic localization: B1 cells arise from fetal liver precursors and are enriched in mucosal tissues and the pleural and peritoneal cavities. B2 cells arise from bone marrow–derived precursors and are enriched in secondary lymphoid organs [4]. Marginal zone (MZ) and follicular (FO) B cells are differentiated from B2 cells in human spleen and lymph nodes [2]. B cells of each linage have distinct and overlapping functions in recognizing antigens via T-independent and T-dependent pathways to produce rapid IgM or long-lasting IgG antibody response [2]. Cytokines play a key role in the commitment of naïve B cells to B effector 1 (Be-1) and B effector 2 (Be-2) lineage. Be-2 differentiation is dependent on the engagement of IL4α on B cells [5], while Be-1 cell development is dependent on the activation of the transcription factor T-bet and the IFNγR on B cells [6].

The process of human B cell development is very complicated and is controlled by many transcription factors [7]. Human B cells are generated in bone marrow from progenitor cells that are committed to the B cell linages (pro-B cells). Each pro-B cell undergoes independent rearrangement of diverse variable (V), diversity (D) and joining (J) gene segments of the immunoglobulin heavy (H)-chain locus [8]. Rearrangement of the H-chain locus creates in each B cell a variable exon with a unique upstream of the immunoglobulin constant region exons and drives the expression of H-chain protein and then proliferate and differentiate to commence immunoglobulin light (L)-chain gene recombination. When a B cell expresses L-chain protein, it pairs with the previously arranged H chain and is expressed as membrane immunoglobulin on the cell surface [9]. Human immune system can generate a diversity of specific antibodies in response to antigen stimulation. This process is of fundamental importance to acquired immunity. The human constant H-chain genes are on chromosome 14 containing Cμ, Cδ and two repeated clusters each having two Cγ genes and Cε genes (Cγ3, Cγ1, pseudo-ε, Cα1 and Cγ2, Cγ4, Cε, Cα2).

In this chapter, I will briefly introduce the roles of germinal centers (GCs) and the steps of immunoglobulin class switch recombination (CSR) in human B cells in GCs. I will discuss the potential functional roles of the newly identified genes from the results of our experiments for global transcript profiling in CSR. I will also discuss the future direction of the researches on CSR in human B cells.

2. Germinal centers and immunoglobulin CSR

Germinal centers (GCs) are the sites within secondary lymphoid organs such as lymph nodes and the spleen where mature B cells can proliferate, differentiate and mutate their antibody genes and switch the class of their antibodies (e.g., from IgM to IgE) during a normal immune response to antigens [10]. In the GCs, naïve B cells can have clonal expansion, somatic hypermutation, affinity maturation, development of B cell memory and long-life plasma cells [11–13]. B cell activation is initiated in the follicle in GCs when it encounters specific antigen [14], and then the B cells are relocated to the periphery of the follicle [15]. The inter-follicular zone in GCs is the site where B cell and T follicular helper cell differential initiates [16]. They develop dynamically after the activation of follicular B cells by T-dependent antigen. B cells in GCs proliferate and can class-switch the BCR constant region from IgM/IgD to IgG, IgA and IgE (discussed later). Additionally, the IgV region genes of B cells in GCs can undergo somatic hypermutation to change the affinity of the encoded BCR for its cognate antigens, allowing subsequent antigen-driven selection and clonal expansion of high-affinity B cells [17]. Human B cells in GCs, in vitro–activated naïve B cells, and those with specific and rapid recall responses to previously encountered antigen express cell-surface CD27. B cells with CD27 expression correlated with greater cell sizes, proliferative capacity, antigen presentation capacity and differentiation into antibody secreting cells [18–20].

In order to generate antibodies, two somatic DNA recombination events of the genetic elements take place in B cells. Firstly, V(D)J recombination generates the functional variable regions of the Ig heavy-chain (IgH) and light-chain genes. Initiation of V(D)J recombination requires the products of recombination activating genes (RAG) 1 and 2 [21, 22]. Lymphoid-specific expression of RAG 1 and 2 limits V(D)J recombination to B and T lymphocytes. Following activation, mature B cells can undergo CSR, linking the IgH variable regions with one of the downstream CH genes, changing the effector function of the antibody [23]. CSR and the other main diversification event, somatic hypermutation (SHM), are both dependent on activation-induced cytidine deaminase (AID), a protein expressed only in activated germinal center B cells [24]. The basic steps of CSR include creating double-strand DNA breaks (DSBs) for CSR and joining donor and acceptor S regions. Class switch recombination occurs between switch (S) regions located upstream of each of the CH regions except Cδ and results in a change from IgM and IgD expression in naïve B cells to express one of the downstream isotypes such as IgG subclasses, IgA and IgE. AID plays a critical role in the vertebrate adaptive immune response [24, 25]. It initiates the conversion of several dC bases to dU bases in each S region, dU bases are then excised by uracil DNA glycosylase (UNG), and the resulting abasic sites are nicked by apurinic/apyrimidic endonuclease (APE), creating single strand breaks (SSBs), that can spontaneously form DSBs if they are near each other on opposite DNA strands. After formation of the DSB in the donor and acceptor S regions, the S regions are recombined by ubiquitous proteins that perform nonhomologous end-joining (NHEJ) [26]. VDJ recombination and early B cell development takes place in the bone morrow. Immature B cells expressing IgM on the surface migrate to peripheral lymphoid tissue in the spleen, lymph nodes and gut-associated lymphoid tissue. CSR and SHM happen in the germinal centers of secondary lymphoid tissues but also in germinal center–like structures in local (nonlymphoid) tissues [27]. CSR is induced by both T lymphocyte–dependent (TD) antigens and T lymphocyte–independent (TI) antigens. TD antigen stimulation can be mimicked in vitro by culturing B cells in the presence of anti-CD40 antibodies along with specific cytokines. IL-4 and anti-CD40 induce isotype switching to IgG1 and IgE [28]. Chromatin structure also contributes to the regulation of CSR. Ig heavy-chain constant genes and 3-regulatory regions are in an active chromatin conformation (acetylated H3 and H4 and lysine 4 trimethylation H3) in unstimulated human B cells, and these modifications can spread to the S region after cytokine stimulation [29]. AID is exclusively expressed in the germinal centers [21]. The basic AID-mediated mechanisms of CSR are quite well studied and defined, but the global regulation of the CSR, accompanying networks of AID and other well-known regulators, remains relatively unclear.

3. The global gene regulation of CSR in human B cells

In vitro, IL4 and anti-CD40 signals can mimic signals from T cell in GCs to induce a strong activation of NF-κB leading human B cells to a proliferative burst and CSR to IgE and IgG [30]. These costimulation signals were applied in the naïve B cells isolated from healthy tonsils and profiled the transcripts at 6 time points for 12 days (0, 12, 36, 72, 120 and 288 h). More than one thousand genes were observed to have significantly differentiated expression after IL4 and anti-CD40 stimulation [31]. The significantly differentiated genes can be formed in 4 cluster groups including 13 temporal profiles. Each cluster contains many new genes that were not known to have roles in CSR before.

3.1. Cluster A group

Cluster A group represented the gene expression on (Cluster A1) or off (Cluster A2) in naïve human B cells after IL4 and anti-CD40 stimulation.

3.1.1. Cluster A1

Cluster A1 was immediately upregulated after IL4 and anti-CD40 cosignal stimulation and the expressions did not change during the course of 12 days for the experiments. The cluster contains 153 genes. The analysis of transcription factor–binding sites for the cluster showed that genes from this cluster were enriched to transcription factors BACH1 and BACH2. BACH1 and BACH2 promote B cell development by repressing the myeloid program [32]. They belong to the basic region–leucine zipper family and are transcription repressors binding to Maf-recognition elements (MAREs) [33]. BACH2 has critical roles in both acquired immunity and innate immunity, including immunoglobulin CSR, the somatic hypermutation of immunoglobulin-encoding genes [34, 35]. BACH2 expression is activated by E2A, Foxo1 and Pax5 in pro-B cells. BACH2 may have a role in early B cell development [36]. BACH1 structure is closely related to BACH2, but its role in B cell development and hematopoiesis largely remains unclear [33]. BACH2 expression frequently preceded that of Ebf1 and Pax5 in the common lymphoid progenitors (CLPs). BACH factors directly repressed various myeloid genes in CLPs and this repression restricted the fate of CLPs to the B cell lineage [32].

In this cluster, chemokine genes *CCL22* and *CCL17* were the most significantly differentiated genes during naïve B cell activation after IL4 and anti-CD40 signal stimulation. CCL22 and CCL17 are both ligands for the chemokine receptor CCR4. *CCR4* gene was also showed in Cluster C6 to have a transient induction after IL4 and anti-CD40 signal stimulation. All three transcripts were within the top 20 differentially expressed genes during the activation of immunoglobulin class switching in human activated B cells. CCL22 and CCL17 are NF-kappa B (NF-kB) target genes, indicating a central role for the NF-kB pathway in the activation of CSR stimulated by IL4 and anti-CD40. The top differentially expressed genes also contained another NF-kB target gene, the TNF receptor-associated factor (*TRAF1*) [37], which was also profiled in Cluster A1. There were many clinical reports that indicated both chemokines might be involved in human immunoglobulin class switching. A significantly higher increase in CCL17, CCL22 and IL-4 serum levels in grass pollen–exposed subjects was observed [38]. Sensitized children with allergic symptoms showed higher CCL17 and CCL22 levels and higher ratios between these Th2-associated chemokines and the Th1-associated chemokine CXCL10 than nonsensitized children without allergic symptoms [39]. Using human dendritic cells (DCs), in vitro exposure to house dust mite (HDM) of DCs from HDM-allergic patients but not healthy controls caused CCL17 and CCL22 release that resulted in chemoattraction of polarized human Th2 cells in a CCR4-dependent way [40]. Both CCL22 and CCL17 have been suggested as biomarkers for disease activity in atopic dermatitis (AD), and raised cord blood (CB) levels of CCL22 predict subsequent allergic sensitization, while raised CCL17 in GC predicts the later development of allergic symptoms, including asthma. Consistent with these observations, allergen exposure in sensitized individuals leads to a dynamic increase in CCL17 and CCL22 [38]. High-affinity neutral ligands have been developed for CCL22 and CCL17 and attenuate levels of CCL22, CCL17 and IgE in a mouse model of atopic dermatitis as well as improve skin inflammatory symptoms [31]. *CCL17* was also shown to have exon retention during B cell activation [31]. All the evidence indicated both chemokines and their receptor CCR4 play important roles in immunoglobulin class switching.

3.1.2. Cluster A2

Cluster A2 was immediately downregulated after IL4 and anti-CD40 cosignal stimulation and the expressions did not change during the course of 12 days of CSR. Cluster A2 contains 83 genes that present downregulating genes during B cell activation. These genes expressed significantly lower in activated B cells than in naïve B cells during the time course of IL4 and anti-CD40 stimulation. The analysis of gene ontology indicated the genes in this cluster were involved with immune system process.

FOSB and *FOS* were the most significantly downregulated genes in Cluster A2 during CSR in naïve B cells after IL4 and anti-CD40 stimulation. *FOS* genes encode leucine zipper proteins that can dimerize with proteins of the JUN family and form transcription factor complex activating protein-1 (AP-1) [41]. The FOS family consists of 4 members: FOS, FOSB, FOSL1 and FOSL2. Activating protein-1 (AP-1) is a dimeric transcription factor composed of Jun, FOS or activating transcription factor (ATF) subunits that bind to a common DNA site, the AP-1–binding site [42]. The different AP-1 factors may regulate different target genes and thus execute distinct biological functions [43]. In addition to regulation by heterodimerization among Jun, FOS and ATF proteins, AP-1 activity is regulated through interactions with specific protein kinases and a variety of transcriptional coactivators [44–46]. Nitrogen oxide (NO) is the radical inhibiting IgE/Ag-induced IL-4, IL-6 and TNF production. It inhibits phosphorylation of phospholipase Cγ1 and the AP-1 transcription factor protein c-Jun. NO further completely abrogated IgE/Ag-induced DNA-binding activity of the nuclear AP-1 proteins FOS and Jun to regulate allergic inflammation [47]. FOS-interacting protein (FIP) is a transcription factor that binds to c-FOS. The aggregation of the mast cell's high-affinity receptor for IgE induced the synthesis of FIP and increased its DNA-binding activity. Moreover, downregulation of the isoenzyme protein kinase C-β (PKC-β) resulted in profound inhibition of FIP-FOS DNA-binding activity [48].

3.2. Cluster B group

Cluster B group showed gradually sustained induction during CSR in B cells. Cluster B1 is the most interesting cluster that sustained induction earlier than Cluster B2.

3.2.1. *Cluster B1*

Cluster B1 was the first group to show gradually sustained expression after IL4 and anti-CD40 cosignal stimulation. Cluster B1 contains 126 genes and the analysis of gene ontology showed that genes in this cluster were majorly involved in the cellular amine metabolic process. The analysis of transcription factor–binding sites indicated the genes in this cluster were enriched to transcription factors RSRFC4 and STAT. Both transcription factors were involved with allergic and airway epithelia inflammations [49, 50]. RSRF-binding sites were found in the regulatory sequences of a number of growth factor–inducible and muscle-specific genes [51]. It was showed that engagement of the B cell antigen receptor could activate STAT through Lyn in a JAK-independent pathway [52].

There were several well-known genes to regulate B cell differentiation in germinal center including *AICDA* [24], *IRF4* [53], *XBP1* [54], *BATF3* [55] and *NFIL3* [56] in this cluster. The cluster showed other genes exhibiting synchronic, coordinated expression with the well-documented regulation genes. *IL17RB* and *BHLHE40 genes* were the most significantly differentiated in the cluster. *IL17RB* encodes a cytokine receptor that specifically binds to IL17B and IL17E but does not bind to IL17 and IL17C. IL17RB has been shown to mediate the activation of NF-κB [57]. *IL17RB* showed highly synchronic expression with *AICDA* in the cluster. IL17RB abundance has previously been shown to increase upon allergen challenge in patients with seasonal allergic rhinitis [58], IgE [59] and asthma [60]. The result indicated that the increase in IL17RB formed an early component of the transcriptional cascade that initiated the germinal center response in B cells. *BHLHE40* encodes a basic helix-loop-helix protein expressed in various tissues and is an environmentally inducible moderator of circadian rhythms and cellular differentiation. *BHLHE40* was profiled at its core of the B1 Cluster. BHLHE40 was recently shown to operate as a master regulator of germinal center activities, modulating the expression of more than 100 target genes [61]. Circadian oscillations in symptom severity are a prominent feature of atopic diseases including atopic dermatitis, asthma, chronic urticarial and allergic rhinitis [62–64]. The variation in IgE/mast cell allergic reactions was recently demonstrated to depend on the circadian clock in mice [65]. Mice deficient for the BHLHE40 ortholog display a variety of immune features including abnormal IgG1 and IgE levels and defective elimination of activated B cells, as well as exhibiting circadian rhythm phenomena [66]. Like *BHLHE40, NFIL3* in this cluster also participates in signaling pathways relating to the circadian clock [67], and together, these data suggest there may be a circadian component to class switch recombination and that this may be of relevance to time-of-day phenomena in IgE-driven diseases.

3.2.2. *Cluster B2*

The genes in Cluster B2 were also gradually sustained induction but they come later in time than Cluster B1 during CSR in human B cell. The cluster contains 112 genes. The most significantly differentiated genes were *EPHB1* and *TNFSF4*.

Erythropoietin-producing hepatocellular carcinoma (Eph) receptors are a subfamily of receptor tyrosine kinases (RTKs*)* [68, 69]. The receptors and their ligands, the ephrins, mediate numerous developmental processes, particularly in the nervous system [70]. Tyrosine phosphorylation of EphB1 requires presentation of ephrin-B1 in either clustered or membrane-attached forms [71]. Eph receptors and ephrin ligands have been shown to be differentially expressed on leucocytes. Ephrin-B3 binds to B lymphocytes, most likely via a nonclassical receptor, and induces migration of the memory B cell subpopulation [72]. *NFSF4* encodes a cytokine of the tumor necrosis factor (TNF) ligand family. The encoded protein functions in T cell and antigen-presenting cell (APC) interact and mediate adhesion of activated T cells to endothelial cells. The tumor necrosis factor ligand superfamily member 4 gene (TNFSF4, OX40L), which encodes for the costimulatory molecule OX40 ligand, has been identified as a susceptibility gene for systemic lupus erythematosus (SLE) in multiple studies [73, 74].

3.3. Cluster C group

Cluster C group has six profiling clusters to show transient induction during CSR in B cells according to the time they were inducted.

3.3.1. Cluster C1

Cluster C1 was the first group to be inducted transcendently during CSR. It has 79 genes and the analysis of gene ontology indicated the genes in this cluster were involved in ribonucleoprotein complex biogenesis. Heterogeneous nuclear ribonucleoproteins (hnRNPs) are a large family of RNA-binding proteins that are important for multiple aspects of nucleic acid metabolism [75]. *TFEC* and *RRP12* were the most significantly introduced genes in this cluster.

Transcription factor EC (TFEC) acts as a repressor or an activator. TFEC works as a transcriptional repressor on minimal promoter containing element F in an E-box sequence-specific manner [76]. It can act as a transcriptional transactivator on the proximal promoter region of the tartrate-resistant acid phosphatase (TRAP) E-box containing promoter. It also acts as a transcriptional repressor on minimal promoter containing mu E3 enhancer sequence [77]. Gain-of-function assays indicated that TFEC was capable of expanding hematopoietic stem cells–derived hematopoiesis. TFEC mutants were showed to reduce hematopoiesis in the caudal hematopoietic tissue, leading to anemia. It mediated these changes by increasing the expression of several cytokines in caudal endothelial cells [78]. Ribosomal RNA Processing 12 Homolog (RRP12) is a protein that may have a function to bind to poly(A) RNA. Rrp12 and the exportin Crm1 participate in late assembly events in the nucleolus during 40S ribosomal subunit biogenesis [79], but there is little knowledge of TFEC and RR12 regulating B cell growth.

3.3.2. Cluster C2

Cluster C2 was the second group to be inducted transcendently during CSR in human B cells and this cluster contains 112 genes. *LMNB2* and *B4GALT5* were the most significantly introduced in this cluster.

LMNB2 encodes a B-type nuclear lamin. The nuclear lamina consists of a two-dimensional matrix of proteins located next to the inner nuclear membrane. Lamin proteins are thought to be involved in nuclear stability, chromatin structure and gene expression. B-type lamins play a role in DNA replication, the formation of the mitotic spindle, chromatin organization and regulation of gene expression [80]. *B4GALT5* encodes one of seven beta-1,4-galactosyltransferase. It is the type II membrane-bound glycoproteins that appear to have exclusive specificity for the donor substrate UDP-galactose; B4GALT5 was found to have a change in a statin-induced experiment in gene expression in EBV-transformed and native B cells [81].

3.3.3. Cluster C3

Cluster C3 was the third group to be inducted transcendently during CSR in B cells and the cluster has 105 genes. The analysis of gene ontology indicated the genes in this cluster were involved with DNA metabolic process. *UHRF1* and *CHEK1* were the most significantly introduced in this group.

UHRF1 gene encodes a member of a subfamily of RING-finger–type E3 ubiquitin ligases. The protein binds to specific DNA sequences and recruits a histone deacetylase to regulate gene expression. Its expression peaks at late G1 phase and continues during G2 and M phases of the cell cycle. Colonization of germ-free mice with gut microbiota showed increasing expression of Uhrf1 in Treg cells. Uhrf1 deficiency resulted in de-repression of the gene (Cdkn1a) [77]. *CHEK1* encodes a protein belonging to the Ser/Thr protein kinase family. It is required for checkpoint-mediated cell cycle arrest in response to DNA damage or the presence of unreplicated DNA. Activated CHEK1 can phosphorylate and modulate the activity of a number of proteins including p53, providing a link between sensing of DNA damage and p53 checkpoint activity. BCL6 can directly bind to a DNA consensus element in the CHEK1 promoter and repress its expression in normal and malignant B cell [82].

3.3.4. Cluster C4

Cluster C4 was the fourth group to be inducted transcendently during CSR and it has 151 genes. The analysis of gene ontology showed that the genes in this cluster were majorly involved in the M phase. The analysis of transcription factor enrichment indicated the genes in this cluster were enriched to nuclear transcription factor Y (NF-Y). NF-Y in eukaryotes consists of three different subunits, NF-YA, NF-YB and NF-YC, which are all necessary for the formation of NF-Y complexes and binding to CCAAT boxes in promoters of their target genes. Recent studies demonstrated novel contributions of NF-Y to apoptosis and apoptosis-induced proliferation and in photoreceptor cell differentiation during the development of the Drosophila compound eye [83].

KIF14 and *PRC1* were the most significantly differential expression genes in the cluster. *KIF14* encodes a member of the kinesin-3 superfamily of microtubule motor proteins. These proteins are involved in numerous processes including vesicle transport, chromosome segregation, mitotic spindle formation and cytokinesis. Knockdown of this gene results in failed cytokinesis with endoreplication. This gene was identified as a likely oncogene in breast, lung and ovarian cancers, as well as in retinoblastomas and gliomas [84]. Protein regulator of cytokinesis 1 (*PRC1*) gene is a crucial regulator of cytokinesis [85]. Its suppression may result in mitotic failure and its involvement in various cancers [86]. PRC1 is a key regulator of cytokinesis that cross-links antiparallel microtubules. Multiple mitotic kinesins and microtubule-associated proteins (MAPs) act in concert to direct cytokinesis [87]. The MAP and microtubule-bundling protein PRC1 is one of the key molecules required for the integrity of this structure. Endogenous PRC1 can be interacted with KIF14. KIF14 targets the central spindle via its interaction with PRC1 and has an essential function in cytokinesis [88].

3.3.5. Cluster C5

Cluster C5 was the fifth group to be inducted transcendently and it has 99 genes. *MCM10* and *PCNA* genes were the most differentially expressed in the cluster.

MCM10 encodes one of the highly conserved mini-chromosome maintenance proteins (MCM) that are involved in the initiation of eukaryotic genome replication. Human MCM10 regulates the catalytic subunit of DNA polymerase-α and prevents DNA damage during replication [89]. MCM10 interacts with RECQ4 (RecQ helicases 4) and is important for efficient replication [90, 91]. PCNA encodes a cofactor of DNA polymerase delta in nucleus. The protein acts as a homotrimer and helps increase the processivity of leading strand synthesis during DNA replication. PCNA was well studied in plants and had the ability to stimulate the activity of DNA polymerase δ and the ability to interact with p21, a regulator of the cell cycle [92].

3.3.6. Cluster C6

Cluster C6 was the sixth group to be inducted transcendently and it contains 128 genes. *CCR4* and *HIST1H1C* genes were the most differentially expressed in the whole process during naïve B cell activation with IL4 and anti-CD40 signal stimulation.

CCR4 is the receptor of CCL17 and CCL22. It is later inducted, which means that the three may work in late stage of CSR. CCR4 was previously detected in nongerminal center cells. The possible functional roles in CSR were discussed in Section 3.1.1. Histone H1 has previously been shown to influence mast cell–mediated type-I hyperreactivity in mice [93].

3.4. Cluster D group

Cluster D group has three profiling clusters to show transient downregulation during CSR according to the time of downregulation.

3.4.1. Cluster D1

Cluster D1 was the first group to be inducted transcendently and it contains 99 genes. *GPR18* and *TP53INP1* genes were the most differentially expressed in the cluster.

GPR18 encodes G protein–coupled receptor 18. The activity of this receptor is mediated by G proteins, which inhibit adenylyl cyclase [94], and it contributes to regulation of the immune system. GPR18 also mediates NAGly-induced process of reorganization of actin filaments and induction of acrosomal exocytosis. Stimulation of human spermatozoa with the GPR18 ligand N-arachidonoylglycine induced the phosphorylation of 12 protein kinases. N-arachidonoylglycine affects the cytoskeleton by changing levels of F-actin and inducing the acrosome reaction in human spermatozoa in a concentration-dependent manner. GPR18 might be involved in physiological processes of human spermatozoa [95]. Tumor protein 53-induced nuclear protein 1 (TP53INP1) is a tumor suppressor. It was described as a p53 target gene involved in cell death, cell-cycle arrest and cellular migration [96]. TP53INP1 is also able to interact with ATG8-family proteins to induce autophagy-dependent cell death by caspase-dependent autophagy [97].

3.4.2. Cluster D2

Cluster D2 was the second group to be inducted transcendently during CSR in B cells. It contains 69 genes. *RAB6B* and *PM20D1* genes were the most differentially expressed.

RAB6B (RAB6B, member RAS oncogene family) has the ability for GTP binding and myosin V binding. Members of the RAB subfamily of small GTPases play an important role in the regulation of intracellular transport routes [98]. RAB6B is predominantly expressed in brain and the neuroblastoma cell line SK-N-SH. In brain, RAB6B was found to be specifically expressed in microglia, pericytes and Purkinje cells. Endogenous RAB6B localizes to the Golgi apparatus and to ERGIC-53–positive vesicles. RAB6B displayed lower GTP-binding activities, and in overexpression studies, the protein is distributed over Golgi and ER membranes [99]. A secreted enzyme, peptidase M20 domain containing 1 (PM20D1), is enriched in UCP1(+) versus UCP1(−) adipocytes. These data identify an enzymatic node and a family of metabolites that regulate energy homeostasis [99].

3.4.3. Cluster D3

Cluster D3 was the third group to be inducted transcendently in CSR of human B cells and the cluster has 113 genes. *IKZF2* and *ADCY1* genes were the most differentially expressed.

IKZF2 encodes a member of the Ikaros family of zinc-finger proteins. Three members of this protein family (Ikaros, Aiolos and Helios) are hematopoietic-specific transcription factors involved in the regulation of lymphocyte development. This protein forms homo- or heterodimers with other Ikaros family members and has a function predominantly in early hematopoietic development. Helios is preferentially expressed at the mRNA level by regulatory T cells (Treg cells) and is potentially a specific marker of thymic-derived Treg cells. It raises the possibility that a significant percentage of Foxp3+ Treg cells are generated extrathymically [100]. *ADCY1* gene encodes a member of the adenylate cyclase family that is primarily expressed in the brain. This protein is regulated by calcium/calmodulin concentration. Cyclic AMP (cAMP) production, which is important for mechanotransduction within the inner ear, is catalyzed by adenylate cyclases (AC). ADCY1 has an evolutionarily conserved role in hearing, and cAMP signaling is important to hair cell function within the inner ear [101].

The most significantly differential genes in each cluster and major pathways in each cluster are listed in **Table 1**. The most interesting clusters are Cluster A1 and Cluster B1 and the full gene names of these two clusters are listed in **Tables 2** and **3**.

Cluster	Numbers	Activation during CSR	Most significant genes	Pathways involved	References
A1	153	Expression on	*CCL22; CCL17; TRAF; BCL2L1; MYB; VIM; TRIP10; FAS; PTGIR; EBI3; AHR; NCF2*	ERK signaling, TRAF pathway; insulin pathway; NF-kB pathway	[105–108]
A2	83	Expression off	*MARCH1; FOSB; DUSP1; FOS; CR1; CR2; RGS2; PLD4; CCR6; RASGRP2; MOP-1; FCRLA*	Toll-like receptor signaling pathways, MAPK signaling pathway; innate immune system pathway	[109–111]

Cluster	Numbers	Activation during CSR	Most significant genes	Pathways involved	References
B1	126	Sustained induction	*BHLHE40; IL17RB; NFIL3; HOMER2; AICDA; BATF3; ARID5A; DUSP4; CD80; TNFAIP2; XBP1; MTHFD2*	Circadian rhythm pathway; IL-17 family signaling pathways; IL4-mediated signaling pathway	[57, 112, 113]
B2	112	Sustained induction	*EPHB1; TNFSF4; DPYSL2; RPS6KA2; SLC41A1; AMICA1; MIIP; RGS9; CISH; LRRC32; AUH; SLC37A3*	EPH-Ephrin signaling; TNF superfamily pathway; transport of glucose pathway	[114–116]
C1	79	Transient induction	*TFEC; RRP12; SLC29A1; GPATCH4; SSRP1; BCL2A1; CYB561; NME1; TTLL12; FASN; NETO2; SLC27A4*	C-MYB transcription factor network; apoptosis modulation and signaling	[117, 118]
C2	112	Transient induction	*LMNB2; B4GALT5; SLC43A3; ESPL1; EZH2; PSMC3; SUV39H2; MREG; FSCN1; SRC; PHOSPHO2-KLHL23*	Apoptosis pathway; glycosaminoglycan metabolism pathway	[119, 120]
C3	105	Transient induction	*UHRF1; CHEK1; FANCI; CHAF1B; DTL; CDC6; EXO1; MCM6; CHAF1A; CDC45; TCF19*	Chromatin regulation/ acetylation pathway; DNA double-strand break repair pathway	[121, 122]
C4	151	Transient induction	*KIF14; PRC1; NDC80; NUF2; HMMR; DEPDC1; AURKA; ARHGAP11B; BRCA1; FAM72B; HIST1H4L; DLGAP5; HIST1H1B*	Signaling by Rho GTPases; cell cycle pathway; DNA double-strand break repair pathway	[85, 123, 124]
C5	99	Transient induction	*MCM10; PCNA; TCFL5; HELLS; ZC3HAV1L; PHF19; CARM1; VDR; LIMA1; MYH10; SEMA4A; TMOD1*	Telomere C-strand synthesis pathway; apoptosis modulation and signaling; chromatin regulation/ acetylation	[125–127]
C6	128	Transient induction	*CCR4; HIST1H1C; CHRNA6; HIST1H3I; CCL1; GPR55; SYT11; PSTPIP2; KIAA1549L; HIST1H1D; PSAT1; TFDP2*	Signaling by GPCR; apoptosis induced DNA fragmentation; nicotine pathway	[128–130]
D1	69	Transient downregulation	*GPR18; TP53INP1; IFIT2; RNASET2; LBH; DOK3; FGD3; CD69; OAS1; ABCG1; PNOC; PARP15*	Signaling by GPCR; p53 pathway, innate immune system; B cell development pathway	[96, 131–133]
D2	69	Transient downregulation	*RAB6B; PM20D1; CYP2C19; CPNE4; TNFSF8; HIST1H2BD; METTL7A; ADHFE1; TMEM140; JMJD7; KLHL24; POU2AF1*	Vesicle-mediated transport; drug metabolism; ERK signaling	[134–136]
D3	113	Transient downregulation	*IKZF2; ADCY1; APOBEC3H; VAMP5; PDCD1LG2; CYP2C18; ILDR1; ADRB1; TM6SF1; GCSAM; CHAC1; ENPP3*	mRNA editing—C to U conversion; NF-kB signaling; cytochrome P450 pathway	[137–139]

Table 1. The most significantly differential genes and pathways in each cluster during CSR.

Cluster A1: 153 genes									
CCL22	*CCL17*	*TRAF1*	*BCL2L1*	*MYB*	*VIM*	*TRIP10*	*FAS*	*PTGIR*	*EBI3*
AHR	*NCF2*	*BCAT1*	*MGLL*	*SEMA4C*	*SIRPA*	*TFPI2*	*ARNTL2*	*STAT5A*	*HYOU1*
ADA	*ICAM1*	*CFLAR*	*MYO1C*	*IGSF3*	*CCR7*	*SEPT11*	*WSB2*	*IL13RA1*	*CDK2AP1*
CLIP2	*NFKB2*	*PGD*	*HIPK2*	*CD58*	*MARCKS*	*SNX8*	*TNFAIP3*	*TNIP1*	*SLAMF7*
SLC43A2	*FADS1*	*FAM129A*	*RAP2A*	*YWHAG*	*CYFIP1*	*LOC101929479*	*GNG8*	*IRF5*	*TMEM120A*
FCER2	*IPO7*	*CBX6*	*CDK6*	*BLVRA*	*AP1S3*	*XPO5*	*PIK3R5*	*LSP1*	*FNBP1*
TAGLN2	*RBBP9*	*SPINT2*	*FYTTD1*	*GPR137B*	*PEF1*	*PPA1*	*RANGAP1*	*LSM11*	*RHOF*
WDR91	*ATP1A1*	*MIR17HG*	*SUPT16H*	*USP14*	*CPNE8*	*MMP7*	*EEF2K*	*PPME1*	*ANXA7*
EHD4	*CDR2*	*SRPK1*	*BLMH*	*UBE2Z*	*KDM2B*	*PPP1R7*	*CAPRIN1*	*SF3B6*	*TALDO1*
LMNA	*MCOLN2*	*SCD*	*PCGF5*	*HERPUD1*	*NFKB1*	*CHURC1-FNTB*	*ERH*	*TJP2*	*BSG*
VOPP1	*KEAP1*	*CEP85*	*NAE1*	*UBTD2*	*TKT*	*GOT2*	*SZRD1*	*APOL1*	*NSUN4*
CHMP4B	*TRIM28*	*KCNN4*	*SLC16A1*	*SLC9A7*	*SLC20A1*	*MAP4*	*ZNF48*	*ECE1*	*ADCY3*
STX11	*LARP4*	*OTUD7B*	*GPR183*	*PSMD8*	*ZAK*	*SLC35F2*	*COA7*	*ANXA5*	*IDE*
SLC39A1	*MDFIC*	*GSTP1*	*OGFOD1*	*SEC23B*	*IMPDH2*	*HDLBP*	*HTT*	*KIF13B*	*GTF3C4*
ACSL4	*MPC1*	*PITPNB*	*TNIP2*	*EXOC3*	*MDH1*	*PLEKHA7*	*UBE2D4*	*JADE3*	*POR*
PEA15	*PIK3CD*	*TP53BP2*							

Table 2. The lists of Cluster A1.

Cluster B1: 126 genes									
BHLHE40	*IL17RB*	*NFIL3*	*HOMER2*	*AICDA*	*BATF3*	*ARID5A*	*DUSP4*	*CD80*	*TNFAIP2*
XBP1	*MTHFD2*	*CD86*	*CD59*	*CAMK4*	*MFHAS1*	*SLC1A5*	*SRGN*	*USP46*	*CHDH*
HDGFR3	*PIGX*	*FLT1*	*RNF19B*	*LTA*	*NOD2*	*ZNF788*	*AARS*	*ATXN1*	*RFC5*
WARS	*PXDC1*	*PPP1R14A*	*DENND5A*	*QSOX1*	*STK38L*	*PRR5L*	*RGS10*	*SLC7A5*	*SCCPDH*
RRAGD	*LY75-CD302*	*ADAMDEC1*	*YARS*	*GPHN*	*TRIM16L*	*IRF4*	*NINJ1*	*SLC7A1*	*SOCS1*
CD274	*ECHDC3*	*NECAP2*	*TSPAN33*	*SEC11C*	*LOXL3*	*AHRR*	*RALB*	*ARID3A*	*RDX*
CSF1	*THG1L*	*SLC39A8*	*SAMSN1*	*TXNL1*	*STK35*	*DARS*	*TARS*	*CLDND1*	*C12orf5*
SEL1L	*CARS*	*FAM162A*	*VCL*	*SEPHS1*	*XPOT*	*ACSL1*	*GOT1*	*PFKM*	*NSMCE1*
RBM47	*CEP19*	*ATXN2L*	*DHRS3*	*RAB39B*	*DCTN2*	*PABPC4*	*HIVEP1*	*CCDC126*	*ACADVL*
MTX2	*AEN*	*TFG*	*RBPJ*	*SLC25A20*	*ETFDH*	*COPA*	*NR4A3*	*GPX4*	*ITFG3*
DUSP22	*CTNS*	*IL2RA*	*RAP1A*	*TNFAIP1*	*PAM*	*SLC37A1*	*DCTN6*	*AKAP2*	*RIPK2*
RAB21	*RPS23*	*KIAA1279*	*MARS*	*ZNF267*	*CLCN5*	*NFKBID*	*PRPSAP1*	*NEDD1*	*ZNF382*
CDKN1A	*PRRT3*	*LYSMD1*	*NCK2*	*AZIN1*	*KIF5B*				

Table 3. The lists of Cluster B1.

4. The future research on CSR in human B cells

A total of 1399 genes were shown to have differential expression during CSR in human B cells, and the novel genes have the roles in immune system process, cellular amine and DNA process and cell cycle phase or ribonucleoprotein biogenesis. Understanding the precisely functional roles of these novel genes in CSR in human B cells will bring new insights into the mechanisms of CSR and find potential therapeutic targets for human immune disorders such as allergic asthma and autoimmune diseases.

The next stage of research will also focus on determining how the naïve B cells turn into the specific IgE-, IgA- or IgG-releasing cells after T cell cytokines signal stimulation. The different stages of CSR in human B cell may contain unique transcription regulators for the destiny for each single cell. The development of single-cell sequencing provides a unique opportunity to explore the subsets of the human B cells to generate IgE, IgA and IgG. Obtaining high-quality single-cell sequencing data from B cells depends on efficient isolation of individual cells and amplifications of the genome or transcriptome of single cell to acquire sufficient materials for downstream analysis, identifying true variations from technological biases [102]. One of the major challenges of analyzing single-cell genomics data is to develop tools that differentiate technical artifacts and noise introduced during single-cell isolation, whole genome amplification, whole transcriptome amplification and sequencing from true biological variation. There are many factors that can influence the single-cell analysis. During single-cell isolation, the population of cells can be biased through the selection of cells based on size, viability or propensity to enter the cell cycle. Cells from cell lines as control may be problematic as they may not be diploid, and they can be highly aneuploid or even polyploidy. These will affect experimental performance [102]. Our understanding of human B cell function in CSR will derive from comparisons between healthy individuals and those with particular immunological diseases, and among groups of patients having the same disease with different clinical outcomes. For example, human SLE is clinically heterogeneous [103], making treatment decision challenging. It is important to know which B cell subsets are responsible for which functions in immune diseases, in addition to identifying how a "signature" profile for an individual subject's collection of subsets may correlate with disease outcome that could eventually allow greater optimization of targeted therapies [104].

Abbreviation

AC	adenylate cyclases
AID	activation-induced cytidine deaminase
AP-1	activating protein-1
APC	antigen-presenting cell
APE	apurinic/apyrimidic endonuclease
BCRs	B cell receptors
Be-1	B effector 1
Be-2	B effector 2
CB	cord blood
CLPs	common lymphoid progenitors
CSR	class switch recombination
DCs	dendritic cells
DSBs	double-strand DNA breaks
Eph	erythropoietin-producing hepatocellular
FIP	FOS-interacting protein
FO	follicular
GCs	germinal centers
HDM	house dust mite
hnRNPs	heterogeneous nuclear ribonucleoproteins
IgH	Ig heavy-chain
MAPs	microtubule-associated proteins

MAREs	Maf-recognition elements
MCM	mini-chromosome maintenance proteins
MZ	marginal zone
NF-kB	NF-kappa B
NHEJ	nonhomologous end-joining
NO	nitrogen oxide
PKC-β	protein kinase C-β
PRC1	protein regulator of cytokinesis 1
RAG	recombination activating gene
RTKs	receptor tyrosine kinases
SLE	systemic lupus erythematosus
TD	T lymphocyte dependent
TFEC	transcription factor EC
TI	T lymphocyte independent
TNF	tumor necrosis factor
TRAF	TNF receptor associated factor
TRAP	tartrate-resistant acid phosphatase
UNG	uracil DNA glycosylase

Author details

Youming Zhang

Address all correspondence to: y.zhang@imperial.ac.uk

Functional Genomics Group, Genomic Medicine Section, National Heart and Lung Institute, Imperial College London, London, England

References

[1] Lund FE, Cytokine-producing B. Lymphocytes-key regulators of immunity. Current Opinion in Immunology. 2008;**20**(3):332-338

[2] Hoffman W, Lakkis FG, Chalasani GB. Cells, antibodies, and more. Clinical Journal of the American Society of Nephrology: CJASN. 2016;**11**(1):137-154

[3] Ribatti D, Crivellato E, Vacca A. The contribution of Bruce Glick to the definition of the role played by the bursa of Fabricius in the development of the B cell lineage. Clinical and Experimental Immunology. 2006;**145**(1):1-4

[4] Welner RS, Pelayo R, Kincade PW. Evolving views on the genealogy of B cells. Nature Reviews Immunology. 2008;**8**(2):95-106

[5] Harris DP, Goodrich S, Mohrs K, Mohrs M, Lund FE. Cutting edge: The development of IL-4-producing B cells (B effector 2 cells) is controlled by IL-4, IL-4 receptor alpha, and Th2 cells. Journal of Immunology. 2005;**175**(11):7103-7107

[6] Harris DP, Goodrich S, Gerth AJ, Peng SL, Lund FE. Regulation of IFN-gamma production by B effector 1 cells: Essential roles for T-bet and the IFN-gamma receptor. Journal of Immunology. 2005;**174**(11):6781-6790

[7] Lin YC, Jhunjhunwala S, Benner C, Heinz S, Welinder E, Mansson R, et al. A global network of transcription factors, involving E2A, EBF1 and Foxo1, that orchestrates B cell fate. Nature Immunology. 2010;**11**(7):635-643

[8] Tonegawa S. Somatic generation of antibody diversity. Nature. 1983;**302**(5909):575-581

[9] Nemazee D. Mechanisms of central tolerance for B cells. Nature Reviews Immunology. 2017;**17**(5):281-294

[10] Pascual V, Liu YJ, Magalski A, de Bouteiller O, Banchereau J, Capra JD. Analysis of somatic mutation in five B cell subsets of human tonsil. The Journal of Experimental Medicine. 1994;**180**(1):329-339

[11] Allen CD, Okada T, Cyster JG. Germinal-center organization and cellular dynamics. Immunity. 2007;**27**(2):190-202

[12] Good-Jacobson KL, Shlomchik MJ. Plasticity and heterogeneity in the generation of memory B cells and long-lived plasma cells: The influence of germinal center interactions and dynamics. Journal of Immunology. 2010;**185**(6):3117-3125

[13] Hauser AE, Junt T, Mempel TR, Sneddon MW, Kleinstein SH, Henrickson SE, et al. Definition of germinal-center B cell migration in vivo reveals predominant intrazonal circulation patterns. Immunity. 2007;**26**(5):655-667

[14] Batista FD, Harwood NE. The who, how and where of antigen presentation to B cells. Nature Reviews Immunology. 2009;**9**(1):15-27

[15] Okada T, Miller MJ, Parker I, Krummel MF, Neighbors M, Hartley SB, et al. Antigen-engaged B cells undergo chemotaxis toward the T zone and form motile conjugates with helper T cells. PLoS Biology. 2005;**3**(6):e150

[16] Kerfoot SM, Yaari G, Patel JR, Johnson KL, Gonzalez DG, Kleinstein SH, et al. Germinal center B cell and T follicular helper cell development initiates in the interfollicular zone. Immunity. 2011;**34**(6):947-960

[17] Kaminski DA, Wei C, Qian Y, Rosenberg AF, Sanz I. Advances in human B cell phenotypic profiling. Frontiers in Immunology. 2012;**3**:302

[18] Wirths S, Lanzavecchia A. ABCB1 transporter discriminates human resting naive B cells from cycling transitional and memory B cells. European Journal of Immunology. 2005;**35**(12):3433-3441

[19] Good KL, Avery DT, Tangye SG. Resting human memory B cells are intrinsically programmed for enhanced survival and responsiveness to diverse stimuli compared to naive B cells. Journal of Immunology. 2009;**182**(2):890-901

[20] Tangye SG, Avery DT, Hodgkin PDA. Division-linked mechanism for the rapid generation of Ig-secreting cells from human memory B cells. Journal of Immunology. 2003;**170**(1):261-269

[21] Oettinger MA, Schatz DG, Gorka C, Baltimore D. RAG-1 and RAG-2, adjacent genes that synergistically activate V(D)J recombination. Science. 1990;**248**(4962):1517-1523

[22] Schatz DG, Oettinger MA, Baltimore D. The V(D)J recombination activating gene, RAG-1. Cell. 1989;**59**(6):1035-1048

[23] Stavnezer J, Guikema JE, Schrader CE. Mechanism and regulation of class switch recombination. Annual Review of Immunology. 2008;**26**:261-292

[24] Muramatsu M, Kinoshita K, Fagarasan S, Yamada S, Shinkai Y, Honjo T. Class switch recombination and hypermutation require activation-induced cytidine deaminase (AID), a potential RNA editing enzyme. Cell. 2000;**102**(5):553-563

[25] Okazaki IM, Kinoshita K, Muramatsu M, Yoshikawa K, Honjo T. The AID enzyme induces class switch recombination in fibroblasts. Nature. 2002;**416**(6878):340-345

[26] Fear DJ. Mechanisms regulating the targeting and activity of activation induced cytidine deaminase. Current Opinion in Immunology. 2013;**25**(5):619-628

[27] Dudley DD, Chaudhuri J, Bassing CH, Alt FW. Mechanism and control of V(D)J recombination versus class switch recombination: Similarities and differences. Advances in Immunology. 2005;**86**:43-112

[28] Manis JP, Tian M, Alt FW. Mechanism and control of class-switch recombination. Trends in Immunology. 2002;**23**(1):31-39

[29] Chowdhury M, Forouhi O, Dayal S, McCloskey N, Gould HJ, Felsenfeld G, et al. Analysis of intergenic transcription and histone modification across the human immunoglobulin heavy-chain locus. Proceedings of the National Academy of Sciences of the United States of America. 2008;**105**(41):15872-15877

[30] Jeppson JD, Patel HR, Sakata N, Domenico J, Terada N, Gelfand EW. Requirement for dual signals by anti-CD40 and IL-4 for the induction of nuclear factor-kappa B, IL-6, and IgE in human B lymphocytes. Journal of Immunology. 1998;**161**(4):1738-1742

[31] Zhang Y, Fear DJ, Willis-Owen SA, Cookson WO, Moffatt MF. Global gene regulation during activation of immunoglobulin class switching in human B cells. Scientific Reports. 2016;**6**:37988

[32] Itoh-Nakadai A, Hikota R, Muto A, Kometani K, Watanabe-Matsui M, Sato Y, et al. The transcription repressors Bach2 and Bach1 promote B cell development by repressing the myeloid program. Nature Immunology. 2014;**15**(12):1171-1180

[33] Oyake T, Itoh K, Motohashi H, Hayashi N, Hoshino H, Nishizawa M, et al. Bach proteins belong to a novel family of BTB-basic leucine zipper transcription factors that interact with MafK and regulate transcription through the NF-E2 site. Molecular and Cellular Biology. 1996;**16**(11):6083-6095

[34] Muto A, Tashiro S, Nakajima O, Hoshino H, Takahashi S, Sakoda E, et al. The transcriptional programme of antibody class switching involves the repressor Bach2. Nature. 2004;**429**(6991):566-571

[35] Muto A, Ochiai K, Kimura Y, Itoh-Nakadai A, Calame KL, Ikebe D, et al. Bach2 represses plasma cell gene regulatory network in B cells to promote antibody class switch. The EMBO Journal. 2010;**29**(23):4048-4061

[36] McManus S, Ebert A, Salvagiotto G, Medvedovic J, Sun Q, Tamir I, et al. The transcription factor Pax5 regulates its target genes by recruiting chromatin-modifying proteins in committed B cells. The EMBO Journal. 2011;**30**(12):2388-2404

[37] Schwenzer R, Siemienski K, Liptay S, Schubert G, Peters N, Scheurich P, et al. The human tumor necrosis factor (TNF) receptor-associated factor 1 gene (TRAF1) is up-regulated by cytokines of the TNF ligand family and modulates TNF-induced activation of NF-kappaB and c-Jun N-terminal kinase. The Journal of Biological Chemistry. 1999;**274**(27):19368-19374

[38] Werfel T, Heratizadeh A, Niebuhr M, Kapp A, Roesner LM, Karch A, et al. Exacerbation of atopic dermatitis on grass pollen exposure in an environmental challenge chamber. The Journal of Allergy and Clinical Immunology. 2015;**136**(1):96-103 e9

[39] Abelius MS, Ernerudh J, Berg G, Matthiesen L, Nilsson LJ, Jenmalm MC. High cord blood levels of the T-helper 2-associated chemokines CCL17 and CCL22 precede allergy development during the first 6 years of life. Pediatric Research. 2011;**70**(5):495-500

[40] Perros F, Hoogsteden HC, Coyle AJ, Lambrecht BN, Hammad H. Blockade of CCR4 in a humanized model of asthma reveals a critical role for DC-derived CCL17 and CCL22 in attracting Th2 cells and inducing airway inflammation. Allergy. 2009;**64**(7):995-1002

[41] Hai T, Curran T. Cross-family dimerization of transcription factors Fos/Jun and ATF/CREB alters DNA binding specificity. Proceedings of the National Academy of Sciences of the United States of America. 1991;**88**(9):3720-3724

[42] Lee W, Mitchell P, Tjian R. Purified transcription factor AP-1 interacts with TPA-inducible enhancer elements. Cell. 1987;**49**(6):741-752

[43] Zhou H, Zarubin T, Ji Z, Min Z, Zhu W, Downey JS, et al. Frequency and distribution of AP-1 sites in the human genome. DNA Research: An International Journal for Rapid Publication of Reports on Genes and Genomes. 2005;**12**(2):139-150

[44] Karin M, Liu Z, Zandi E. AP-1 function and regulation. Current Opinion in Cell Biology. 1997;**9**(2):240-246

[45] Gustems M, Woellmer A, Rothbauer U, Eck SH, Wieland T, Lutter D, et al. c-Jun/c-Fos heterodimers regulate cellular genes via a newly identified class of methylated DNA sequence motifs. Nucleic Acids Research. 2014;**42**(5):3059-3072

[46] Chiu R, Boyle WJ, Meek J, Smeal T, Hunter T, Karin M. The c-Fos protein interacts with c-Jun/AP-1 to stimulate transcription of AP-1 responsive genes. Cell. 1988;**54**(4):541-552

[47] Davis BJ, Flanagan BF, Gilfillan AM, Metcalfe DD, Coleman JW. Nitric oxide inhibits IgE-dependent cytokine production and Fos and Jun activation in mast cells. Journal of Immunology. 2004;**173**(11):6914-6920

[48] Lewin I, Jacob-Hirsch J, Zang ZC, Kupershtein V, Szallasi Z, Rivera J, et al. Aggregation of the Fc epsilon RI in mast cells induces the synthesis of Fos-interacting protein and increases its DNA binding-activity: The dependence on protein kinase C-beta. The Journal of Biological Chemistry. 1996;**271**(3):1514-1519

[49] Zhao J, Harper R, Barchowsky A, Di YP. Identification of multiple MAPK-mediated transcription factors regulated by tobacco smoke in airway epithelial cells. American Journal of Physiology Lung Cellular and Molecular Physiology. 2007;**293**(2):L480-L490

[50] Papin JA, Palsson BO. The JAK-STAT signaling network in the human B-cell: An extreme signaling pathway analysis. Biophysical Journal. 2004;**87**(1):37-46

[51] Pollock R, Treisman R. Human SRF-related proteins: DNA-binding properties and potential regulatory targets. Genes & Development. 1991;**5**(12A):2327-2341

[52] Wang L, Kurosaki T, Corey SJ. Engagement of the B-cell antigen receptor activates STAT through Lyn in a Jak-independent pathway. Oncogene. 2007;**26**(20):2851-2859

[53] Mittrucker HW, Matsuyama T, Grossman A, Kundig TM, Potter J, Shahinian A, et al. Requirement for the transcription factor LSIRF/IRF4 for mature B and T lymphocyte function. Science. 1997;**275**(5299):540-543

[54] Todd DJ, McHeyzer-Williams LJ, Kowal C, Lee AH, Volpe BT, Diamond B, et al. XBP1 governs late events in plasma cell differentiation and is not required for antigen-specific memory B cell development. The Journal of Experimental Medicine. 2009;**206**(10):2151-2159

[55] Ise W, Kohyama M, Schraml BU, Zhang T, Schwer B, Basu U, et al. The transcription factor BATF controls the global regulators of class-switch recombination in both B cells and T cells. Nature Immunology. 2011;**12**(6):536-543

[56] Kashiwada M, Levy DM, McKeag L, Murray K, Schroder AJ, Canfield SM, et al. IL-4-induced transcription factor NFIL3/E4BP4 controls IgE class switching. Proceedings of the National Academy of Sciences of the United States of America. 2010;**107**(2):821-826

[57] Bie Q, Jin C, Zhang B, Dong H. IL-17B: A new area of study in the IL-17 family. Molecular Immunology. 2017;**90**:50-56

[58] Wang H, Mobini R, Fang Y, Barrenas F, Zhang H, Xiang Z, et al. Allergen challenge of peripheral blood mononuclear cells from patients with seasonal allergic rhinitis increases IL-17RB, which regulates basophil apoptosis and degranulation. Clinical and Experimental Allergy: Journal of the British Society for Allergy and Clinical Immunology. 2010;**40**(8):1194-1202

[59] Hunninghake GM, Chu JH, Sharma SS, Cho MH, Himes BE, Rogers AJ, et al. The CD4+ T-cell transcriptome and serum IgE in asthma: IL17RB and the role of sex. BMC Pulmonary Medicine. 2011;**11**:17

[60] Jung JS, Park BL, Cheong HS, Bae JS, Kim JH, Chang HS, et al. Association of IL-17RB gene polymorphism with asthma. Chest. 2009;**135**(5):1173-1180

[61] Lefebvre C, Rajbhandari P, Alvarez MJ, Bandaru P, Lim WK, Sato M, et al. A human B-cell interactome identifies MYB and FOXM1 as master regulators of proliferation in germinal centers. Molecular Systems Biology. 2010;**6**:377

[62] Reinberg A, Gervais P, Levi F, Smolensky M, Del Cerro L, Ugolini C. Circadian and circannual rhythms of allergic rhinitis: An epidemiologic study involving chronobiologic methods. The Journal of Allergy and Clinical Immunology. 1988;**81**(1):51-62

[63] Kelly EA, Houtman JJ, Jarjour NN. Inflammatory changes associated with circadian variation in pulmonary function in subjects with mild asthma. Clinical and Experimental Allergy: Journal of the British Society for Allergy and Clinical Immunology. 2004; **34**(2):227-233

[64] Maurer M, Ortonne JP, Zuberbier T. Chronic urticaria: An internet survey of health behaviours, symptom patterns and treatment needs in European adult patients. The British Journal of Dermatology. 2009;**160**(3):633-641

[65] Nakamura Y, Harama D, Shimokawa N, Hara M, Suzuki R, Tahara Y, et al. Circadian clock gene Period2 regulates a time-of-day-dependent variation in cutaneous anaphylactic reaction. The Journal of Allergy and Clinical Immunology. 2011;**127**(4):1038-45 e1-3.

[66] Sun H, Lu B, Li RQ, Flavell RA, Taneja R, Defective T. Cell activation and autoimmune disorder in Stra13-deficient mice. Nature Immunology. 2001;**2**(11):1040-1047

[67] Yu X, Rollins D, Ruhn KA, Stubblefield JJ, Green CB, Kashiwada M, et al. TH17 cell differentiation is regulated by the circadian clock. Science. 2013;**342**(6159):727-730

[68] Nakada M, Hayashi Y, Hamada J. Role of Eph/ephrin tyrosine kinase in malignant glioma. Neuro-Oncology. 2011;**13**(11):1163-1170

[69] Gucciardo E, Sugiyama N, Lehti K. Eph- and ephrin-dependent mechanisms in tumor and stem cell dynamics. Cellular and Molecular Life Sciences: CMLS. 2014;**71**(19):3685-3710

[70] Wei W, Wang H, Ji S. Paradoxes of the EphB1 receptor in malignant brain tumors. Cancer Cell International. 2017;**17**:21

[71] Davis S, Gale NW, Aldrich TH, Maisonpierre PC, Lhotak V, Pawson T, et al. Ligands for EPH-related receptor tyrosine kinases that require membrane attachment or clustering for activity. Science. 1994;**266**(5186):816-819

[72] Holen HL, Zernichow L, Fjelland KE, Evenroed IM, Tveit H, Aasheim HC. Ephrin-B3 binds specifically to B lymphocytes in blood and induces migration. Scandinavian Journal of Immunology. 2011;**74**(2):144-154

[73] Cunninghame Graham DS, Graham RR, Manku H, Wong AK, Whittaker JC, Gaffney PM, et al. Polymorphism at the TNF superfamily gene TNFSF4 confers susceptibility to systemic lupus erythematosus. Nature Genetics. 2008;**40**(1):83-89

[74] Gourh P, Arnett FC, Tan FK, Assassi S, Divecha D, Paz G, et al. Association of TNFSF4 (OX40L) polymorphisms with susceptibility to systemic sclerosis. Annals of the Rheumatic Diseases. 2010;**69**(3):550-555

[75] Sun X, Haider Ali MSS, Moran M. The role of interactions of long non-coding RNAs and heterogeneous nuclear ribonucleoproteins in regulating cellular functions. The Biochemical Journal. 2017;**474**(17):2925-2935

[76] Chung MC, Kim HK, Kawamoto S. TFEC can function as a transcriptional activator of the nonmuscle myosin II heavy chain—A gene in transfected cells. Biochemistry. 2001;**40**(30):8887-8897

[77] Zhao GQ, Zhao Q, Zhou X, Mattei MG, de Crombrugghe B. TFEC, a basic helix-loop-helix protein, forms heterodimers with TFE3 and inhibits TFE3-dependent transcription activation. Molecular and Cellular Biology. 1993;**13**(8):4505-4512

[78] Mahony CB, Fish RJ, Pasche C, Bertrand JY. tfec controls the hematopoietic stem cell vascular niche during zebrafish embryogenesis. Blood. 2016;**128**(10):1336-1345

[79] Moriggi G, Nieto B, Dosil M. Rrp12 and the Exportin Crm1 participate in late assembly events in the nucleolus during 40S ribosomal subunit biogenesis. PLoS Genetics. 2014;**10**(12):e1004836

[80] Yang SH, Jung HJ, Coffinier C, Fong LG, Young SG. Are B-type lamins essential in all mammalian cells? Nucleus. 2011;**2**(6):562-569

[81] Bolotin E, Armendariz A, Kim K, Heo SJ, Boffelli D, Tantisira K, et al. Statin-induced changes in gene expression in EBV-transformed and native B-cells. Human Molecular Genetics. 2014;**23**(5):1202-1210

[82] Ranuncolo SM, Polo JM, Melnick A. BCL6 represses CHEK1 and suppresses DNA damage pathways in normal and malignant B-cells. Blood Cells, Molecules & Diseases. 2008;**41**(1):95-99

[83] Ly LL, Yoshida H, Yamaguchi M. Nuclear transcription factor Y and its roles in cellular processes related to human disease. American Journal of Cancer Research. 2013;**3**(4):339-346

[84] Corson TW, Huang A, Tsao MS, Gallie BL. KIF14 is a candidate oncogene in the 1q minimal region of genomic gain in multiple cancers. Oncogene. 2005;**24**(30):4741-4753

[85] Jiang W, Jimenez G, Wells NJ, Hope TJ, Wahl GM, Hunter T, et al. PRC1: A human mitotic spindle-associated CDK substrate protein required for cytokinesis. Molecular Cell. 1998;**2**(6):877-885

[86] Tang H, Xiao G, Behrens C, Schiller J, Allen J, Chow CW, et al. A 12-gene set predicts survival benefits from adjuvant chemotherapy in non-small cell lung cancer patients.

Clinical Cancer Research: An Official Journal of the American Association for Cancer Research. 2013;**19**(6):1577-1586

[87] Glotzer M. The molecular requirements for cytokinesis. Science. 2005;**307**(5716):1735-1739

[88] Gruneberg U, Neef R, Li X, Chan EH, Chalamalasetty RB, Nigg EA, et al. KIF14 and citron kinase act together to promote efficient cytokinesis. The Journal of Cell Biology. 2006;**172**(3):363-372

[89] Chattopadhyay S, Bielinsky AK. Human Mcm10 regulates the catalytic subunit of DNA polymerase-alpha and prevents DNA damage during replication. Molecular Biology of the Cell. 2007;**18**(10):4085-4095

[90] Xu X, Rochette PJ, Feyissa EA, TV S, Liu Y. MCM10 mediates RECQ4 association with MCM2–7 helicase complex during DNA replication. The EMBO Journal. 2009;**28**(19): 3005-3014

[91] Kliszczak M, Sedlackova H, Pitchai GP, Streicher WW, Krejci L, Hickson ID. Interaction of RECQ4 and MCM10 is important for efficient DNA replication origin firing in human cells. Oncotarget. 2015;**6**(38):40464-40479

[92] Strzalka W, Ziemienowicz A. Proliferating cell nuclear antigen (PCNA): A key factor in DNA replication and cell cycle regulation. Annals of Botany. 2011;**107**(7):1127-1140

[93] Nakano T, Kamei R, Fujimura T, Takaoka Y, Hori A, Lai CY, et al. Impact of histone H1 on the progression of allergic rhinitis and its suppression by neutralizing antibody in mice. PLoS One. 2016;**11**(4):e0153630

[94] Kohno M, Hasegawa H, Inoue A, Muraoka M, Miyazaki T, Oka K, et al. Identification of N-arachidonylglycine as the endogenous ligand for orphan G-protein-coupled receptor GPR18. Biochemical and Biophysical Research Communications. 2006;**347**(3):827-832

[95] Flegel C, Vogel F, Hofreuter A, Wojcik S, Schoeder C, Kiec-Kononowicz K, et al. Characterization of non-olfactory GPCRs in human sperm with a focus on GPR18. Scientific Reports. 2016;**6**:32255

[96] Shahbazi J, Lock R, Liu T. Tumor protein 53-induced nuclear protein 1 enhances p53 function and represses tumorigenesis. Frontiers in Genetics. 2013;**4**:80

[97] Seillier M, Peuget S, Gayet O, Gauthier C, N'Guessan P, Monte M, et al. TP53INP1, a tumor suppressor, interacts with LC3 and ATG8-family proteins through the LC3-interacting region (LIR) and promotes autophagy-dependent cell death. Cell Death and Differentiation. 2012;**19**(9):1525-1535

[98] Del Nery E, Miserey-Lenkei S, Falguieres T, Nizak C, Johannes L, Perez F, et al. Rab6A and Rab6A' GTPases play non-overlapping roles in membrane trafficking. Traffic. 2006; **7**(4):394-407

[99] Opdam FJ, Echard A, Croes HJ, van den Hurk JA, van de Vorstenbosch RA, Ginsel LA, et al. The small GTPase Rab6B, a novel Rab6 subfamily member, is cell-type specifically expressed and localised to the Golgi apparatus. Journal of Cell Science. 2000;**113**(Pt 15): 2725-2735

[100] Thornton AM, Korty PE, Tran DQ, Wohlfert EA, Murray PE, Belkaid Y, et al. Expression of Helios, an Ikaros transcription factor family member, differentiates thymic-derived from peripherally induced Foxp3+ T regulatory cells. Journal of Immunology. 2010;**184**(7): 3433-3441

[101] Santos-Cortez RL, Lee K, Giese AP, Ansar M, Amin-Ud-Din M, Rehn K, et al. Adenylate cyclase 1 (ADCY1) mutations cause recessive hearing impairment in humans and defects in hair cell function and hearing in zebrafish. Human Molecular Genetics. 2014;**23**(12):3289-3298

[102] Gawad C, Koh W, Quake SR. Single-cell genome sequencing: Current state of the science. Nature Reviews Genetics. 2016;**17**(3):175-188

[103] Bertsias GK, Salmon JE, Boumpas DT. Therapeutic opportunities in systemic lupus erythematosus: State of the art and prospects for the new decade. Annals of the Rheumatic Diseases. 2010;**69**(9):1603-1611

[104] Sanz I, Lee FEB. Cells as therapeutic targets in SLE. Nature Reviews Rheumatology. 2010;**6**(6):326-337

[105] Inoue M, Yamada J, Aomatsu-Kikuchi E, Satoh K, Kondo H, Ishisaki A, et al. SCRG1 suppresses LPS-induced CCL22 production through ERK1/2 activation in mouse macrophage Raw264.7 cells. Molecular Medicine Reports. 2017;**15**(6):4069-4076

[106] Oeckinghaus A, Hayden MS, Ghosh S. Crosstalk in NF-kappaB signaling pathways. Nature Immunology. 2011;**12**(8):695-708

[107] Das UN, Rao AA. Gene expression profile in obesity and type 2 diabetes mellitus. Lipids in Health and Disease. 2007;**6**:35

[108] Suhasini M, Pilz RB. Transcriptional elongation of c-myb is regulated by NF-kappaB (p50/RelB). Oncogene. 1999;**18**(51):7360-7369

[109] Kawai T, Akira S. TLR signaling. Cell Death and Differentiation. 2006;**13**(5):816-825

[110] Kondoh K, Nishida E. Regulation of MAP kinases by MAP kinase phosphatases. Biochimica et Biophysica Acta. 2007;**1773**(8):1227-1237

[111] Dunkelberger JR, Song WC. Complement and its role in innate and adaptive immune responses. Cell Research. 2010;**20**(1):34-50

[112] Li JZ, Bunney BG, Meng F, Hagenauer MH, Walsh DM, Vawter MP, et al. Circadian patterns of gene expression in the human brain and disruption in major depressive disorder. Proceedings of the National Academy of Sciences of the United States of America. 2013;**110**(24):9950-9955

[113] Pone EJ, Zhang J, Mai T, White CA, Li G, Sakakura JK, et al. BCR-signalling synergizes with TLR-signalling for induction of AID and immunoglobulin class-switching through the non-canonical NF-kappaB pathway. Nature Communications. 2012;**3**:767

[114] Coulthard MG, Morgan M, Woodruff TM, Arumugam TV, Taylor SM, Carpenter TC, et al. Eph/Ephrin signaling in injury and inflammation. The American Journal of Pathology. 2012;**181**(5):1493-1503

[115] Lee SJ, Park SS, Cho YH, Park K, Kim EJ, Jung KH, et al. Activation of matrix metalloproteinase-9 by TNF-alpha in human urinary bladder cancer HT1376 cells: The role of MAP kinase signaling pathways. Oncology Reports. 2008;**19**(4):1007-1013

[116] Mastrototaro L, Tietjen U, Sponder G, Vormann J, Aschenbach JR, Kolisek M. Insulin modulates the Na+/Mg2+ exchanger SLC41A1 and influences Mg2+ efflux from intracellular stores in transgenic HEK293 cells. The Journal of Nutrition. 2015;**145**(11):2440-2447

[117] Miller AJ, Levy C, Davis IJ, Razin E, Fisher DE. Sumoylation of MITF and its related family members TFE3 and TFEB. The Journal of Biological Chemistry. 2005;**280**(1):146-155

[118] Pecina-Slaus N. Wnt signal transduction pathway and apoptosis: A review. Cancer Cell International. 2010;**10**:22

[119] Yang SH, Chang SY, Yin L, Tu Y, Hu Y, Yoshinaga Y, et al. An absence of both lamin B1 and lamin B2 in keratinocytes has no effect on cell proliferation or the development of skin and hair. Human Molecular Genetics. 2011;**20**(18):3537-3544

[120] Shi YF, Fong CC, Zhang Q, Cheung PY, Tzang CH, RS W, et al. Hypoxia induces the activation of human hepatic stellate cells LX-2 through TGF-beta signaling pathway. FEBS Letters. 2007;**581**(2):203-210

[121] Du J, Johnson LM, Jacobsen SE, Patel DJDNA. Methylation pathways and their crosstalk with histone methylation. Nature Reviews Molecular Cell Biology. 2015;**16**(9):519-532

[122] Khanna KK, Jackson SP. DNA double-strand breaks: Signaling, repair and the cancer connection. Nature Genetics. 2001;**27**(3):247-254

[123] Tseliou M, Al-Qahtani A, Alarifi S, Alkahtani SH, Stournaras C, Sourvinos G. The role of RhoA, RhoB and RhoC GTPases in cell morphology, proliferation and migration in human cytomegalovirus (HCMV) infected glioblastoma cells. Cellular Physiology and Biochemistry: International Journal of Experimental Cellular Physiology, Biochemistry, and Pharmacology. 2016;**38**(1):94-109

[124] Katsha A, Belkhiri A, Goff L, El-Rifai W. Aurora kinase A in gastrointestinal cancers: Time to target. Molecular Cancer. 2015;**14**:106

[125] Moldovan GL, Pfander B, Jentsch S. PCNA the maestro of the replication fork. Cell. 2007;**129**(4):665-679

[126] Huen MS, Chen J. The DNA damage response pathways: At the crossroad of protein modifications. Cell Research. 2008;**18**(1):8-16

[127] Mjelle R, Hegre SA, Aas PA, Slupphaug G, Drablos F, Saetrom P, et al. Cell cycle regulation of human DNA repair and chromatin remodeling genes. DNA Repair. 2015;**30**:53-67

[128] Shi GX, Harrison K, Han SB, Moratz C, Kehrl JH. Toll-like receptor signaling alters the expression of regulator of G protein signaling proteins in dendritic cells: Implications for G protein-coupled receptor signaling. Journal of Immunology. 2004;**172**(9):5175-5184

[129] Millan-Arino L, Islam AB, Izquierdo-Bouldstridge A, Mayor R, Terme JM, Luque N, et al. Mapping of six somatic linker histone H1 variants in human breast cancer cells uncovers specific features of H1.2. Nucleic Acids Research. 2014;**42**(7):4474-4493

[130] Wen L, Yang Z, Cui W, Li MD. Crucial roles of the CHRNB3-CHRNA6 gene cluster on chromosome 8 in nicotine dependence: Update and subjects for future research. Translational Psychiatry. 2016;**6**(6):e843

[131] Yin H, Chu A, Li W, Wang B, Shelton F, Otero F, et al. Lipid G protein-coupled receptor ligand identification using beta-arrestin PathHunter assay. The Journal of Biological Chemistry. 2009;**284**(18):12328-12338

[132] Perwitasari O, Cho H, Diamond MS, Gale M Jr. Inhibitor of kappaB kinase epsilon (IKK (epsilon)), STAT1, and IFIT2 proteins define novel innate immune effector pathway against West Nile virus infection. The Journal of Biological Chemistry. 2011;**286**(52):44412-44423

[133] Acquati F, Monti L, Lualdi M, Fabbri M, Sacco MG, Gribaldo L, et al. Molecular signature induced by RNASET2, a tumor antagonizing gene, in ovarian cancer cells. Oncotarget. 2011;**2**(6):477-484

[134] Schlager MA, Kapitein LC, Grigoriev I, Burzynski GM, Wulf PS, Keijzer N, et al. Pericentrosomal targeting of Rab6 secretory vesicles by Bicaudal-D-related protein 1 (BICDR-1) regulates neuritogenesis. The EMBO Journal. 2010;**29**(10):1637-1651

[135] Zanger UM, Schwab M. Cytochrome P450 enzymes in drug metabolism: Regulation of gene expression, enzyme activities, and impact of genetic variation. Pharmacology & Therapeutics. 2013;**138**(1):103-141

[136] Ward-Kavanagh LK, Lin WW, Sedy JR, Ware CF. The TNF receptor superfamily in co-stimulating and co-inhibitory responses. Immunity. 2016;**44**(5):1005-1019

[137] Li MM, Emerman M. Polymorphism in human APOBEC3H affects a phenotype dominant for subcellular localization and antiviral activity. Journal of Virology. 2011;**85**(16): 8197-8207

[138] Steidl C, Gascoyne RD. The molecular pathogenesis of primary mediastinal large B-cell lymphoma. Blood. 2011;**118**(10):2659-2669

[139] Elliot DJ, Suharjono LBC, Gillam EM, Birkett DJ, Gross AS, et al. Identification of the human cytochromes P450 catalysing the rate-limiting pathways of gliclazide elimination. British Journal of Clinical Pharmacology. 2007;**64**(4):450-457

Chapter 10

The Interplay between Transcription Factors and Epigenetic Modifications in Th2 Cells

Atsushi Onodera, Kota Kokubo and
Toshinori Nakayama

Additional information is available at the end of the chapter

http://dx.doi.org/10.5772/intechopen.73027

Abstract

Functionally polarized CD4 T helper (Th) cells, such as Th1, Th2, and Th17 cells, are essential for the regulation of acquired immunity. Differentiation of naïve CD4 T cells into Th2 cells is characterized by chromatin remodeling and the induced expression of a set of Th2-specific genes, which include Th2 cytokine genes. In the first stage of this differentiation, a Th2 skewing cytokine environment, especially IL-4, induces STAT6 activation. Activated STAT6 increases the expression of GATA3, a master regulator of Th2 cell differentiation, via direct binding to the *Gata3* gene locus. This transcriptional induction of *Gata3* mRNA during Th2 cell differentiation is accompanied by dynamic changes in the binding patterns of two epigenetic modification proteins such as Polycomb and Trithorax complexes. Consequently, expressed GATA3 epigenetically modifies and upregulates Th2-specific genes to establish Th2 cell identity. This identity is maintained by high-level expression of the *Gata*3 gene controlled by Menin, which is a member of the Trithorax proteins, after cycles of cultivation *in vitro* and a long-term resting state *in vivo*. Thus, the Menin-GATA3 axis handles the Th2-specific gene regulatory network.

Keywords: Th2, GATA3, STAT6, Menin

1. Introduction

Naïve CD4-positive (CD4+) T cells can differentiate into several effector T cell subsets, mainly known as Th1, Th2, and Th17 cells [1]. Th1 cells perform the crucial function of protecting against viruses and intracellular pathogens. Th17 cells similarly work against extracellular bacteria or fungi. Th2 cells are required for the removal of extracellular parasites. Each effector subset exerts its protective functions through the secretion of unique cytokines. Th1 cells mainly produce IFN-γ, which activates macrophages and CD8 T cells. Th17 cells secrete IL-17A, which propagates cascades of events that lead to neutrophil recruitment, inflammation, and host defense [2]. Th2 cells activate B cells to induce immunoglobulin class switching through IL-4, and enhance mucus production from epithelial cells by IL-13. In addition, Th2 cells recruit eosinophils to induce an inflammatory response through IL-5. However, the responses caused by these subsets are sometimes excessive and result in immunological diseases. For example, an excess amount of Th2 cytokines is known to induce allergic disease, such as asthma [3].

Each subset-specific cytokine enhances differentiation toward the corresponding Th subset, and environmental cytokines decide the differentiation fate of CD4 T cells. For example, IL-12-induced STAT4 activation in Th1 cells and IL-4-induced STAT6 activation in Th2 cells are essential for their respective differentiation [4, 5]. These STAT signals are commonly used for CD4 T cell differentiation into each subset and induce the upregulation of master transcription factors, T-bet in Th1 and GATA3 in Th2 [6, 7]. The master transcription factors directly bind to DNA and regulate the expression of each subset-specific gene, causing epigenetic modification of the DNA, which stabilizes the differentiation program. Due to this epigenetic modification, fully differentiated effector T cells are rarely converted to other Th subsets and are able to maintain their identity during the transition from effector to memory cells.

The Th2 master transcription factor GATA3 collaborates with the epigenetic regulator Menin to induce and stabilize the complex gene regulatory network. Th2-specific genes, which have been identified by gene expression profiling [8, 9], participate in this regulatory network and are controlled by neither, either or both GATA3 and Menin [10]. In fact, GATA3 or Menin deletion results in the loss of Th2 identity [10, 11]. Clarifying the interplay between the transcription factors and epigenetic modifiers is required to comprehend the Th2 cell biology and to identify new therapeutic targets for Th2-mediated immunological diseases [3].

2. STAT6 and GATA3: important transcription factors for Th2 cells

2.1. STAT6 is activated by IL-4 signaling

The most essential pathway promoting the Th2 fate is the IL-4 signaling cascade, followed by activating the transcription factor STAT6 [12–14]. When IL-4 is recognized by its receptor (type-I IL-4R), which consists of IL-4 receptor alpha chain (IL-4Rα) and a common gamma chain (γc), IL-4 can transmit a signal into a cell. Binding of IL-4 induces dimerization of IL-4Rα and γc, resulting in the phosphorylation of tyrosine residues within the intracellular portion of IL-4Rα by Janus Kinases. This phosphorylated intracellular portion of IL-4Rα recruits and phosphorylates signal transducer and activator of transcription (STAT)6, which then forms a dimer and translocates into the nucleus where the dimerized STAT6 regulates the expression of IL-4 target genes. STAT6 recognizes the DNA sequence TTCNNNNGAA, whereas other STAT family proteins prefer the DNA sequence TTCNNNGAA [15].

Like other STAT proteins, a major role of STAT6 is to activate the expression of its target genes, which is how it received its name ("signal transducer and activator of transcription"). The best-known target gene of STAT6 is the *Gata3* gene, and the detailed mechanisms underlying the STAT6-dependent regulation of the *Gata3* gene are described in Section 4. However, some studies have reported that STAT6 also exerts an inhibitory function by occupying overlapping binding sites of other transcription factors and blocking their binding [16, 17]. It is now well known that STAT-mediated repression is important for the lineage commitment of Th subsets [18]. For example, STAT6 binds to the genomic loci of Th1-associated genes and inhibits their expression, and STAT4, a key transcription factor of Th1, acts on Th2-associated genes in a similar way [19].

It has been proposed that the IL-4/STAT6 cascade is necessary for the Th2 phenotype. This fact is also demonstrated by a series of knockout studies. In these studies, IL-4 deficient mice showed impaired Th2 responses, attributed to a reduced Th2 effector cytokine production, loss of IgE class switching, and reduced eosinophilia upon infection with *Nippostrongylus brasiliensis* [20]. A similar but more significant phenotype is observed in STAT6 knockout mice. In addition, STAT6 appears to be highly specific to Th2 functions, as the phenotype of STAT6-deficient mice is largely related to the loss of the Th2 cell function, and deficient mice show normal development with ordinary numbers of T cells [21, 22]. Other STAT signaling cascades are also involved in Th2 polarization. STAT5A and STAT3, which are activated by IL-2 [23] and IL-6 [24], respectively, are also reported to induce the Th2 phenotype. However, STAT5 and STAT3 are activated not only in Th2 but also in other CD4+ T cell subsets. Therefore, only STAT6 exclusively promotes Th2 differentiation.

2.2. GATA3 plays roles in various tissues as well as the immune system

The GATA family proteins (GATA1–6) are conserved transcription factors that contain one or two C2-C2-type zinc-finger motif that recognize the consensus DNA sequence WGATAR [25–27]. Each member of the GATA family has different expression patterns in the body and can be grouped into hematopoietic factors (GATA1–3) and endodermal factors (GATA4–6). Among hematopoietic cells, immune cells, particularly developing and mature T cells, natural killer (NK) cells, and CD1-restricted NKT cells, mainly express GATA-binding protein 3 (GATA3) [6, 28, 29]. Mature mast cells express GATA1 and GATA2 but not GATA3 [30]. Outside of the immune system, GATA3 is also expressed in many embryonic and adult tissues, including the adrenal glands, kidneys, central nervous system, inner ear, hair follicles and skin, and breast tissue [27].

In the immune system, GATA3 is predominantly expressed in T lymphocytes and is essential for the development of CD4 single-positive (SP) cells in the thymus [31–33]. GATA3 exerts an important function at the β-selection checkpoint, which is involved in the CD4 versus CD8 lineage choice in the thymus [34]. It is continuously expressed in peripheral naïve CD4 T cells at a basal level, where the activation of STAT6 induced by the IL-4/IL-4 receptor signaling pathway upregulates *Gata3* mRNA expression during Th2 cell differentiation [35]. GATA3 is thought to be necessary as the master regulator of Th2 differentiation [6, 7], since enforced GATA3 expression induces Th2 differentiation even when the cells are cultured under Th1-skewing conditions [35]. Enforced expression of GATA3 has also been reported to endogenously upregulate GATA3 expression [36]. In addition, the amount of GATA3 protein in Th2 cells is regulated by various posttranscriptional mechanisms [37–39]. Furthermore, high-level expression of GATA3 is essential for the production of large amounts of Th2 cytokines in established Th2 cells [11, 40–42]. The detailed mechanisms underlying the GATA3-dependent regulation of its target genes are described in Section 5.

3. Polycomb and Trithorax proteins: fundamental epigenetic regulators for cell differentiation

3.1. Polycomb and Trithorax proteins epigenetically modify chromatin in a different way

Huge numbers of genes involved in epigenetic regulation have been identified. Many of them encode histone-modifying enzymatic proteins and their interaction partners. Among them, members of the Polycomb group (PcG) and Trithorax group (TrxG) complexes have been recognized as key epigenetic regulators [3, 43–46]. PcG and TrxG proteins were originally identified in *Drosophila*; however, they also play essential roles in controlling mammalian gene expression in various normal and tumor tissues. It has long been thought that PcG and TrxG proteins antagonize each other for turning target gene expression off or on, respectively. PcG proteins mediate gene silencing by controlling the repressive histone mark H3K27me3 (trimethylated histone H3 lysine 27), whereas TrxG proteins mediate gene activation by modifying the permissive histone mark H3K4me3. Both histone-modifying complexes are often found to regulate the same genes at different stages of development [47]. In addition, emerging evidence shows that PcG and TxrG proteins participate in complex regulatory mechanisms in mammalian tissues [48].

PcG complexes are classified into two canonical types such as Polycomb repressive complex 1 (PRC1) and PRC2. Both of them are involved in transcriptional repression. A sequential recruiting mechanism is proposed for the binding of PRC2 and PRC1 to genomic DNA. First, enhancer of zeste (EZH), the enzymatically active subunit of PRC2, methylates H3K27. Next, the PRC1 complex recognizes trimethylated H3K27, resulting in its co-localization with PRC2. In addition, the ring finger protein 1 (RING1), a subunit of PRC1, has a ubiquitin ligase activity for histone H2AK119 [49]. In CD4+ T cells, Ezh2 appeared to directly bind and facilitate the correct expression of the *Gata3* gene during differentiation into effector Th2 cells [50, 51]. In our previous study, Ezh2 bound much more strongly to transcription factor genes, including the *Gata3* gene, than to the cytokine or cytokine receptor genes. Genome-wide, in the genes encoding transcription factors, the Ezh2 binding levels appear to be higher in non-expressed genes than in expressed genes [52].

In contrast, mixed lineage leukemia (MLL) family proteins, which are major subunits of the TrxG complex, have H3K4 methyltransferase activity that induces a change in the chromatin structure to a form permissive for transcription. In mammals, six H3K4 methylases (MLL1–4, SET1A, and SET1B) have been discovered [53]. The H3K4 methylase complexes containing MLL1 or MLL2 are associated with a unique subunit named Menin (encoded by the *Men1* gene in mice). A mutation of *MEN1* has been found in patients with multiple endocrine neoplasia type 1 (MEN1) syndrome [54, 55]. Menin can act as a tumor suppressor and is required for TrxG complex binding to DNA [53]. Menin is also indicated to have essential roles in the immune system, as Menin has been shown to be important for the Th2 cell function both in mice and humans [51, 56]. The MLL3- or MLL4-containing complex associates with the H3K27 demethylase UTX (encoded by the *Kdm6a* gene in mice) and induces demethylation. H3K4 trimethylation appears to be mediated by these MLL-associated complexes in a gene-specific manner. The SET1A- or SET1B-containing complexes have the unique WD repeat-containing 82 (WDR82). TrxG proteins activate target gene expression and/or keep them active, indicating that these proteins are associated with more than simple gene activation [53]. TrxG proteins have more diverse binding molecules than PcG proteins with which they form complexes.

3.2. Spatial interplay between Polycomb and Trithorax complexes

Although many studies have been performed on the nature of PcG proteins and TrxG proteins individually, few have successfully defined how transcriptional counter-regulation is organized by the PcG and TrxG complexes. One pioneering work demonstrated the dynamic transformations of histone modifications during T cell development [57]. In addition, in our previous study, we successfully analyzed how the global signature of PcG and TrxG co-occupied genes changed during the developmental process. This study showed that a binding pattern in which Ezh2 binds upstream and Menin binds downstream of the transcription start site was frequently found at highly expressed genes, and a binding pattern in which Ezh2 and Menin bind to opposite positions was frequently found at low-expressed genes in T lymphocytes. Interestingly, genes showing a binding pattern in which Ezh2 and Menin occupied the same position displayed greatly enhanced sensitivity to Ezh2 deletion [3, 58].

4. STAT6 induces dynamic changes in epigenetic states at the *Gata3* gene locus

4.1. The *Gata3* gene is epigenetically regulated during Th2 cell differentiation

Epigenetic changes at the *Gata3* gene locus in T cells are essential for the acquisition and maintenance of the Th2 cell identity [3, 51, 59]. During Th2 cell differentiation, PcG and TrxG proteins dynamically change their binding patterns at the *Gata3* gene locus. In addition, these epigenetic changes result in GATA3 protein upregulation that consequently induces chromatin remodeling at the Th2 cytokine gene loci, including *Il4, Il5,* and *Il13* [51, 59]. The *Gata3* gene is known to have distal and proximal promoters. Both basal transcription in naïve CD4 T cells and induced transcription in differentiated Th2 cells are controlled by the proximal promoter [51, 60]. In naïve CD4 T cells, PcG complexes bind upstream and TrxG complexes bind downstream of the *Gata3* proximal promoter [51]. During Th2 cell differentiation, PcG proteins dissociate upstream of the *Gata3* proximal promoter, and the binding of TrxG proteins spreads into this region. Consequently, rapid alterations in the binding patterns of PcG and TrxG proteins are observed in the region between the *Gata3* distal and proximal promoters in this period. Histone modification patterns basically exhibit the same behavior; H3K27me3 levels are decreased at the upstream region of the *Gata3* proximal promoter, and H3K4me3 spreads into this region. In contrast, changes in DNA methylation pattern are only observed at exon 2, in which DNA is methylated in naïve CD4 T cells and demethylated in Th2 cells [61]. At present, the mechanism underlying this demethylation process remains unclear.

4.2. STAT6 directly modifies epigenetic states at the *Gata3* gene locus

We identified two functional STAT6 binding sites within the intronic regions of the *Gata3* gene locus [51]. A chromatin immunoprecipitation followed by massively parallel sequencing (ChIP-seq) analysis also identified one STAT6 binding site at the same region [62]. In the absence of STAT6, displacement of PcG by TrxG is not observed. These results indicate that STAT6 directly binds to the *Gata3* gene locus and induces PcG/TrxG displacement, although the precise mechanism is still unclear. A study of human Th2 cells indicated that STAT6 binding was hardly detected at the *GATA3* gene locus, although *STAT6* knockdown was effective for reducing the *GATA3* expression [18]. Interestingly, our ChIP-seq analysis detected one GATA3 binding peak close to one of the STAT6 binding sites at the *Gata3* gene locus [8, 51] and one of the strong peaks on the assay for transposase-accessible chromatin sequencing (ATAC-seq) [63]. This GATA3 binding site may be important for cis-regulation via GATA3-dependent auto activation of the *Gata3* gene [36]. Although STAT6 induces TrxG spreading into the promoter region, the T cell-specific deletion of Menin, a component of the TrxG complex, does not affect Th2 cell differentiation. This suggests that the induction of high-level expression of *Gata3* (i.e. the acquisition of the Th2 cell identity) is dependent on STAT6 and not the Menin/TrxG complex [51]. However, the maintenance of the *Gata3* expression is dependent on the Menin/TrxG complex and independent of IL-4 and STAT6 in Th2 cells. A similar molecular mechanism was found to underlie the *Gata3* expression *in vivo* [10, 64]. In human memory Th2 cells, MLL and Menin form a core transcriptional complex and regulate the *GATA3* expression [65]. Therefore, TrxG proteins represent an essential mechanism underlying transcriptional maintenance in the memory Th2 cell response [3].

4.3. PRC2 components prevent hyperactivation of the *Gata3* gene

In contrast to TrxG proteins, PcG proteins are proposed to maintain their *Gata3* expression at an appropriate level in CD4 T cells [3]. T cell-specific deletion of Ezh2 enhances the sensitivity of IL-4 and results in *Gata3* upregulation and hyper-production of Th2 cytokines [50]. A ChIP-seq analysis revealed that the Ezh2 binding levels were high at the *Gata3* gene locus but very low at the Th2 cytokine gene loci, indicating that Ezh2 controls the Th2 cytokine expression via direct binding to the *Gata3* gene locus. However, measurable levels of H3K27me3 were detected at the *Il4* and *Il13* genes loci, and direct regulation of H3K27me3 by Ezh2 at these genes has also been proposed as important for transcriptional silencing in Th1 cells [66]. In contrast, SUV39H1-dependent H3K9me3 has been found to maintain the silencing of Th1 cell-related genes in Th2 cells [67].

5. GATA3-dependent epigenetic and transcriptional regulation in the Th2 cytokine gene loci

5.1. Chromatin remodeling induced by GATA3 at the Th2 cytokine gene loci

Induction of changes in histone modifications has been reported at the *Il4*, *Il5*, and *Il13* gene loci (so-called the Th2 cytokine gene loci) during Th2 differentiation [12, 59, 68]. Particularly, histone H3K4 methylation and H3K9 acetylation play an important role in forming the open chromatin structure. Thus, the regions that acquire these histone modifications become accessible to transcription factors and are frequently associated with DNase I hypersensitive (HS) sites. Chromatin remodeling at the Th2 cytokine gene loci is necessary for the efficient expression of IL-4, IL-5, and

http://dx.doi.org/10.5772/intechopen.73027

IL-13 in Th2 cells, and GATA3 has been proposed to regulate chromatin remodeling at these genes. Notably, the H3K9 acetylation levels are higher around the GATA3 binding sites at the Th2 cytokine gene loci than the regions without GATA3 binding [8]. However, genome-wide surveys on GATA3 binding and histone modifications suggest that GATA3 binding do not perfectly coincide with changes in permissive histone modifications, which correlate highly with the states of transcription [62, 69]. In fact, some studies suggest that GATA3 acts not only as an activator but also as a repressor in both Th1 and Th2 cells [8]. Although GATA3 is recognized as a master regulator of Th2 cell differentiation, the transcription of many Th2-specific genes is not regulated by GATA3 itself; therefore, GATA3 is not the only essential factor for Th2 differentiation.

5.2. Interaction between GATA3 and regulatory elements

It has been reported that GATA3 interacts with some regulatory elements at Th2 cytokine gene loci, including conserved non-coding sequence (CNS)-1, HSVa, the conserved GATA response element (CGRE), and HSII in intron 2 of the *Il4* gene [12, 68, 70–74]. CNS-1 is located at the intergenic region between the *Il4* and *Il13* genes and was originally described as Th2-specific HS sites (HSS1 and HSS2) [75, 76]. To characterize the function of CNS-1, mice lacking this genomic region was generated [77]. Genetic deletion of the CNS-1 region resulted in a reduction of Th2 cells producing IL-4, IL-5, and IL-13. In this mutant mouse, IL-4 production *in vivo* was also abrogated [77]. However, CNS-1-deficieny had no effect on IL-4 production in bone marrow-derived mast cells [78]. This is consistent with the observation of no HS sites in CNS-1 of mast cells. Although an electrophoresis mobility shift assay showed that GATA3 binds to HSS2 *in vitro* [70, 71], two independent genome-wide GATA3 ChIP-seq data analyses failed to detect significant GATA3 binding peak in the CNS-1 region (**Figure 1**) [8, 79].

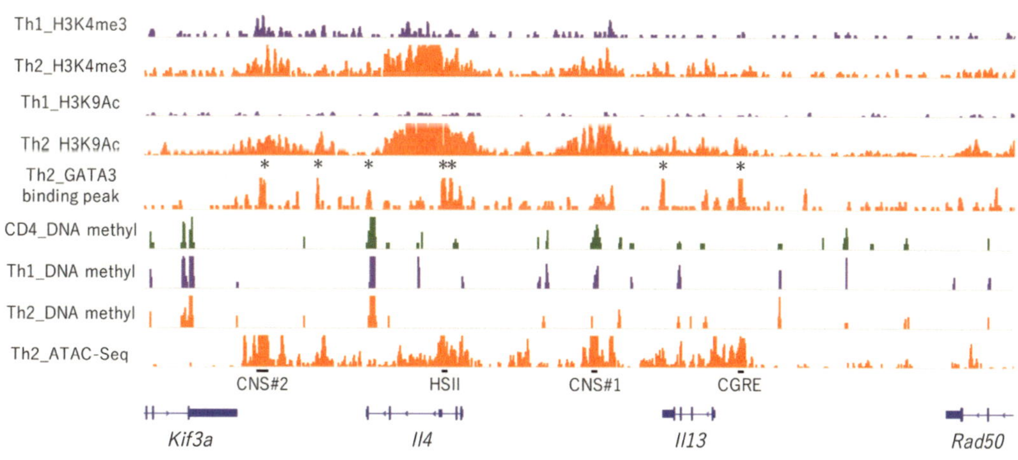

Figure 1. GATA3-dependent epigenetic and transcriptional regulation in the Th2 cytokine gene loci. Epigenetic permissive histone marks (H3K9 acetylation and H3K4 tri-methylation) in the Th2 cytokine loci are shown in Th1 and Th2 cells (GSE28292) using the IGV genome browser (http://www.broadinstitute.org/igv/). GATA3 ChIP-seq data with statistically significant peaks (asterisks) are also shown in Th2 cells. DNA methylation data are shown in CD4+ naïve T, Th1, and Th2 cells (GSE25688). Data from an assay for transposase-accessible chromatin sequencing (ATAC-Seq), which identifies opened chromatin regions, were obtained for lung Th2 cells (GSE77695).

Taken together with the fact that histone acetylation levels are increased with progressive DNA demethylation in the CNS-1 region [61, 80], this region may recruit other critical transcription factors that induce epigenetic modifications and promote IL-4 production in Th2 cells.

HSVa is a TCR re-stimulation-dependent HS site, whose DNase I hypersensitiveness is induced in Th2 cells upon stimulation [72]. HSVa is located 5 kbp downstream of the 3′ end of the *Il4* coding region. Th2 cells generated from the mice in which the genomic region containing both HSVa and HSV (CNS-2) has been deleted display a reduced IL-4 production [81]. Another study reported on the phenotypes of mice with genomes containing the specific deletion of the CNS-2 region [82]. Mice lacking CNS-2 display marked defects in Th2 humoral immune responses. However, the effector Th2 cells involved in tissue responses were not likely to be dependent on CNS-2. In this region, increased histone acetylation levels are observed. In contrast, changes in DNA methylation state are not induced, as DNA is demethylated even in naïve CD4 T cells [80]. By using a conventional ChIP technique, both GATA3 and nuclear factor of activated T cells 1 (NFAT1) have been shown to bind to HSVa in Th2 cells [72]. We and others have performed a GATA3 ChIP-seq analysis and detected GATA3 binding peaks at the HSVa [8, 79], implying that HSVa functions as an important regulatory element through which GATA3 and NFAT1 collaborate to induce IL-4 production in stimulated Th2 cells.

As we reported in 2002, CGRE was originally identified as a region with a 71-bp sequence located 1.6 kbp upstream of the *Il13* gene [73]. The location of CGRE corresponds approximately to the site of HSI. CGRE contains four putative GATA-binding sequences conserved across species [73]. Strong signals of GATA3 binding have been detected by both conventional ChIP assay and ChIP-seq analyses at the CGRE [8, 9, 79]. Interestingly, CGRE is also located at the 5′ edge of the region of histone hyperacetylation, suggesting that GATA3 binds to the CGRE and induces histone acetylation toward the 3′ region of the *Il13* gene. Indeed, GATA3 associates with RNA polymerase II and CBP/p300, which contain histone acetyltransferase activity at this region [73]. In addition, CGRE is located at the 5′ edge of the accessible DNA region detected by ATAC-seq [63]. Thus, the CGRE region may play an important role in *Il13* transcription and in chromatin remodeling at the *Il13* locus. Notably, the Th2 cells generated from CGRE-deficient mice exhibit diminished IL-13 but not IL-4 or IL-5 production [74].

Among several GATA3 binding sites found in the *Il4* gene locus, the strongest GATA3 binding signal was detected at the HSII site located in intron 2 of the *Il4* gene [8]. This region also contains binding sites for STAT5, which has been reported to be important for the maintenance of DNA accessibility of this region in Th2 cells [23, 83]. Correspondingly, a strong ATAC-seq peak was detected at this region in Th2 cells [63]. Recently, a group reported that genetic deletion of HSII resulted in a reduction in IL-4 but not IL-13 production, implying its role in regulating IL-4 production [74]. In addition to histone hyperacetylation induced in this region, H3K4me3 was strongly induced at HSII in Th2 but not Th1 cells [84], suggesting that GATA3 may work together with STAT5 and remodel the chromatin structure at this region. Parallel to changes in histone modifications, progressive DNA demethylation was observed across the *Il4* gene locus. In naïve CD4 T cells, only the promoter region of the *Il4* gene is demethylated, and DNA demethylation extends into the *Il4* gene body during Th2 cell differentiation [80].

http://dx.doi.org/10.5772/intechopen.73027

5.3. GATA3-dependent transcriptional regulation of Th2 signature genes

In addition to regulating chromatin remodeling, GATA3 may induce *Il5* and *Il13* transcription by directly binding to the promoters of these cytokine genes upon TCR re-stimulation [7, 85–87]. In fact, *Gata3* siRNA knockdown just before TCR re-stimulation resulted in reduced expression of *Il5* and *Il13* in established Th2 cells (**Figure 2**). The role of GATA3 in *Il5* and *Il13* transcription was also reported using genetic deletion of the *Gata3* gene. While GATA3 deletion during Th2 differentiation abolished the expression of all Th2 cytokines, GATA3 deletion in established Th2

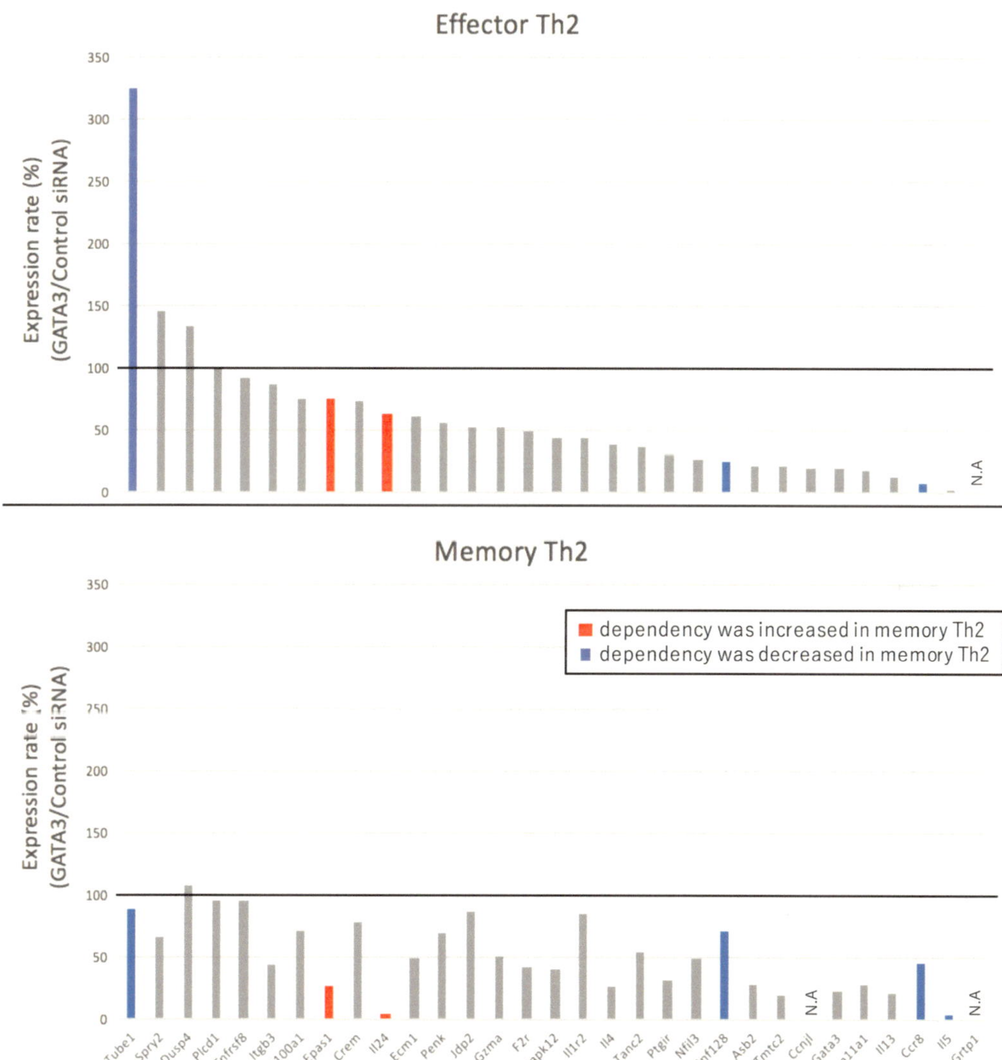

Figure 2. The effects of GATA3 knockdown on the Th2-specific genes in effector and memory Th2 cells. The effects of GATA3 knockdown on effector Th2 (upper) and memory Th2 (lower) were determined with qRT-PCR (originally published in *PLoS ONE*. Sasaki et al. [9]). The relative expression (GATA3/control siRNA) is rank-ordered and shown as a percentage. The genes indicated in the red bar showed increased GATA3 dependency in memory Th2 cells, while those in blue showed decreased GATA3 dependency.

cells strongly influenced the expression of both IL-5 and IL-13 and induced only a modest reduction in IL-4 production [42]. GATA3 is also crucial for the expression of the Th2 cytokine genes in memory Th2 cells, as *Gata3* siRNA knockdown reduces the transcription of those genes [9]. Furthermore, GATA3 is involved in the transcriptional regulation of other Th2 signature genes in both effector and memory Th2 cells (**Figure 2**). Approximately half of the Th2-specific genes (16 out of 31) showed a significant reduction in their expression in effector Th2 cells (*F2r, Mapk12, Il1r2, Il4, Tanc2, Ptgir, Nfil3, Rnf128, Asb2, Tmtc2, Ccnjl, Gata3, Cyp11a1, Il13, Ccr8,* and *Il5*) by GATA3 knockdown. In contrast, only the *Tube1* gene showed a significant increase in its expression. These results suggest that a major role of GATA3 is the activation of its target gene transcription.

Interestingly, changes in GATA3 dependency are observed during transition from effector to memory cells. In a previous study [9], we compared the GATA3 dependency in Th2-specific genes between effector Th2 cells and *in vivo*-generated memory Th2 cells by *Gata3* siRNA knockdown. GATA3 dependency increased by more than twofold in the *Epas1* and *Il24* genes in memory Th2 cells compared to the effector Th2 cells. In addition, for the *Tube1, Rnfl28, Ccr8,* and *Il5* genes, the GATA3 dependency decreased by more than twofold. These results indicate that each Th2-specific gene differentially changes its dependency on GATA3 during maturation to memory Th2 cells from effector Th2 cells. The changes in GATA3 dependency, however, do not correlate with dependency itself. For example, *Il5* is a gene with high dependency on GATA3 that shows a decreased dependency in memory Th2 cells. Taken together, these findings indicate that GATA3 is important for maintaining the transcriptional signatures in established Th2 cells.

6. A gene regulatory network in fully developed Th2 cells: the interplay between GATA3 and Menin, a component of the Trithorax complex

As described in Section 4.2, although Menin deficiency had little effect on the ordinary induction of Th2 differentiation, 'Th2 cells' lost their Th2 identity after several cycles of cultivation in the absence of Menin. Our study also revealed that Menin directly bound and epigenetically regulated the *Gata3* gene, suggesting that constant expression of Menin and its binding to the *Gata3* locus is necessary for the maintenance of the Th2 identity. Similar results were obtained with *in vivo*-generated memory Th2 cells, indicating that Menin maintains the memory Th2 cell function during the long-term resting phase. Indeed, Menin-deficient memory Th2 cells show an impaired ability to recruit eosinophils to the lung, causing the attenuation of airway inflammation induced by memory Th2 cells [52].

Since Th2 cells derived from Menin-deficient mice have defects in both Menin and GATA3 expression, whether the lack of Menin, decreased expression of GATA3, or both are responsible for the dysregulation of the Th2-specific gene expression in Menin-deficient cells remains unclear. In a recent study [52], we addressed this point using differentiated Th2 cells with two additional cycles of cultivation (Th2-3rd cells). Consequently, the gene expression profiles under three conditions (i.e. genetic deletion of Menin, *Gata3* siRNA treatment, and retroviral gene transduction of h*GATA3*) were used to classify the Th2-specific genes into four groups (**Figure 3**). *Asb2, Ccr8, Gzma, Il4, Il5, Il13, Il24, Mapk12, Tanc2,* and *Tube1* were assigned to Group 1, being controlled by both GATA3 and Menin. Interestingly, only *Gzma* was negatively regulated by Menin, while the other nine genes were positively regulated. Although *Gata3* siRNA treatment downregulated the *Gzma* expression, the forced expression of h*GATA3* also reduced the *Gzma* expression for some unknown reason. Seven genes (*Crem, Cyp11a1, F2r, Nfil3, Ptgir, Rnf128,* and *Tmtc2*) were found to be positively controlled by GATA3 and not affected by Menin deficiency (Group 2). Group 3 consisted of *Spry2* and *S100a*, which were found to be controlled in a Menin-dependent and GATA3-independent manner. For the other 11 genes (*Ccnjl, Dusp4, Ecm1, Epas1, Grtp1, Il1r2, Itgb3, Jdp2, Penk, Plcd1,* and *Tnfrsf8*), neither *Gata3* knockdown nor Menin deficiency had a significant effect on the gene expression (Group 4).

In our ChIP-seq analysis, the direct binding of Menin was observed in most of the 31 Th2-specific genes, except for *Asb2, Mapk12, Ecm1, Grtp1,* and *Plcd1*. Nine of the Menin target genes (*Ccr8, Gata3, Il4, Il5, Il13, Il24, S100a1, Tanc2,* and *Tube1*) were positively regulated by Menin, whereas two targets (*Gzma* and *Spry2*) were negatively regulated. No significant effect of Menin deficiency was observed on the other 15 targets (*Ccnjl, Crem, Cyp11a1, Dusp4, Epas1, F2r, Il1r2, Itgb3, Jdp2, Nfil3, Ptgir, Penk, Rnf128, Tmtc2,* and *Tnfrsf8*). Several questions remain to be addressed regarding this regulatory network: Are any other factors involved? What recruits Menin to these gene loci? Why does Menin exert a suppressive effect on some target genes? (**Table 1**).

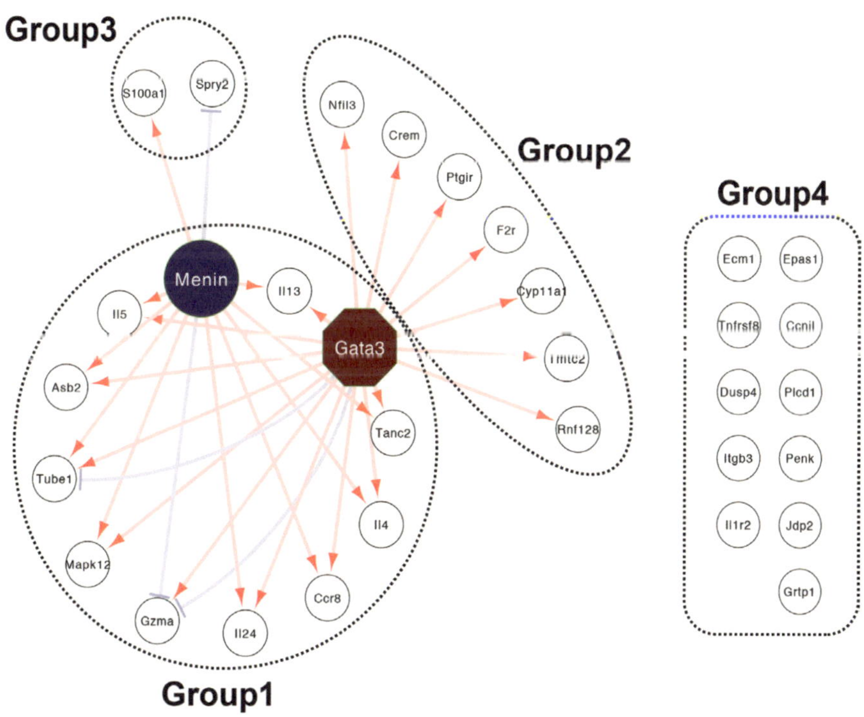

Figure 3. Th2-specific gene regulatory network. The regulatory network formed by Menin- and Th2-specific genes, including GATA3 (originally published in *The Journal of Immunology*. Onodera et al. [10]). Group 1 contains genes that are controlled by both GATA3 and Menin. Genes in Groups 2 and 3 are controlled by either GATA3 or Menin, respectively. Group 4 includes genes that are affected by neither GATA3 knockdown nor Menin knockout. Red arrows indicate the regulatory interactions that activate the target gene expression, whereas blue lines indicate the suppressive effects for targets.

RefSeq ID	Gene symbol	Group	GO term (function, process, or component)
NM_008355	Il13	1	Cytokine activity
NM_010558	Il5	1	Cytokine activity [88]
NM_023049	Asb2	1	Contributes to ubiquitin protein ligase activity [89]
NM_028006	Tube1	1	GTPase activity
NM_013871	Mapk12	1	MAP kinase activity
NM_010370	Gzma	1	Serine-type peptidase activity [90]
NM_053095	Il24	1	Cytokine activity [91]
NM_007720	Ccr8	1	C-C chemokine receptor activity [92]
NM_021283	Il4	1	Cytokine activity [93]
NM_181071	Tanc2	1	In utero embryonic development [94]
NM_017373	Nfil3	2	RNA polymerase II core promoter sequence-specific DNA binding [95]
NM_013498	Crem	2	Core promoter sequence-specific DNA binding [96]
NM_008967	Ptgir	2	G-protein coupled receptor activity
NM_010169	F2r	2	G-protein alpha-/beta-subunit binding [97]
NM_019779	Cyp11a1	2	Cholesterol monooxygenase (side-chain-cleaving) activity [98]
NM_177368	Tmtc2	2	Calcium ion homeostasis
NM_023270	Rnf128	2	Ubiquitin protein ligase activity [99]
NM_011309	S100a1	3	Protein binding [100]
NM_011897	Spry2	3	Negative regulation of ERK1 and ERK2 cascade [101]
NM_007899	Ecm1	4	Interleukin-2 receptor binding [102]
NM_009401	Tnfsf8	4	Tumor necrosis factor-activated receptor activity
NM_176933	Dusp4	4	MAP kinase tyrosine/serine/threonine phosphatase activity
NM_016780	Itgb3	4	Alpha9-beta1 integrin-ADAM8 complex [103]
NM_010555	Il1r2	4	Interleukin-1 receptor activity [104]
NM_010137	Epas1	4	DNA binding transcription factor activity [105]
NM_001045530	Ccnjl	4	Nucleus component
NM_019676	Plcd1	4	Phosphatidylinositol phosphate binding [106]
NM_001002927	Penk	4	Aggressive behavior [107]
NM_030887	Jdp2	4	RNA polymerase II proximal promoter sequence-specific DNA binding [108]
NM_025768	Grtp1	4	Rab GTPase binding

Table 1. Summary of the target genes of the GATA3 and Menin with functions of the encoded proteins (based on https://www.ncbi.nlm.nih.gov/gene).

http://dx.doi.org/10.5772/intechopen.73027

7. Conclusions

Since the human genome project was completed in 2003, the human genomic DNA database has become accessible to researchers [109]. Open access to the reference genomes of humans, mice, and other organisms encourages scientists to develop elegant technologies, including ChIP-seq and high-throughput sequencing of RNA (RNA-seq) [110]. This technique enables us to analyze the epigenetic status of each population of cells on a genome-wide scale. Many scientists have tried to use this technique to clarify the functional roles of epigenetic modifications in gene expression, particularly in the fields of developmental biology and immunology [47].

Recently, we identified several important principles between the binding positions of PcG and TrxG proteins and the gene expression [52]; a binding pattern in which PcG binds upstream and TrxG binds downstream of the transcription start site is frequently found at highly expressed genes, and a binding pattern in which PcG and TrxG bind to opposite positions is frequently found at low-expressed genes in T lymphocytes. We hope that these findings will prove useful for understanding how CD4+ T cells acquire effector functions and identifying new therapeutic targets for treating allergic diseases, such as asthma, allergic rhinitis, food allergy, and atopic dermatitis. A recently developed epigenetic editing technique using the CRISPR/Cas9 system now allows us to modify epigenetic marks in a site-specific manner [111]. In the future, we may use this technique to treat various diseases cause by epigenetic alternations.

Abbreviations

ATAC-Seq	assay for transposase-accessible chromatin sequencing
ChIP-Seq	chromatin immunoprecipitation followed by massively parallel sequencing
CNS	conserved non-coding sequence
H3K27me3	trimethylated histone H3 lysine 27
H3K4me3	trimethylated histone H3 lysine 4
HS	DNase I hypersensitive site
IL	interleukin
PcG	Polycomb group
PRC	Polycomb repressive complex
STAT	signal transducer and activator of transcription
Th	helper T cell
TrxG	Trithorax group

Author details

Atsushi Onodera[1,2], Kota Kokubo[1] and Toshinori Nakayama[1*]

*Address all correspondence to: tnakayama@faculty.chiba-u.jp

1 Department of Immunology, Graduate School of Medicine, Chiba University, Chuo-ku, Chiba, Japan

2 Institue for Global Prominent Research, Chiba University, Inage-ku, Chiba, Japan

References

[1] Zhu J, Yamane H, Paul WE. Differentiation of effector CD4 T cell populations (*). Annual Review of Immunology. 2010;**28**:445-489

[2] Gu C, Wu L, Li X. IL-17 family: Cytokines, receptors and signaling. Cytokine. 2013;**64**(2): 477-485

[3] Nakayama T, Hirahara K, Onodera A, Endo Y, Hosokawa H, Shinoda K, et al. Th2 cells in health and disease. Annual Review of Immunology. 2017;**35**:53-84

[4] Szabo SJ, Kim ST, Costa GL, Zhang X, Fathman CG, Glimcher LH. A novel transcription factor, T-bet, directs Th1 lineage commitment. Cell. 2000;**100**(6):655-669

[5] Kaplan MH, Schindler U, Smiley ST, Grusby MJ. Stat6 is required for mediating responses to IL-4 and for development of Th2 cells. Immunity. 1996;**4**(3):313-319

[6] Zheng W, Flavell RA. The transcription factor GATA-3 is necessary and sufficient for Th2 cytokine gene expression in CD4 T cells. Cell. 1997;**89**(4):587-596

[7] Zhang DH, Cohn L, Ray P, Bottomly K, Ray A. Transcription factor GATA-3 is differentially expressed in murine Th1 and Th2 cells and controls Th2-specific expression of the interleukin-5 gene. The Journal of Biological Chemistry. 1997;**272**(34):21597-21603

[8] Horiuchi S, Onodera A, Hosokawa H, Watanabe Y, Tanaka T, Sugano S, et al. Genome-wide analysis reveals unique regulation of transcription of Th2-specific genes by GATA3. Journal of Immunology. 2011;**186**(11):6378-6389

[9] Sasaki T, Onodera A, Hosokawa H, Watanabe Y, Horiuchi S, Yamashita J, et al. Genome-wide gene expression profiling revealed a critical role for GATA3 in the maintenance of the Th2 cell identity. PLoS One. 2013;**8**(6):e66468. DOI: 10.1371/journal.pone.0066468

[10] Onodera A, Kiuchi M, Kokubo K, Kato M, Ogino T, Horiuchi S, et al. Menin controls the memory Th2 cell function by maintaining the epigenetic integrity of Th2 cells. Journal of Immunology. 2017;**199**(3):1153-1162. Copyright © [2017] The American Association of Immunologists, Inc

[11] Pai SY, Truitt ML, Ho IC. GATA-3 deficiency abrogates the development and maintenance of T helper type 2 cells. Proceedings of the National Academy of Sciences of the United States of America. 2004;**101**(7):1993-1998

[12] Goenka S, Kaplan MH. Transcriptional regulation by STAT6. Immunologic Research. 2011;**50**(1):87-96

[13] Hebenstreit D, Wirnsberger G, Horejs-Hoeck J, Duschl A. Signaling mechanisms, interaction partners, and target genes of STAT6. Cytokine & Growth Factor Reviews. 2006;**17**(3): 173-188

[14] Maier E, Duschl A, Horejs-Hoeck J. STAT6-dependent and -independent mechanisms in Th2 polarization. European Journal of Immunology. 2012;**42**(11):2827-2833

[15] Ehret GB, Reichenbach P, Schindler U, Horvath CM, Fritz S, Nabholz M, et al. DNA binding specificity of different STAT proteins. Comparison of in vitro specificity with natural target sites. The Journal of Biological Chemistry. 2001;**276**(9):6675-6688

[16] Nguyen VT, Benveniste EN. IL-4-activated STAT-6 inhibits IFN-gamma-induced CD40 gene expression in macrophages/microglia. Journal of Immunology. 2000;**165**(11): 6235-6243

[17] Bennett BL, Cruz R, Lacson RG, Manning AM. Interleukin-4 suppression of tumor necrosis factor alpha-stimulated E-selectin gene transcription is mediated by STAT6 antagonism of NF-kappaB. The Journal of Biological Chemistry. 1997;**272**(15):10212-10219

[18] Elo LL, Jarvenpaa H, Tuomela S, Raghav S, Ahlfors H, Laurila K, et al. Genome-wide profiling of interleukin-4 and STAT6 transcription factor regulation of human Th2 cell programming. Immunity. 2010;**32**(6):852-862

[19] O'Shea JJ, Lahesmaa R, Vahedi G, Laurence A, Kanno Y. Genomic views of STAT function in CD4+ T helper cell differentiation. Nature Reviews. Immunology. 2011;**11**(4):239-250

[20] Kopf M, Le Gros G, Bachmann M, Lamers MC, Bluethmann H, Kohler G. Disruption of the murine IL-4 gene blocks Th2 cytokine responses. Nature. 1993;**362**(6417):245-248

[21] Wurster AL, Tanaka T, Grusby MJ. The biology of Stat4 and Stat6. Oncogene. 2000;**19**(21): 2577-2584

[22] Takeda K, Tanaka T, Shi W, Matsumoto M, Minami M, Kashiwamura S, et al. Essential role of Stat6 in IL-4 signalling. Nature. 1996;**380**(6575):627-630

[23] Cote-Sierra J, Foucras G, Guo L, Chiodetti L, Young HA, Hu-Li J, et al. Interleukin 2 plays a central role in Th2 differentiation. Proceedings of the National Academy of Sciences of the United States of America. 2004;**101**(11):3880-3885

[24] Stritesky GL, Muthukrishnan R, Sehra S, Goswami R, Pham D, Travers J, et al. The transcription factor STAT3 is required for T helper 2 cell development. Immunity. 2011;**34**(1): 39-49

[25] Mosmann TR, Coffman RL. TH1 and TH2 cells: Different patterns of lymphokine secretion lead to different functional properties. Annual Review of Immunology. 1989;**7**:145-173

[26] Reiner SL, Locksley RM. The regulation of immunity to Leishmania major. Annual Review of Immunology. 1995;**13**:151-177

[27] Ho IC, Tai TS, Pai SY. GATA3 and the T-cell lineage: Essential functions before and after T-helper-2-cell differentiation. Nature Reviews. Immunology. 2009;**9**(2):125-135

[28] Korn T, Bettelli E, Oukka M, Kuchroo VK. IL-17 and Th17 cells. Annual Review of Immunology. 2009;**27**:485-517

[29] Szabo SJ, Sullivan BM, Stemmann C, Satoskar AR, Sleckman BP, Glimcher LH. Distinct effects of T-bet in TH1 lineage commitment and IFN-gamma production in CD4 and CD8 T cells. Science. 2002;**295**(5553):338-342

[30] Lee HJ, Takemoto N, Kurata H, Kamogawa Y, Miyatake S, O'Garra A, et al. GATA-3 induces T helper cell type 2 (Th2) cytokine expression and chromatin remodeling in committed Th1 cells. The Journal of Experimental Medicine. 2000;**192**(1):105-115

[31] Pai SY, Truitt ML, Ting CN, Leiden JM, Glimcher LH, Ho IC. Critical roles for transcription factor GATA-3 in thymocyte development. Immunity. 2003;**19**(6):863-875

[32] Hernandez-Hoyos G, Anderson MK, Wang C, Rothenberg EV, Alberola-Ila J. GATA-3 expression is controlled by TCR signals and regulates CD4/CD8 differentiation. Immunity. 2003;**19**(1):83-94

[33] Yamamoto M, Ko LJ, Leonard MW, Beug H, Orkin SH, Engel JD. Activity and tissue-specific expression of the transcription factor NF-E1 multigene family. Genes & Development. 1990;**4**(10):1650-1662

[34] Hosoya T, Maillard I, Engel JD. From the cradle to the grave: Activities of GATA-3 throughout T-cell development and differentiation. Immunological Reviews. 2010;**238**(1):110-125

[35] Ouyang W, Ranganath SH, Weindel K, Bhattacharya D, Murphy TL, Sha WC, et al. Inhibition of Th1 development mediated by GATA-3 through an IL-4-independent mechanism. Immunity. 1998;**9**(5):745-755

[36] Ouyang W, Lohning M, Gao Z, Assenmacher M, Ranganath S, Radbruch A, et al. Stat6-independent GATA-3 autoactivation directs IL-4-independent Th2 development and commitment. Immunity. 2000;**12**(1):27-37

[37] Hosokawa H, Kimura MY, Shinnakasu R, Suzuki A, Miki T, Koseki H, et al. Regulation of Th2 cell development by Polycomb group gene bmi-1 through the stabilization of GATA3. Journal of Immunology. 2006;**177**(11):7656-7664

[38] Shinnakasu R, Yamashita M, Shinoda K, Endo Y, Hosokawa H, Hasegawa A, et al. Critical YxKxHxxxRP motif in the C-terminal region of GATA3 for its DNA binding and function. Journal of Immunology. 2006;**177**(9):5801-5810

[39] Yamashita M, Shinnakasu R, Asou H, Kimura M, Hasegawa A, Hashimoto K, et al. Ras-ERK MAPK cascade regulates GATA3 stability and Th2 differentiation through ubiquitin-proteasome pathway. The Journal of Biological Chemistry. 2005;**280**(33):29409-29419

[40] Yamashita M, Ukai-Tadenuma M, Miyamoto T, Sugaya K, Hosokawa H, Hasegawa A, et al. Essential role of GATA3 for the maintenance of type 2 helper T (Th2) cytokine production and chromatin remodeling at the Th2 cytokine gene loci. The Journal of Biological Chemistry. 2004;**279**(26):26983-26990

[41] Inami M, Yamashita M, Tenda Y, Hasegawa A, Kimura M, Hashimoto K, et al. CD28 costimulation controls histone hyperacetylation of the interleukin 5 gene locus in developing th2 cells. The Journal of Biological Chemistry. 2004;**279**(22):23123-23133

[42] Zhu J, Min B, Hu-Li J, Watson CJ, Grinberg A, Wang Q, et al. Conditional deletion of Gata3 shows its essential function in T(H)1-T(H)2 responses. Nature Immunology. 2004;**5**(11): 1157-1165

[43] Nakayama T, Yamashita M. Critical role of the Polycomb and Trithorax complexes in the maintenance of CD4 T cell memory. Seminars in Immunology. 2009;**21**(2):78-83

[44] Onodera A, Nakayama T. Epigenetics of T cells regulated by Polycomb/Trithorax molecules. Trends in Molecular Medicine. 2015;**21**(5):330-340

[45] Di Croce L, Helin K. Transcriptional regulation by Polycomb group proteins. Nature Structural & Molecular Biology. 2013;**20**(10):1147-1155

[46] Mohan M, Herz HM, Shilatifard A. SnapShot: Histone lysine methylase complexes. Cell. 2012;**149**(2):498-4e1

[47] Steffen PA, Ringrose L. What are memories made of? How Polycomb and Trithorax proteins mediate epigenetic memory. Nature Reviews. Molecular Cell Biology. 2014;**15**(5):340-356

[48] Hopkin AS, Gordon W, Klein RH, Espitia F, Daily K, Zeller M, et al. GRHL3/GET1 and trithorax group members collaborate to activate the epidermal progenitor differentiation program. PLoS Genetics. 2012;**8**(7):e1002829

[49] Wang H, Wang L, Erdjument-Bromage H, Vidal M, Tempst P, Jones RS, et al. Role of histone H2A ubiquitination in Polycomb silencing. Nature. 2004;**431**(7010):873-878

[50] Tumes DJ, Onodera A, Suzuki A, Shinoda K, Endo Y, Iwamura C, et al. The polycomb protein Ezh2 regulates differentiation and plasticity of CD4(+) T helper type 1 and type 2 cells. Immunity. 2013;**39**(5):819-832

[51] Onodera A, Yamashita M, Endo Y, Kuwahara M, Tofukuji S, Hosokawa H, et al. STAT6-mediated displacement of polycomb by trithorax complex establishes long-term maintenance of GATA3 expression in T helper type 2 cells. The Journal of Experimental Medicine. 2010;**207**(11):2493-2506

[52] Onodera A, Tumes DJ, Watanabe Y, Hirahara K, Kaneda A, Sugiyama F, et al. Spatial interplay between polycomb and trithorax complexes controls transcriptional activity in T lymphocytes. Molecular and Cellular Biology. 2015;**35**(22):3841-3853

[53] Schuettengruber B, Martinez AM, Iovino N, Cavalli G. Trithorax group proteins: Switching genes on and keeping them active. Nature Reviews. Molecular Cell Biology. 2011;**12**(12):799-814

[54] Matkar S, Thiel A, Hua X. Menin: A scaffold protein that controls gene expression and cell signaling. Trends in Biochemical Sciences. 2013;**38**(8):394-402

[55] Balogh K, Racz K, Patocs A, Hunyady L. Menin and its interacting proteins: Elucidation of menin function. Trends in Endocrinology and Metabolism. 2006;**17**(9):357-364

[56] Nakata Y, Brignier AC, Jin S, Shen Y, Rudnick SI, Sugita M, et al. C-Myb, Menin, GATA-3, and MLL form a dynamic transcription complex that plays a pivotal role in human T helper type 2 cell development. Blood. 2010;**116**(8):1280-1290

[57] Zhang JA, Mortazavi A, Williams BA, Wold BJ, Rothenberg EV. Dynamic transformations of genome-wide epigenetic marking and transcriptional control establish T cell identity. Cell. 2012;**149**(2):467-482

[58] Margueron R, Reinberg D. The polycomb complex PRC2 and its mark in life. Nature. 2011;**469**(7330):343-349

[59] Ansel KM, Djuretic I, Tanasa B, Rao A. Regulation of Th2 differentiation and Il4 locus accessibility. Annual Review of Immunology. 2006;**24**:607-656

[60] Scheinman EJ, Avni O. Transcriptional regulation of GATA3 in T helper cells by the integrated activities of transcription factors downstream of the interleukin-4 receptor and T cell receptor. The Journal of Biological Chemistry. 2009;**284**(5):3037-3048

[61] Deaton AM, Webb S, Kerr AR, Illingworth RS, Guy J, Andrews R, et al. Cell type-specific DNA methylation at intragenic CpG islands in the immune system. Genome Research. 2011;**21**(7):1074-1086

[62] Wei L, Vahedi G, Sun HW, Watford WT, Takatori H, Ramos HL, et al. Discrete roles of STAT4 and STAT6 transcription factors in tuning epigenetic modifications and transcription during T helper cell differentiation. Immunity. 2010;**32**(6):840-851

[63] Shih HY, Sciume G, Mikami Y, Guo L, Sun HW, Brooks SR, et al. Developmental acquisition of regulomes underlies innate lymphoid cell functionality. Cell. 2016;**165**(5):1120-1133

[64] Yamashita M, Hirahara K, Shinnakasu R, Hosokawa H, Norikane S, Kimura MY, et al. Crucial role of MLL for the maintenance of memory T helper type 2 cell responses. Immunity. 2006;**24**(5):611-622

[65] Liu J, Cao L, Chen J, Song S, Lee IH, Quijano C, et al. Bmi1 regulates mitochondrial function and the DNA damage response pathway. Nature. 2009;**459**(7245):387-392

[66] Koyanagi M, Baguet A, Martens J, Margueron R, Jenuwein T, Bix M. EZH2 and histone 3 trimethyl lysine 27 associated with Il4 and Il13 gene silencing in Th1 cells. The Journal of Biological Chemistry. 2005;**280**(36):31470-31477

[67] Allan RS, Zueva E, Cammas F, Schreiber HA, Masson V, Belz GT, et al. An epigenetic silencing pathway controlling T helper 2 cell lineage commitment. Nature. 2012;**487**(7406): 249-253

[68] Yagi R, Zhu J, Paul WE. An updated view on transcription factor GATA3-mediated regulation of Th1 and Th2 cell differentiation. International Immunology. 2011;**23**(7):415-420

[69] Yu M, Riva L, Xie H, Schindler Y, Moran TB, Cheng Y, et al. Insights into GATA-1-mediated gene activation versus repression via genome-wide chromatin occupancy analysis. Molecular Cell. 2009;**36**(4):682-695

[70] Takemoto N, Kamogawa Y, Jun Lee H, Kurata H, Arai KI, O'Garra A, et al. Cutting edge: Chromatin remodeling at the IL-4/IL-13 intergenic regulatory region for Th2-specific cytokine gene cluster. Journal of Immunology. 2000;**165**(12):6687-6691

[71] Takemoto N, Arai K, Miyatake S. Cutting edge: The differential involvement of the N-finger of GATA-3 in chromatin remodeling and transactivation during Th2 development. Journal of Immunology. 2002;**169**(8):4103-4107

[72] Agarwal S, Avni O, Rao A. Cell-type-restricted binding of the transcription factor NFAT to a distal IL-4 enhancer in vivo. Immunity. 2000;**12**(6):643-652

[73] Yamashita M, Ukai-Tadenuma M, Kimura M, Omori M, Inami M, Taniguchi M, et al. Identification of a conserved GATA3 response element upstream proximal from the interleukin-13 gene locus. The Journal of Biological Chemistry. 2002;**277**(44):42399-42408

[74] Tanaka S, Motomura Y, Suzuki Y, Yagi R, Inoue H, Miyatake S, et al. The enhancer HS2 critically regulates GATA-3-mediated Il4 transcription in T(H)2 cells. Nature Immunology. 2011;**12**(1):77-85

[75] Takemoto N, Koyano-Nakagawa N, Yokota T, Arai N, Miyatake S, Arai K. Th2-specific DNase I-hypersensitive sites in the murine IL-13 and IL-4 intergenic region. International Immunology. 1998;**10**(12):1981-1985

[76] Lee GR, Kim ST, Spilianakis CG, Fields PE, Flavell RA. T helper cell differentiation: Regulation by cis elements and epigenetics. Immunity. 2006;**24**(4):369-379

[77] Mohrs M, Blankespoor CM, Wang ZE, Loots GG, Afzal V, Hadeiba H, et al. Deletion of a coordinate regulator of type 2 cytokine expression in mice. Nature Immunology. 2001;**2**(9):842-847

[78] Monticelli S, Lee DU, Nardone J, Bolton DL, Rao A. Chromatin-based regulation of cytokine transcription in Th2 cells and mast cells. International Immunology. 2005;**17**(11): 1513-1524

[79] Wei G, Abraham BJ, Yagi R, Jothi R, Cui K, Sharma S, et al. Genome-wide analyses of transcription factor GATA3-mediated gene regulation in distinct T cell types. Immunity. 2011;**35**(2):299-311

[80] Lee DU, Agarwal S, Rao A. Th2 lineage commitment and efficient IL-4 production involves extended demethylation of the IL-4 gene. Immunity. 2002;**16**(5):649-660

[81] Solymar DC, Agarwal S, Bassing CH, Alt FW, Rao A. A 3′ enhancer in the IL-4 gene regulates cytokine production by Th2 cells and mast cells. Immunity. 2002;**17**(1):41-50

[82] Vijayanand P, Seumois G, Simpson LJ, Abdul-Wajid S, Baumjohann D, Panduro M, et al. Interleukin-4 production by follicular helper T cells requires the conserved Il4 enhancer hypersensitivity site V. Immunity. 2012;**36**(2):175-187

[83] Zhu J, Cote-Sierra J, Guo L, Paul WE. Stat5 activation plays a critical role in Th2 differentiation. Immunity. 2003;**19**(5):739-748

[84] Wei G, Wei L, Zhu J, Zang C, Hu-Li J, Yao Z, et al. Global mapping of H3K4me3 and H3K27me3 reveals specificity and plasticity in lineage fate determination of differentiating CD4+ T cells. Immunity. 2009;**30**(1):155-167

[85] Lee HJ, O'Garra A, Arai K, Arai N. Characterization of cis-regulatory elements and nuclear factors conferring Th2-specific expression of the IL-5 gene: A role for a GATA-binding protein. Journal of Immunology. 1998;**160**(5):2343-2352

[86] Schwenger GT, Fournier R, Kok CC, Mordvinov VA, Yeoman D, Sanderson CJ. GATA-3 has dual regulatory functions in human interleukin-5 transcription. The Journal of Biological Chemistry. 2001;**276**(51):48502-48509

[87] Kishikawa H, Sun J, Choi A, Miaw SC, Ho IC. The cell type-specific expression of the murine IL-13 gene is regulated by GATA-3. Journal of Immunology. 2001;**167**(8):4414-4420

[88] Iseki M, Takaki S, Takatsu K. Molecular cloning of the mouse APS as a member of the Lnk family adaptor proteins. Biochemical and Biophysical Research Communications. 2000;**272**(1):45-54

[89] Bello NF, Lamsoul I, Heuze ML, Metais A, Moreaux G, Calderwood DA, et al. The E3 ubiquitin ligase specificity subunit ASB2beta is a novel regulator of muscle differentiation that targets filamin B to proteasomal degradation. Cell Death and Differentiation. 2009;**16**(6):921-932

[90] Zhang M, Park SM, Wang Y, Shah R, Liu N, Murmann AE, et al. Serine protease inhibitor 6 protects cytotoxic T cells from self-inflicted injury by ensuring the integrity of cytotoxic granules. Immunity. 2006;**24**(4):451-461

[91] Schaefer G, Venkataraman C, Schindler U. Cutting edge: FISP (IL-4-induced secreted protein), a novel cytokine-like molecule secreted by Th2 cells. Journal of Immunology. 2001;**166**(10):5859-5863

[92] Zingoni A, Soto H, Hedrick JA, Stoppacciaro A, Storlazzi CT, Sinigaglia F, et al. The chemokine receptor CCR8 is preferentially expressed in Th2 but not Th1 cells. Journal of Immunology. 1998;**161**(2):547-551

[93] Casey LS, Lichtman AH, Boothby M. IL-4 induces IL-2 receptor p75 beta-chain gene expression and IL-2-dependent proliferation in mouse T lymphocytes. Journal of Immunology. 1992;**148**(11):3418-3426

[94] Han S, Nam J, Li Y, Kim S, Cho SH, Cho YS, et al. Regulation of dendritic spines, spatial memory, and embryonic development by the TANC family of PSD-95-interacting proteins. The Journal of Neuroscience. 2010;**30**(45):15102-15112

[95] Motomura Y, Kitamura H, Hijikata A, Matsunaga Y, Matsumoto K, Inoue H, et al. The transcription factor E4BP4 regulates the production of IL-10 and IL-13 in CD4+ T cells. Nature Immunology. 2011;**12**(5):450-459

[96] Zmrzljak UP, Korencic A, Kosir R, Golicnik M, Sassone-Corsi P, Rozman D. Inducible cAMP early repressor regulates the period 1 gene of the hepatic and adrenal clocks. The Journal of Biological Chemistry. 2013;**288**(15):10318-10327

[97] McCoy KL, Traynelis SF, Hepler JR. PAR1 and PAR2 couple to overlapping and distinct sets of G proteins and linked signaling pathways to differentially regulate cell physiology. Molecular Pharmacology. 2010;**77**(6):1005-1015

[98] O'Shaughnessy PJ, Mannan MA. Development of cytochrome P-450 side chain cleavage mRNA levels in neonatal ovaries of normal and hypogonadal (hpg) mice. Molecular and Cellular Endocrinology. 1994;**104**(2):133-138

[99] Borchers AG, Hufton AL, Eldridge AG, Jackson PK, Harland RM, Baker JC. The E3 ubiquitin ligase GREUL1 anteriorizes ectoderm during Xenopus development. Developmental Biology. 2002;**251**(2):395-408

[100] Tarabykina S, Kriajevska M, Scott DJ, Hill TJ, Lafitte D, Derrick PJ, et al. Heterocomplex formation between metastasis-related protein S100A4 (Mts1) and S100A1 as revealed by the yeast two-hybrid system. FEBS Letters. 2000;**475**(3):187-191

[101] Gross I, Bassit B, Benezra M, Licht JD. Mammalian sprouty proteins inhibit cell growth and differentiation by preventing ras activation. The Journal of Biological Chemistry. 2001;**276**(49):46460-46468

[102] Li Z, Zhang Y, Liu Z, Wu X, Zheng Y, Tao Z, et al. ECM1 controls T(H)2 cell egress from lymph nodes through re-expression of S1P(1). Nature Immunology. 2011;**12**(2):178-185

[103] Rao H, Lu G, Kajiya H, Garcia-Palacios V, Kurihara N, Anderson J, et al. Alpha9beta1: A novel osteoclast integrin that regulates osteoclast formation and function. Journal of Bone and Mineral Research. 2006;**21**(10):1657-1665

[104] Zheng Y, Humphry M, Maguire JJ, Bennett MR, Clarke MC. Intracellular interleukin-1 receptor 2 binding prevents cleavage and activity of interleukin-1alpha, controlling necrosis-induced sterile inflammation. Immunity. 2013;**38**(2):285-295

[105] Elvert G, Kappel A, Heidenreich R, Englmeier U, Lanz S, Acker T, et al. Cooperative interaction of hypoxia-inducible factor-2alpha (HIF-2alpha) and Ets-1 in the transcriptional activation of vascular endothelial growth factor receptor-2 (Flk-1). The Journal of Biological Chemistry. 2003;**278**(9):7520-7530

[106] Kim NY, Ahn SJ, Kim MS, Seo JS, Kim BS, Bak HJ, et al. PLC-delta1-lf, a novel N-terminal extended phospholipase C-delta1. Gene. 2013;**528**(2):170-177

[107] Konig M, Zimmer AM, Steiner H, Holmes PV, Crawley JN, Brownstein MJ, et al. Pain responses, anxiety and aggression in mice deficient in pre-proenkephalin. Nature. 1996;**383**(6600):535-538

[108] Jin C, Ugai H, Song J, Murata T, Nili F, Sun K, et al. Identification of mouse Jun dimerization protein 2 as a novel repressor of ATF-2. FEBS Letters. 2001;**489**(1):34-41

[109] Collins FS, Green ED, Guttmacher AE, Guyer MS. A vision for the future of genomics research. Nature. 2003;**422**(6934):835-847

[110] Barski A, Cuddapah S, Cui K, Roh TY, Schones DE, Wang Z, et al. High-resolution profiling of histone methylations in the human genome. Cell. 2007;**129**(4):823-837

[111] Thakore PI, D'Ippolito AM, Song L, Safi A, Shivakumar NK, Kabadi AM, et al. Highly specific epigenome editing by CRISPR-Cas9 repressors for silencing of distal regulatory elements. Nature Methods. 2015;**12**(12):1143-1149

Chapter 11

Post-Transcriptional and Translational Mechanisms of Regulation of Gene Expression in T Cell Subsets

Roman Istomine and Ciriaco A. Piccirillo

Additional information is available at the end of the chapter

http://dx.doi.org/10.5772/intechopen.73319

Abstract

The immune system is under strict regulatory control to ensure homeostasis of inflammatory responses, lying dormant when not needed but quick to act when called upon. Small changes in gene expression can lead to drastic changes in lineage commitment, cellular function, and immunity. Conventional assessment of these changes centered on the analysis of mRNA levels through a variety of methodologies, including microarrays. However, mRNA synthesis does not always correlate directly to protein synthesis and downstream functional activity. Work conducted in recent years has begun to shed light on the various post-transcriptional changes that occur in response to a dynamic external environment in which a given immune cell type encounters. In this chapter, we provide a critical review of key post-transcriptional and translational mechanisms of regulation of gene expression in the immune system, with an emphasis of these regulatory processes in various CD4+ T cell subsets and their related effector functions.

Keywords: inflammation, CD4+ T cells, transcriptional, translatome, immune regulation, immunity

1. Introduction

CD4+ T cells are key players in the adaptive immune response, capable of adapting their function depending on the immune challenge being faced. CD4+ T cells employ a wide variety of signaling pathways to integrate environmental cues and translate them into the requisite gene expression programs required to carry out their effector functions. These gene expression programs are enacted by a complex network of factors, involving the direct action of transcription factors to drive mRNA synthesis, epigenetic modification of DNA accessibility to modulate gene expression, as well as a variety of post-transcriptional mechanisms including RNA-binding proteins and microRNA that influence the stability and translation of synthesized mRNA. This complexity ensures that CD4+ T cells can mount an appropriate and adequate response to a wide variety of pathogens.

2. Transcriptional regulation of CD4+ T cell activation

Complex transcriptional changes are required for CD4+ T cell generation and egress from the thymus (reviewed in [1]). Recent thymic emigrant naïve CD4+ T cells are maintained in the periphery through the action of important cytokines, like IL-7, which support cell survival. Naïve CD4+ T cells maintain high levels of the IL-7 receptor (CD127), which is maintained in part through the action of the transcription factor, ETS-1 [2]. ETS-1 has been shown to directly bind the *il7ra* promoter to maintain expression on the cell surface, with levels of ETS-1 being shown to directly correlate with the levels of CD127 expression. Runx1 is another transcription factor that is required for CD127 expression in naïve CD4+ T cells, possessing a binding site in close proximity to ETS-1 in the *il7ra* promoter [3]. Signaling through CD127 is necessary to trigger phosphorylation of STAT5 and the expression of the antiapoptotic proteins BCL-2, BCL-xL, and MCL-1, all necessary for the survival of naïve CD4+ T cells during homeostatic expansion. This results in the maintenance of the pool of naïve cells prior to antigen engagement of the T cell receptor (TCR) [4]. The recognition of the cognate antigen by the TCR is responsible for the initial changes to the T cell transcriptional program through the activation of the Nuclear Factor of Activated T Cells (NFAT) transcription factor family. In naïve CD4+ T cells, NFAT is maintained in a phosphorylated and inactive state through the action of the kinases GSK3 and CK1 [5, 6]; however, the TCR signaling cascade and subsequent calcium influx result in the dephosphorylation of NFAT by calcineurin allowing for nuclear translocation of NFAT to enact its transcriptional program [7]. The nature of this transcriptional program is dependent on the presence of the NFAT binding partner, AP-1. The AP-1 complex consists of the FOS and JUN transcription factors and is assembled upon activation of the CD28 co-stimulatory pathway [8]. The cooperative action of NFAT and AP-1 drives the transcription of IL-2, which acts in an autocrine and paracrine fashion, and drives the proliferation of CD4+ T cells via phosphorylation of STAT5. STAT5 signaling is responsible for enhancing the transcription of genes necessary for the proliferation and survival of CD4+ T cells following activation, including promoting the expression of the high-affinity component of its own receptor CD25 (IL-2Rα chain), while reducing the transcription of CD127 [9, 10]. Co-engagement of the TCR and CD28 co-stimulatory molecule also promotes the activation of the NF-κB family of transcription factors, necessary to prevent activation-induced cell death and apoptosis [11]. While NFAT and NF-κB are necessary during the initial stages of T cell activation, they are also necessary for the differentiation o CD4+ T cells into distinct Th cell subset each endowed with its cytokine signature and specific effector functions [12, 13]. The CD4+ T cell lineage choice is determined largely by the extracellular milieu and presence of various cytokines that trigger the expression of a diverse network of transcription factors upon activation of the cytokine signaling pathways. This lineage choice is determined by a number of factors including the nature of the pathogen and genetic background of the host. Several Th cell subsets have been identified and include Th1 effector T (T_{EFF}) cells arise to enhance cytotoxic activity of immune cells against intracellular bacterial and viral infections, Th2 cells facilitating antibody generation, and Th17 cells protecting against extracellular pathogens including parasites and fungi, while regulatory T cells (T_{REG}) are necessary for the resolution of inflammation and to control aberrant T cell responses in the periphery to promote self-tolerance [14].

2.1. Transcription factor networks regulating CD4+ T cell differentiation

Th cell lineage commitment is dependent on the expression and function of lineage-specifying transcriptional factors. The transcription factor TBX21 (T-bet) is thought to be the main driver of the Th1 transcriptional program, which is initiated through the activation of STAT pathways by Interferon gamma (IFNγ) and IL-12 secreted by antigen-presenting cells (APCs) [15]. IFNγ-activated STAT1 binds the *Tbx21* promoter to drive the first round of T-bet expression [16]. This prompts the expression of the IL-12 receptor β2 subunit, allowing IL-12 present in the extracellular milieu to activate STAT4, which further drives T-bet expression [17]. T-bet also activates the transcription of the transcription factors H2.0-like homeobox (HLX) and runt-related transcription factor 3 (RUNX3) [18, 19]. T-bet can bind the IFNγ promoter facilitating chromatin looping, allowing for T-bet binding partners HLX and RUNX3 to drive IFNγ expression in Th1 cells [20]. IFNγ acts in a feed-forward loop to drive continued T-bet expression through STAT1. The production of IFNγ is also regulated by the NF-κB family member, RelA, with RelA deficiency being shown to reduce IFNγ expression. Additionally, the recruitment of RelA to the *ifng* locus is dependent on T-bet expression [21]. NFAT has also been shown to act synergistically with T-bet by binding the 5′ enhancer region of the *ifng* gene [22]. However, the NFAT enhancing activity is not limited to the Th1 cell differentiation, as it has been linked to the promotion of a variety of activation-induced genes in CD4+ T cells, with activation of these genes being blocked by calcineurin inhibitors [23]. T-bet is responsible for activating the majority of Th1-related genes including the chemokine receptors CXCR3 and CCR5 as well as the requisite ligand CCL3 and CCL4 for attracting other Th1 cells to the site of inflammation [24]. The T-bet-mediated Th1 transcriptional program also drives the expression of other Th1 cytokines including TNFα and lymphotoxin-α [25].

The Th2 transcriptional program is largely mediated through the action of GATA3. While GATA3 expression is already present in naive CD4+ T cells, it is insufficient to drive Th2 polarization [26]. Enhanced expression of GATA3 in Th2 cells can occur in response to two distinct pathways. IL-4 activates STAT6 to activate the transcription of GATA3 while signaling through the Notch pathway can activate GATA3 transcription independent of STAT6 [27, 28]. Activation of GATA3 induces its partner transcription factor c-MAF [29]. Together, they induce the expression of IL-4, which acts as an enhancer of Th2 differentiation in an autocrine loop through STAT6 leading to increased GATA3 expression [30]. GATA3 and STAT6 act in conjunction to activate transcription of Th2 cytokine genes *il5 and il13,* as well as further transcription of *il4* [26]. The transcription factor BCL3 has also been shown to transactivate the GATA3 promoter [31]. The NF-κB family member p50 is important for Th2 function, as mice lacking p50 are unable to transcribe *il4*, *il5,* and *il13* [32]. NFAT is also known to act as an enhancer for

GATA3 binding to *il4* locus to further cement Th2 lineage commitment due to an IL-4 feed-forward loop [33]. While GATA3 drives the Th2 transcriptional program, it can also restrict Th1 differentiation by repressing the transcription of IFNγ and STAT4 [34]. Conversely, T-bet in conjunction with RUNX3 can suppress *il4* transcription by competing with GATA3 for binding to the *il4* promoter [19].

Th17 cells arise in specific conditions where Th1 and Th2 differentiation can be inhibited as the presence of the Th1 or Th2 transcriptional program can repress Th17 differentiation. The transcription factor RORγT (encoded by the *rorc* gene) is responsible for driving Th17 differentiation and effector function [35]. RORγT induction is dependent on the Transforming Growth Factor β (TGF-β) signaling pathway, which inhibits both Th1 and Th2 differentiation [36, 37]. TGF-β signaling on its own favors the development of T_{REG} cells; however, the presence of exogenous IL-6 redirects cells toward a Th17 fate. IL-6 mediated activation of STAT3 is responsible for blocking expression of the master regulatory transcription factor of T_{REG} cells, Foxp3 [38, 39]. In the absence of Foxp3, TGF-β induces the transcription of RORγT that activates the transcription of Th17-related cytokines including IL-17A/F, IL-21, and IL-22 [35]. IL-21 amplifies STAT3 activity through an autocrine loop to further enhance Th17 differentiation [40]. RORγT is also responsible for inducing the expression of the IL-23R to allow for enhanced maintenance of RORγT expression [37]. Exogenous IL-23 and autocrine IL-21 act in concert with TGF-β to activate further transcription of RORγT, enhancing commitment to the Th17 lineage. The transcription factor DDx5 partner with RORγT to drive Th17 cytokine expression; however, it is dispensable for RORγT induction [41]. DDX5 and RORγT co-localize to the *il17a and il17f* loci to enhance Th17 effector function. The transcription factor BATF is another important early regulator of the Th17 transcriptional program. BATF-deficient mice possess normal Th1 and Th2 differentiation; however, Th17 induction in these mice was severely impaired as they failed to induce the expression of IL-21 and RORγT [42].

T_{REG} cells are central to the maintenance of peripheral tolerance and the resolution of inflammation. T_{REG} cells can differentiate in the thymus or under unique stimulatory conditions in the periphery. As such, The T_{REG} cell pool consists of thymic-derived T_{REG} cells (tT_{REG}) as well as peripherally induced T_{REG} cells (pT_{REG}) cells [43]. Foxp3 expression in tT_{REG} cells has been shown to be dependent on the binding of several transcription factors to both the *foxp3* promoter and conserved noncoding sequences (CNS), which function as enhancers of *foxp3* transcription [44]. The NFAT and AP-1 complexes bind to the *foxp3* promoter following TCR stimulation in the thymus to drive Foxp3 expression [44]. The NF-κB family member c-Rel is responsible for enhancing tT_{REG} generation through binding to CNS3, while the Foxo family member proteins, Foxo1 and Foxo3, enhance expression through binding to the *foxp3* promoter as well as to CNS2 [45, 46]. In the periphery, induction of Foxp3 in pT_{REG} cells is dependent on the action of key cytokines like TGF-β. TGF-β signaling activates Mothers Against Decapentaplegic Homologues 2 and 3 (SMAD2/3), which act in concert with NFAT to drive Foxp3 expression by binding to CNS1 [47]. Foxp3 has been shown to interact with ~361 binding partners that allow it to enable the T_{REG} transcriptional program. Foxp3 acts mostly as a transcriptional repressor preventing the expression of Th1 and Th2 characteristic cytokines including IFNγ, IL-2, and IL-4. This repressive activity is dependent on the interaction of Foxp3 and NFAT and Eos [48–50]. Repression of IL-2 expression and production means that T_{REG} cells, anergic by nature, are entirely dependent on exogenous sources of IL-2 for proliferation and survival. However, this need is in part met by enhanced CD25 transcription by Foxp3. Moreover, upregulation of CD25 in T_{REG} cells allows them to receive the requisite STAT5 signals for the mediation of their suppressive effector function [43]. The transcriptional program enacted by Foxp3 is also responsible for upregulating the expression of genes that give T_{REG} cells their suppressive capacity. This includes the anti-inflammatory cytokine, IL-10, as well as surface proteins such as CTLA4 for contact-dependent inhibition of APCs, and CD39/CD73 to shift the extracellular milieu from an ATP-driven inflammatory state through conversion of ATP to adenosine [48, 51, 52]. T_{REG} cells have also been shown to depend on co-expression of T-bet, GATA3, and RORγT to mediate suppression of the CD4+ Th cell subsets, in turn enabling them to express distinct chemokine receptors to allow T_{REG} cells to traffic to inflammatory sites and suppress the corresponding T_{EFF} cell type [53]. T_{REG} cells are also known to downregulate Foxp3 expression resulting in their reprogramming into highly pro-inflammatory cells under certain inflammatory contexts [54]. However, the nature of environmental triggers, stability, and reversibility of this transformation remains a topic of intense investigation.

3. Epigenetic control of transcriptional programs in Th cell subsets

The transcriptional programs described thus far shed light on the mechanism leading to the differentiation of various CD4+ T cell subsets (**Figure 1**). However, the ability of transcription factors to drive their relative gene expression programs is dependent on several key factors including transcription factor abundance, their location, any posttranslational modifications, and importantly, whether the enhancer or promoter region they bind to is accessible in the DNA. The accessibility of DNA is dictated by chromatin accessibility dependent on nucleosome modifications as well as the methylation status of the DNA itself.

Methylation of cytosines in cytosine-phosphate-guanine (CpG) dinucleotides in promoter and enhancer regions of the DNA has been shown to directly impact the ability of transcription factors to drive mRNA expression by either directly inhibiting transcription factor binding or through recruitment of methyl-CpG-binding domain proteins [55]. DNA methylation markers are transferred to progeny DNA through the action of DNA methyl transferase 1 (DNMT1), while demethylating enzymes such as Tet2 can facilitate the removal of methyl groups from CpG islands [56, 57]. Unlike DNA methylation, the nucleosome modifications present in chromatin can be dynamic and varied. Nucleosomes can vary in their composition with variant form of histone H2, H3, and linker histones being incorporated or removed from the nucleosome to alter DNA accessibility. Histone modifications include the addition of acetyl or methyl groups as well as sumoyl, ubiquitin, and ADP-ribose to modify DNA-binding sites for regulatory elements that can either enhance or repress transcription [58]. Accessible DNA results in the creation of DNase1 hypersensitivity sites, which has allowed for identification of permissive sites in the DNA [59]. Recent studies have uncovered a wide array of possible histone modifications that take place within mammalian cells; however, a few main types of modifications stand out as being characteristic of silenced, readily accessible, and inactive but ready to be transcribed genes. Silenced genes are characterized by the presence of histone H3 with

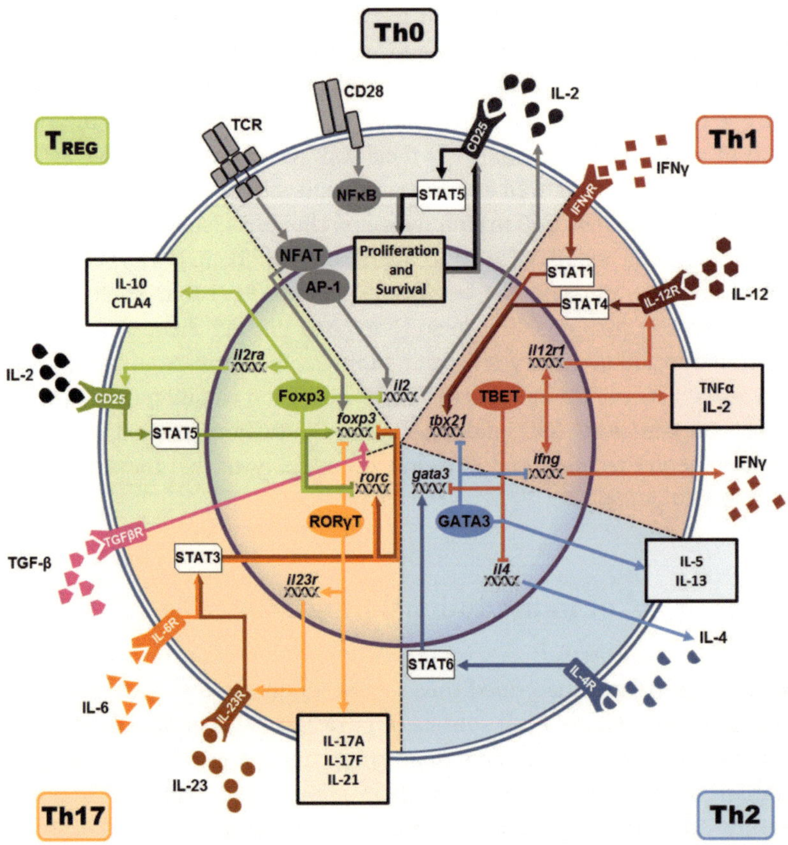

Figure 1. A generalized overview of CD4+ T cell activation and differentiation. Activation of the TCR and CD28 co-stimulation pathways is required for the induction of genes necessary for T cell proliferation and survival, allowing for further differentiation based on requisite signals. Activation of STAT1 and STAT4 pathways, triggered by IFNγ and IL-12 respectively, is required to induce the expression of T-bet resulting in the secretion of IFNγ and other Th1 cytokines. The Th2 lineage is driven by GATA3 upon activation of the STAT6 pathway by IL-4. TGF-β in conjunction with STAT3 activating signals is required to drive a Th17 response via expression of RORγT. Similarly, TGF-β and NFAT can facilitate the conversion of T_{EFF} cells to a T_{REG} phenotype through induction of Foxp3, resulting in the expression of proteins required for T_{REG} suppressive function but making them dependent on exogenous IL-2 for proliferation and survival.

either dimethylation or trimethylation of lysine 9 or 27 (H3K27 and K3 K9), whereas readily accessible and transcribed genes possess single, di-, or tri- methylation of lysine 4 on histone 3 (H3K4) [60]. In addition, the presence of acetyl groups on histones increases the mobility of nucleosomes, allowing enhanced transcription of genes in proximity to acetylated histones. Genes that are inactive but poised and ready to be transcribed possess bivalent modifications incorporating both permissive and silencing modifications. In recently activated naïve CD4+ T cells, the presence of these bivalent modifications at important cytokine loci allows Th subset-dependent factors to make the corresponding loci more accessible while silencing loci associated with alternate lineages. TCR stimulation results in the creation of DNAse-1 hypersensitivity sites in the *ifng* and *il4* loci dependent on the recruitment of NFAT to these loci, as inhibition of TCR activation with CsA ablated the creation of these sites [61].

During Th1 lineage commitment, the *ifng* locus is marked by the presence of both H3K4 and H3K27 modifications; however, progression through Th1 differentiation in response to the initial upregulation of T-bet leads to a significant increase in the presence of permissive H3K4 modifications, while H3K27 modifications are removed throughout the locus [62]. This results in a marked increase of DNase-1 hypersensitivity sites at regulatory elements of the IFNγ locus. STAT4 further contributes to the generation of a permissive environment at this locus through recruitment of chromatin-remodeling complexes to the promoter allowing for increased IFNγ expression [63]. However, while STAT4 signaling is required for enhancing Th1 differentiation, T-bet can drive lineage commitment in the absence of STAT4 signaling due to its ability to bind the *ifng* locus when it is repressively methylated and to recruit histone demethylases to remove repressive H3K27 modifications [64]. Additionally, T-bet is known to recruit methyl-transferases to create permissive H3K4 trimethylation [65]. Thus, T-bet expression can override the repressive modifications to the *ifng* locus during the process of Th2 differentiation.

The epigenetic modifications that arise during Th2 differentiation have been extensively studied in past decades. Unlike the loci for other subset-specific cytokines, the *il4* promoter possesses a reduced degree of CpG methylation allowing low-level transcription of *il4* mRNA following the TCR stimulation, allowing this locus to convert to a more permissive state as the level of Th2 cytokine signaling increases [66, 67]. The increased IL-4 signaling through STAT6 results in the recruitment of histone acetyl transferases to the GATA3 promoter [68]. As the expression of GATA3 increases in Th2 cells, it mediates a variety of epigenetic changes at Th2 cytokine loci. One action of GATA3 is to inhibit the binding of MBD proteins to CpG methyl groups and restrict the action of DNMT1, resulting in a loss of CpG methylation as cells continue to divide under Th2 polarizing conditions [69]. Even in committed Th1 cells, inhibition of DNMT1 results in the ability of Th1 cells to secrete IL-4, demonstrating the importance of GATA3-mediated demethylation of the Th2 cytokine locus in Th2 cell commitment [66]. GATA3 is also able to sustain its own expression through recruitment of methyltransferases to the *gata3* promoter to induce permissive H3K4 modifications, indicating that while STAT6 is necessary for the initiating the conversion of naïve CD4+ T cells to a Th2 phenotype, GATA3 transcriptional activity and epigenetic modifications are responsible for stabilizing commitment to the Th2 cell fate. In addition to maintain Th2 differentiation, GATA3 is known to bind the *ifng* promoter in conjunction with STAT6 to mediate recruitment of methyltransferases to increase the presence of repressive H3K27 modifications, as well as by recruiting histone deacetylase complexes to further repress transcription of the *ifng* locus and suppress Th1 cell commitment [70].

Unlike with Th1 and Th2 differentiation, there is no evidence that the master transcription factor of the Th17 lineage, RORγT, can induce the necessary epigenetic changes to facilitate the Th17 transcriptional program. However, STAT3 is known to recruit histone acetyltransferases to the *il17a* and *il17f* promoters to promote Th17 effector function [71]. Interestingly, analysis of histone modifications in freshly isolated Th17 cells has revealed that they possess bivalent modifications at both the *ifng* and *tbx21* loci, allowing for the generation of IFNγ+IL-17+ Th cells. These loci are thought to become permissive following TCR stimulation, and studies with immunization of OT-II mice with ovalbumin reveal an increase in the amount of double positive cells compared to unimmunized controls with higher levels of *il12rb2* mRNA found within the Th17 cells of immunized mice [72].

The epigenetic landscape of T_{REG} cells is crucial for the induction and stable expression of Foxp3 and ensuing T_{REG} transcriptional program through alterations to the CNS regions of the *foxp3* locus. While the binding of c-REL to CNS3 is important for Foxp3 induction in tT_{REG} cells in the thymus, and the binding of SMAD/NFAT complexes to CNS1 is responsible for the induction of Foxp3 in pT_{REG} cells, CNS2 has been identified as being necessary for sustained Foxp3 expression in the maintenance of the T_{REG} phenotype [73]. This region, termed as the T_{REG}-specific demethylated region (TSDR), contains binding sites for various transcription factors involved in maintaining Foxp3 expression, including ETS-1, STAT5, CREB/ATF, as well as Foxp3 itself [74]. In tT_{REG} cells, this region is devoid of CpG methylation while being highly methylated in induced T_{REG} cells; however, pT_{REG} cells induced *in vivo* possess partially hypomethylated TSDRs resembling that of tT_{REG} cells [75]. Maintenance of the TSDR in T_{REG} cells is achieved in part through regulation of DNMT1 expression. DNMT1 has been shown to be able to disrupt the TSDR in tT_{REG} cells. DNMT1 expression is induced via activation of STAT3 in response to exogenous IL-6, resulting in methylation of the TSDR and downregulation of Foxp3 expression. In addition, the strength of TCR signaling during pT_{REG} induction has been shown to regulate the level of DNMT expression, with high levels of TCR signaling resulting in the impaired induction of Foxp3. Conversely, TGF-β signaling is known to antagonize DNMT1 activity in T_{REG} cells [76, 77]. Furthermore, the MBD protein MBD2 has been demonstrated to be essential for maintenance of the TSDR in tT_{REG} cells. tT_{REG} from MBD2−/− mice were shown to possess demethylated TSDR in the thymus but were unable to maintain the TSDR in the periphery. This is due to impaired recruitment of the demethylase Tet2 to the TSDR in the absence of MBD2, suggesting a role for MBD2 in the active demethylation of the TSDR [78].

4. Regulation of mRNA stability in CD4+ T cell subsets

Thus far, we have examined how transcriptional and epigenetic changes are able to influence various gene expression programs of CD4+ T cell subsets through the induction of mRNA synthesis to enact both lineage commitment and effector function. However, recent studies have demonstrated that the level of mRNA within a cell is dependent not only on the generation of new mRNA transcripts but also on the stability of mRNA in the cytosol allowing for continued protein expression. Several mechanisms have been described that are capable of regulating mRNA stability including RNA-binding proteins (RBP) as well as other RNA molecules.

RBPs are a specialized group of proteins that recognize conserved sequences present in the untranslated regions (UTR) of mRNA. One of the determinants of mRNA stability is the length of the polyadenylated tails with the removal of mRNA poly-a-tails being a precursor to the removal of 5′ CAP and subsequent degradation of mRNA [79]. The RBP CPEB1 has been shown to recognize cytosolic polyacetylation motifs in the UTR of mRNA and can modulate the length of the poly-a-tail depending on its phosphorylation status. Other RBPs such as tristetraprolin (TTP) recognize AU-rich elements (ARE) and are responsible for degrading mRNA synthesized under homeostatic conditions, but can be inactivated in inflammatory contexts to facilitate mRNA translation. Conversely, RBPs-like HuR can stabilize mRNA within the cytosol, allowing for prolonged gene expression [80].

Recent years have seen an emergence in the study of how noncoding RNA molecules can regulate mRNA stability. This group consists of short RNA sequences called micro-RNA (miRNA) as well as longer noncoding sequences (LncRNA). miRNAs are synthesized as longer pre-miRNA; however, processing by various RNAse proteins, such as Drosha, Dicer, and DGCR8, cleaves the miRNA molecule to its mature ~22 nucleotide length consisting of a sequence that is antisense to its mRNA target, with binding sites being found primarily in the UTR regions of target mRNA transcripts. Mature miRNA recruits the RNA-induced silencing complex to target mRNA transcripts, inducing their degradation [81]. On the other hand, LncRNA has been shown to play a variety of roles, including miRNA sponges by providing decoy sites for miRNA binding as well as factors involved in facilitating transcription factor complex formation [82].

These mRNA stability mechanisms play an important role in the activation of naïve CD4+ T cells. The absence of miRNA in T cells through ablation of the processing enzyme DICER resulted in a decrease in the expansion of DICER-deficient CD4+ T cells following TCR stimulation [83]. Importantly, the miR 17~92 cluster has been found to have an important function in facilitating the CD28 co-stimulatory pathway through repression of the inhibitory protein PTEN, allowing for T cell proliferation [84]. miRNA has also been shown to modulate TCR sensitivity, with miR-181a targeting the inhibitory kinases PTPN22 and SHP-2, which act to terminate TCR signaling. Antagonizing miR-181a abolishes CD69 expression, a characteristic marker of recent TCR stimulation [85]. miR-21 also contributes to the epigenetic landscape in T cell by targeting DNMT1 mRNA, creating hypomethylated regions in CD4 + T cells, resulting in aberrant activation and cytokine secretion [86]. On the other hand, several miRNAs are known to restrict CD4+ T cell activation, and miR181c targets IL-2 mRNA to repress expression in naïve CD4+ T cells; however, its expression is downregulated following TCR stimulation allowing for IL-2 secretion [87]. mIR-125b has also been shown to be important in keeping CD4 + T cells in a naïve state by targeting key cytokines and cytokine receptors involved in CD4 + T cell differentiation [88]. However, another study has demonstrated that TCR activation causes lymphocytes to produce mRNA transcripts with shortened UTRs negating some of the inhibitory effect of miRNAs [89]. In addition, expression of the RBP HuR is increased in activated CD4+ T cells, resulting in increased mRNA stability [90].

mRNA stability has been shown to be a contributing factor in regulating Th1/Th2 differentiation. miR-155 facilitates Th1 differentiation by targeting the Th2 accessory transcription factor c-Maf to limit Th2 differentiation, while miR-17 has been shown to restrict expression of the TGF-β receptor subunit 2 to block Th17 and pT_{REG} conversion [91–93]. Other miRNAs have been shown to limit Th1 differentiation. miR-138 has been shown to alter the Th1/Th2 cell balance by targeting RUNX3 mRNA impeding the T-bet-mediated induction of IFNγ [94].

Signaling through STAT1 initiates the transcription of miR-29, which contributes to the restriction of Th1 lineage commitment by directly targeting both T-bet and IFNγ mRNA, preventing the IFNγ-mediated feed-forward loop from driving further T-bet expression [95]. The RNA-binding protein TTP is also known to degrade IFNγ mRNA in activated T cells resulting in a twofold reduction of the half-life of IFNγ-mRNA in CD4+ T cells [96]. TTP has also been shown to facilitate degradation of TNFα mRNA in other cell types, suggesting that a similar mechanism may be present in Th1 cells. The RBP HuR has shown to increase the half-life of *il4* and *il13* mRNA to promote Th2 differentiation. Furthermore, HuR protected GATA3 from TTP-mediated degradation by blocking the ARE element present in GATA3 mRNA [97–99]. miRNA has also been linked to increased Th2 responses. Studies employing the use of asthma models have revealed that miR-19 and mIR-146a are able to enhance Th2 responses with elevated levels being detected in Th2 cytokine-secreting cells [100]. Elevated cytokine secretion was seen in cells that express miR-19 compared to miR-19-deficient cells that express high levels of GATA3. Ablation of miR-146a resulted in a skewing toward Th1/Th17 differentiation [101]. Other miRNAs act to increase the DNA-binding activity of GATA3 with mIR-126 targeting a negative regulator of GATA3 transcriptional activity [102]. Conversely, some miRNAs act to reduce Th2 differentiation directly with miR-340 destabilizing IL-4 mRNA or indirectly with miR-128 resulting in increased ubiquitin-mediated degradation of GATA3 through targeting of BMI1 [103].

Many studies in recent years have also demonstrated the importance of miRNA in regulating Th17 and T_{REG} differentiation and function. miR-21 facilitates TGF-β signaling pathway by targeting the negative regulator SMAD 7, which can enhance the generation of both cell types [104]. The STAT signaling activity in these cells is also under regulation of miR-155. mIR-155 is thought to enhance T_{REG} survival through attenuation of SOCS1, and inhibitor of STAT signaling to enhance STAT5 activity in T_{REG} cells [105]. This miRNA, however, has also been shown to be important for the IFNγ and IL-17 secretion in response to *H. Pylori* infection indicating that miRNA can play a role in both suppressing and driving inflammation [106]. In Th17 cells, miR-155 has not been shown to directly target RORγT or BATF mRNA; however, there is a significant reduction in *il17f, il17a*, and *il22* mRNA transcripts in the absence of miR-155 [107]. miR-326 has an indirect effect in enhancing Th17 differentiation by targeting ETS-1, a known negative regulator of the Th17 lineage [108]. Other miRNAs have been shown to have subset specific functions. Elevated expression of miR-10a is detected in both tT_{REG} and pT_{REG} cells. While ablation of miR-10a results in a slight reduction of Foxp3 levels in tT_{REG} cells, its expression is important in maintaining lineage commitment in pT_{REG} cells through degradation of Bcl-6 mRNA to inhibit conversion of these cells to a follicular T helper (Tfh) phenotype [109]. Other miRNAs are involved in modulating T_{REG} effector function. miR-466 l has been shown to mask ARE elements in the 3′ UTR of IL-10 mRNA to prevent degradation via TTP in other cell types, while the miR-17~92 cluster has been demonstrated to be necessary for the expansion of IL-10 secreting T_{REG} cells [110, 111]. Conversely, miR-210 is involved in the downregulation of Foxp3 expression and miR142-3p and miR-31 are known to target the cAMP generation pathways, inhibiting T_{REG} metabolism [112–114].

The study of mRNA stability has revealed a convoluted network of miRNA and RBPs while adding another layer of complexity to the transcription factor and epigenetic modifications dictating CD4 + T cell subset differentiation and function. Due to the permissive nature of miRNA base pairing, further investigation is necessary to uncover the mechanism by which miRNA targets specific mRNA for degradation depending on the context a cell finds itself in.

5. The emerging role of differential mRNA translation in modulating CD4+ T cell functions

The accessibility of DNA, the activity of necessary transcription factors, and the mechanisms governing how long mRNA lasts in the cytosol are all key factors in determining the total abundance of specific mRNA transcripts within cells. Historically, techniques measuring RNA abundance including RT-PCR and microarrays have been used to identify how specific factors mediate their effect in CD4+ T cells through examination of their RNA signature. These transcriptional signatures have been useful in inferring the genes involved in giving CD4+ T cell subsets their diverse and specific functions in regulating the adaptive immune response to achieve a balance between necessary inflammatory functions for host protection without undue detrimental effects from over activity. However, studies in recent years have revealed discrepancies between mRNA transcript and protein levels within cells, suggesting that mechanisms controlling gene transcription and mRNA stability are insufficient to explain the full scope of regulatory mechanisms governing immune cell function [115, 116]. From a functional standpoint, translational regulation of gene expression offers several advantages in controlling immune responses. Thus, translational regulation of gene expression enables rapid integration of environmental cues to control protein activity, allows rapid onset and reversibility of the response by utilizing the existing mRNA pool within a cell, and forgoes the need for de novo mRNA synthesis. The advent of techniques to measure ribosome loading on individual mRNA transcripts has led to the identification of multiple genes in both the innate and adaptive immune systems that are regulated at the level of mRNA translation.

Studies in CD4+ T cells have shown distinct translational regulation regulating several key components of cell function. IL-2 is translationally repressed in naïve CD4+ T cells through inhibition of ribosome loading to prevent aberrant expression prior to TCR stimulation [117]. The MAPK-signal integrating kinase, Mnk1, has been shown to promote the translation of TNFα via phosphorylation of the translational silencer hnRNP A1, preventing its binding to TNFα mRNA [118]. Additionally, the rate of GATA3 translation is increased following the activation of the CD28 co-stimulatory pathway in CD4+ T cells without direct increase in GATA3 mRNA abundance, while IL-4 signaling can facilitate IL-4 translation in a similar manner [97, 119]. Recently, a genome-wide study examined the role of mRNA translational regulation in CD4+ T cell subsets [120]. The isolation of polyribosome-bound transcripts, enriched with highly translated mRNA transcripts and comparison with total cytosolic mRNA, identified distinct translational signatures differentiating T_{REG} and T_{EFF} cells. While there was little discrepancy in the translational signature of naïve unstimulated cells, TCR stimulation causes these subsets to acquire divergent translational programs. The identified translationally regulated mRNAs were found to be co-regulated in groups corresponding to specific biological processes. Among these, the genes involved in cell cycle progression were found to be translationally silenced in TCR-stimulated T_{REG} cells compared to T_{EFF} cells. Within this group of genes, there was a significant reduction in the translation of the eukaryotic translation initiation factor, eIF4E.

eIF4E is a key component of the eIF4F translation initiation complex responsible for binding the 5′CAP of mRNA to initiate ribosome assembly and mRNA translation. eIF4E is necessary for the translation of many genes encoding for proliferation, survival, and cell cycle progression [121]. During homeostatic conditions, the eIF4E-binding proteins, eIF4E-BP1 and 2, bind and sequester eIF4E. Growth factors, hormones, or cytokines signaling through the PI3K/AKT axis activate the mammalian target of rapamycin (mTOR). Activation of the mTOR pathway results in the phosphorylation of eiF4E-BP and the release of eIF4E into the cytosol, allowing for eIF4E-mediated translation. Consistent with the translational silencing of eIF4E in T_{REG} cells, mTOR gene deficiency or inhibition can abrogate the proliferation and differentiation of Th1, Th2, or Th17 cells, while promoting Foxp3 expression and adopting a T_{REG} phenotype [122]. In line with this, inhibition of eIF4E activity in CD4+ T cells abrogated their proliferation in response to TCR stimulation in the presence of IL-2 [120]. Surprisingly, inhibition of eIF4E activity in activated T_{EFF} cells also resulted in the induction of Foxp3 expression in a subset of cells, suggesting that modulation of eIF4E expression may impact CD4+ T cell lineage identity, with translational silencing of eIF4E being required for T_{REG} stability.

The study of mRNA translation regulation is an emerging concept in the study of CD4+ T cell function, offering a new perspective on the regulation of the complicated gene-expression programs found in CD4+ T cells. Further investigation is necessary to understand how CD4+ T cells can integrate environmental signals to fine tune a transcriptional landscape to modulate function without undoing the complex transcriptional and epigenetic changes necessary to acquire their specialized functions in the first place.

6. Conclusion

Several post-transcriptional mechanisms regulate gene expression for many key aspects of T cell activation, differentiation, and effector functions. During immune responses, the rapid induction and termination of various immune cell effector activities must be controlled in a timely and efficient manner to prevent the adverse consequences of pathologic inflammation. To achieve this fine control of biological responses, transcriptional mechanisms play an essential role for the regulation of gene expression. Moreover, many post-transcriptional mechanisms, including translational control of gene expression, are particularly advantageous to a cell as it integrates inflammatory signals with rapid and context-dependent protein synthesis and effector responses without the energy expenditures associated with time-consuming *de novo* mRNA synthesis. Recent single gene or genome-wide approaches highlight how post-transcriptional mechanisms control gene expression in various innate and adaptive cell types and potentiate a modular regulation of gene expression for a more efficient response to cellular activation and environmental cues.

http://dx.doi.org/10.5772/intechopen.73319

The past decade has witnessed a rapid rise in research on post-transcriptional mechanisms directing gene expression programs in innate immune cells. However, the mechanisms underlying the regulation of adaptive immunity still remain poorly defined. For instance, uncovering the regulatory steps that control gene expression events during cell function in CD4+ T cell subsets, key orchestrators of adaptive immunity, may shed light into the identification of novel immune "checkpoints" and therapeutic applications. Unraveling the molecular definition of key pathways involved in T cell proliferation or differentiation, promotion of Foxp3+ T_{REG} activities in metastatic tumors, or those that induce pathogenic T cell lineages in autoimmune diseases, for example, could allow for the development of novel therapies to restore immune quiescence.

Author details

Roman Istomine[1,2,3] and Ciriaco A. Piccirillo[1,2,3]*

*Address all correspondence to: ciro.piccirillo@mcgill.ca

1 Department of Microbiology and Immunology, McGill University, Montreal, QC, Canada

2 Program in Infectious Disease and Immunity in Global Health, Research Institute of the McGill University Health Center, Montreal, QC, Canada

3 FOCiS Centre of Excellence in Translational Immunology (CETI), Montreal, QC, Canada

References

[1] Shah DK, Zúñiga-Pflücker JC. An overview of the intrathymic intricacies of T Cell development. The Journal of Immunology. 2014;**192**:4017-4023

[2] Grenningloh R, Tai T-S, Frahm N, Hongo TC, Chicoine AT, Brander C, et al. Ets-1 maintains IL-7 receptor expression in peripheral T cells. The Journal of Immunology. 2011;**186**:969-976

[3] Lee H-C, Shibata H, Ogawa S, Maki K, Ikuta K. Transcriptional regulation of the mouse IL-7 receptor α promoter by glucocorticoid receptor. The Journal of Immunology. 2005; **174**:7800-7806

[4] Carrette F, Surh CD. IL-7 signaling and CD127 receptor regulation in the control of T cell homeostasis. Seminars in Immunology. 2012;**24**(3):209-217

[5] Neal JW, Clipstone NA. Glycogen synthase kinase-3 inhibits the DNA binding activity of NFATc. Journal of Biological Chemistry. 2001;**276**(5):3666-3673

[6] Okamura H, Garcia-Rodriguez C, Martinson H, Qin J, Virshup DM, Rao A. A conserved docking motif for CK1 binding controls the nuclear localization of NFAT1. Molecular and cellular biology. 2004;**24**(10):4184-4195

[7] Im S-H, Rao A. Activation and deactivation of gene expression by Ca 2+/calcineurin-NFAT-mediated signaling. Molecules & Cells (Springer Science & Business Media BV). 2004;**18**(1):1-9

[8] McGuire KL, Iacobelli M. Involvement of Rel, Fos, and Jun proteins in binding activity to the IL-2 promoter CD28 response element/AP-1 sequence in human T cells. The Journal of Immunology. 1997;**159**:1319-1327

[9] Nakajima H, Liu X-W, Wynshaw-Boris A, Rosenthal LA, Imada K, Finbloom DS, et al. An indirect effect of Stat5a in IL-2–induced proliferation: A critical role for STAT5A in IL-2–mediated IL-2 receptor α chain induction. Immunity. 1997;**7**(5):691-701

[10] Xue H-H, Kovanen PE, Pise-Masison CA, Berg M, Radovich MF, Brady JN, et al. IL-2 negatively regulates IL-7 receptor α chain expression in activated T lymphocytes. Proceedings of the National Academy of Sciences. 2002;**99**(21):13,759-13,764

[11] Jeremias I, Kupatt C, Baumann B, Herr I, Wirth T, Debatin KM. Inhibition of nuclear factor κB activation attenuates apoptosis resistance in lymphoid cells. Blood. 1998;**91**: 4624-4631

[12] Zhu J, Yamane H, Paul WE. Differentiation of effector CD4 T cell populations. Annual review of immunology. 2010;**28**:445-489

[13] Oh H, Ghosh S. NF-κB: Roles and regulation in different CD4(+) T cell subsets. Immunological Reviews. 2013;**252**(1):41-51

[14] Raphael I, Nalawade S, Eagar TN, Forsthuber TG. T cell subsets and their signature cytokines in autoimmune and inflammatory diseases. Cytokine. 2015;**74**(1):5-17

[15] Szabo SJ, Kim ST, Costa GL, Zhang X, Fathman CG, Glimcher LH. A novel transcription factor, T-bet, directs Th1 lineage commitment. Cell. 2000;**100**(6):655-669

[16] Afkarian M, Sedy JR, Yang J, Jacobson NG, Cereb N, Yang SY, et al. T-bet is a STAT1-induced regulator of IL-12R expression in naive CD4+ T cells. Nature Immunology. 2002;**3**(6)

[17] Schulz EG, Mariani L, Radbruch A, Höfer T. Sequential polarization and imprinting of type 1 T helper lymphocytes by interferon-γ and interleukin-12. Immunity. 2009;**30**(5): 673-683

[18] Mullen AC, Hutchins AS, High FA, Lee HW, Sykes KJ, Chodosh LA, et al. Hlx is induced by and genetically interacts with T-bet to promote heritable TH1 gene induction. Nature Immunology. 2002;**3**(7):652-659

[19] Djuretic IM, Levanon D, Negreanu V, Groner Y, Rao A, Ansel KM. Transcription factors T-bet and Runx3 cooperate to activate Ifng and silence Il4 in T helper type 1 cells. Nature Immunology. 2007;**8**(2):1-11

[20] Sekimata M, Pérez-Melgosa M, Miller SA, Weinmann AS, Sabo PJ, Sandstrom R, et al. CCCTC-binding factor and the transcription factor T-bet orchestrate T helper 1 cell-specific structure and function at the interferon-γ locus. Immunity. 2009;**31**(4):551-564

[21] Balasubramani A, Shibata Y, Crawford GE, Baldwin AS, Hatton RD, Weaver CT. Modular utilization of distal cis-regulatory elements controls ifng gene expression in T cells activated by distinct stimuli. Immunity. 2010;**33**(1):35-47

[22] Lee DU, Avni O, Chen L, Rao A. A Distal Enhancer in the Interferon-γ (IFN-γ) Locus Revealed by Genome Sequence Comparison. Journal of Biological Chemistry. 2004; **279**(6):4802-4810

[23] Feske S, Giltnane J, Dolmetsch R, Staudt LM, Rao A. Gene regulation mediated by calcium signals in T lymphocytes. Nature Immunology. 2001;**2**(4):316-324

[24] Lord GM, Rao RM, Choe H, Sullivan BM, Lichtman AH, Luscinskas FW, et al. T-bet is required for optimal proinflammatory CD4(+) T-cell trafficking. Blood. 2005;**106**(10): 3432-3439

[25] O'Shea JJ, Ma A, Lipsky P. Cytokines and autoimmunity. Nature Reviews Immunology 2002;**2**(1):37-45

[26] Ho IC, Tai T-S, Pai S-Y. GATA3 and the T-cell lineage: essential functions before and after T-helper-2-cell differentiation. Nature Reviews Immunology. 2009;**9**(2):125-135

[27] Zheng W-P, Flavell RA. The transcription factor GATA-3 Is necessary and sufficient for Th2 cytokine gene expression in CD4 T cells. Cell. 1997;**89**(4):587-596

[28] Fang TC, Yashiro-Ohtani Y, Del Bianco C, Knoblock DM, Blacklow SC, Pear WS. Notch directly regulates Gata3 expression during T helper 2 cell differentiation. Immunity. 2007;**27**(1):100-110

[29] Ouyang W, Löhning M, Gao Z, Assenmacher M, Ranganath S, Radbruch A, et al. Stat6-independent GATA-3 autoactivation directs IL-4-independent Th2 development and commitment. Immunity. 2000;**12**(1):27-37

[30] Gilmour J, Lavender P. Control of IL-4 expression in T helper 1 and 2 cells. Immunology. 2008;**124**(4):437-444

[31] Corn RA, Hunter C, Liou H-C, Siebenlist U, Boothby MR. Opposing Roles for RelB and Bcl-3 in Regulation of T-Box Expressed in T Cells, GATA-3, and Th Effector Differentiation. The Journal of Immunology. 2005;**175**(4):2102

[32] Das J, Chen C-H, Yang L, Cohn L, Ray P, Ray A. A critical role for NF-[kappa]B in Gata3 expression and TH2 differentiation in allergic airway inflammation. Nature Immunology. 2001;**2**(1):45-50

[33] Rengarajan J, Mowen KA, McBride KD, Smith ED, Singh H, Glimcher LH. Interferon regulatory factor 4 (IRF4) interacts with NFATc2 to modulate interleukin 4 gene expression. The Journal of Experimental Medicine. 2002;**195**(8):1003-1012

[34] Usui T, Nishikomori R, Kitani A, Strober W. GATA-3 suppresses Th1 development by downregulation of STAT4 and not through effects on IL-12Rβ2 chain or T-bet. Immunity. 2003;**18**(3):415-428

[35] Manel N, Unutmaz D, Littman DR. The differentiation of human TH-17 cells requires transforming growth factor-[beta] and induction of the nuclear receptor ROR[gamma]t. Nature Immunology 2008;**9**(6):641-649

[36] Chen C-H, Seguin-Devaux C, Burke NA, Oriss TB, Watkins SC, Clipstone N, et al. Transforming growth factor β blocks Tec kinase phosphorylation, Ca2+ influx, and NFATc translocation causing inhibition of T cell differentiation. Journal of Experimental Medicine. 2003;**197**(12):1689-1699

[37] Ivanov II, Zhou L, Littman DR. Transcriptional regulation of Th17 cell differentiation. Seminars in immunology. 2007;**19**(6):409-417

[38] Zhou L, Lopes JE, Chong MMW, Ivanov II, Min R, Victora GD, et al. TGF-[bgr]-induced Foxp3 inhibits TH17 cell differentiation by antagonizing ROR[ggr]t function. Nature. 2008;**453**(7192):236-240

[39] Korn T, Mitsdoerffer M, Croxford AL, Awasthi A, Dardalhon VA, Galileos G, et al. IL-6 controls Th17 immunity in vivo by inhibiting the conversion of conventional T cells into Foxp3+ regulatory T cells. Proceedings of the National Academy of Sciences. 2008; **105**(47):18,460-18,465

[40] Zhou L, Ivanov II, Spolski R, Min R, Shenderov K, Egawa T, et al. IL-6 programs TH-17 cell differentiation by promoting sequential engagement of the IL-21 and IL-23 pathways. Nature Immunology. 2007;**8**(9):967-974

[41] Huang W, Thomas B, Flynn RA, Gavzy SJ, Wu L, Kim SV, et al. DDX5 and its associated lncRNA Rmrp modulate Th17 cell effector functions. Nature. 2015;**528**(7583):517-522

[42] Schraml BU, Hildner K, Ise W, Lee W-L, Smith WAE, Solomon B, et al. The AP-1 transcription factor Batf controls T(H)17 differentiation. Nature. 2009;**460**(7253):405-409

[43] Bin Dhuban K, Kornete M, S Mason E, Piccirillo CA. Functional dynamics of Foxp3+ regulatory T cells in mice and humans. Immunological Reviews. 2014;**259**(1):140-158

[44] Maruyama T, Konkel JE, Zamarron BF, Chen W. The molecular mechanisms of Foxp3 gene regulation. Seminars in Immunology. 2011;**23**(6):418-423

[45] Isomura I, Palmer S, Grumont RJ, Bunting K, Hoyne G, Wilkinson N, et al. c-Rel is required for the development of thymic Foxp3⁺ CD4 regulatory T cells. The Journal of Experimental Medicine. 2009;**206**(13):3001

[46] Ouyang W, Beckett O, Ma Q, Paik J-h, DePinho RA, Li MO. Foxo proteins cooperatively control the differentiation of Foxp3+ regulatory T cells. Nature Immunology. 2010;**11**(7): 618-627

[47] Tone Y, Furuuchi K, Kojima Y, Tykocinski ML, Greene MI, Tone M. Smad3 and NFAT cooperate to induce Foxp3 expression through its enhancer. Nature immunology. 2008; **9**(2):194-202

[48] Hori S, Nomura T, Sakaguchi S. Control of regulatory T cell development by the transcription factor Foxp3. Science. 2003;**299**:1057-1061

[49] Wu Y, Borde M, Heissmeyer V, Feuerer M, Lapan AD, Stroud JC, et al. FOXP3 controls regulatory T cell function through cooperation with NFAT. Cell. 2006;**126**(2):375-387

[50] Pan F, Yu H, Dang EV, Barbi J, Pan X, Grosso JF, et al. Eos mediates Foxp3-dependent gene silencing in regulatory T cells. Science (New York, NY). 2009;**325**(5944):1142-1146

[51] Borsellino G, Kleinewietfeld M, Di Mitri D, Sternjak A, Diamantini A, Giometto R, et al. Expression of ectonucleotidase CD39 by Foxp3+ Treg cells: hydrolysis of extracellular ATP and immune suppression. Blood. 2007;**110**(4):1225

[52] Wing K, Onishi Y, Prieto-Martin P, Yamaguchi T, Miyara M, Fehervari Z, et al. CTLA-4 Control over Foxp3⁺ regulatory T cell function. Science. 2008; **322**(5899):271

[53] Josefowicz SZ, Lu L-F, Rudensky AY. Regulatory T cells: Mechanisms of differentiation and function. Annual Review Of Immunology. 2012;**30**:531-564

[54] Zhou X, Bailey-Bucktrout SL, Jeker LT, Penaranda C, Martínez-Llordella M, Ashby M, et al. Instability of the transcription factor Foxp3 leads to the generation of pathogenic memory T cells in vivo. Nature Immunology. 2009;**10**(9):1000-1007

[55] Bird A. DNA methylation patterns and epigenetic memory. Genes & Development. 2002;**16**(1):6-21

[56] Fatemi M, Hermann A, Gowher H, Jeltsch A. Dnmt3a and Dnmt1 functionally cooperate during de novo methylation of DNA. The FEBS Journal. 2002;**269**(20):4981-4984

[57] Kohli RM, Zhang Y. TET enzymes, TDG and the dynamics of DNA demethylation. Nature. 2013;**502**(7472):472

[58] Patel DJ. A Structural Perspective on Readout of Epigenetic Histone and DNA Methylation Marks. Cold Spring Harbor Perspectives in Biology. 2016;**8**(3):a018754

[59] Crawford GE, Holt IE, Mullikin JC, Tai D, Center NIoHIS, Green ED, et al. Identifying gene regulatory elements by genome-wide recovery of DNase hypersensitive sites. Proceedings of the National Academy of Sciences of the United States of America. 2004; **101**(4):992-997

[60] Du J, Johnson LM, Jacobsen SE, Patel DJ. DNA methylation pathways and their crosstalk with histone methylation. Nature Reviews Molecular Cell Biology. 2015;**16**(9):519

[61] Agarwal S, Rao A. Modulation of chromatin structure regulates cytokine gene expression during T cell differentiation. Immunity. 1998;**9**(6):765-775

[62] Thomas RM, Gamper CJ, Ladle BH, Powell JD, Wells AD. De novo DNA methylation is required to restrict T helper lineage plasticity. Journal of Biological Chemistry. 2012; **287**(27):22,900-22,909

[63] Shi M, Lin TH, Appell KC, Berg LJ. Jak3-dependent signals induce chromatin remodeling at the Ifng locus during Th1 differentiation. Immunity. 2008;**28**(6):763-773

[64] Tong Y, Aune T, Boothby M. T-bet antagonizes mSin3a recruitment and transactivates a fully methylated IFN-γ promoter via a conserved T-box half-site. Proceedings of the National Academy of Sciences of the United States of America. 2005; **102**(6):2034-2039

[65] Miller SA, Huang AC, Miazgowicz MM, Brassil MM, Weinmann AS. Coordinated but physically separable interaction with H3K27-demethylase and H3K4-methyltransferase activities are required for T-box protein-mediated activation of developmental gene expression. Genes & Development. 2008;**22**(21):2980-2993

[66] Lee DU, Agarwal S, Rao A. Th2 lineage commitment and efficient IL-4 production involves extended demethylation of the IL-4 gene. Immunity. 2002;**16**(5):649-660

[67] Makar KW, Perez-Melgosa M, Shnyreva M, Weaver WM, Fitzpatrick DR, Wilson CB. Active recruitment of DNA methyltransferases regulates interleukin 4 in thymocytes and T cells. Nature Immunology. 2003;**4**(12):1183-1190

[68] Onodera A, Yamashita M, Endo Y, Kuwahara M, Tofukuji S, Hosokawa H, et al. STAT6-mediated displacement of polycomb by trithorax complex establishes long-term maintenance of GATA3 expression in T helper type 2 cells. The Journal of Experimental Medicine. 2010;**207**(11):2493-2506

[69] Tykocinski L-O, Hajkova P, Chang H-D, Stamm T, SÖzeri O, LÖhning M, et al. A critical control element for interleukin-4 memory expression in T helper lymphocytes. Journal of Biological Chemistry. 2005;**280**(31):28,177-28,185

[70] Hosokawa H, Tanaka T, Suzuki Y, Iwamura C, Ohkubo S, Endoh K, et al. Functionally distinct Gata3/Chd4 complexes coordinately establish T helper 2 (Th2) cell identity. Proceedings of the National Academy of Sciences. 2013;**110**(12):4691-4696

[71] Akimzhanov AM, Yang XO, Dong C. Chromatin remodeling of interleukin-17 (IL-17)-IL-17F cytokine gene locus during inflammatory helper T cell differentiation. Journal of Biological Chemistry. 2007;**282**(9):5969-5972

[72] Bending D, Newland S, Krejčí A, Phillips JM, Bray S, Cooke A. Epigenetic changes at Il12rb2 and Tbx21 in relation to plasticity behavior of Th17 Cells. The Journal of Immunology. 2011;**186**(6):3373-3382

[73] Polansky JK, Kretschmer K, Freyer J, Floess S, Garbe A, Baron U, et al. DNA methylation controls Foxp3 gene expression. European Journal of Immunology. 2008;**38**(6): 1654-1663

[74] Povoleri GAM, Scottà C, Nova-Lamperti EA, John S, Lombardi G, Afzali B. Thymic versus induced regulatory T cells–who regulates the regulators? Frontiers in Immunology. 2013;**4**:169

[75] Ohkura N, Hamaguchi M, Morikawa H, Sugimura K, Tanaka A, Ito Y, et al. T cell receptor stimulation-induced epigenetic changes and Foxp3 expression are independent and complementary events required for Treg cell development. Immunity. 2012;**37**(5): 785-799

[76] Zheng Q, Xu Y, Liu Y, Zhang B, Li X, Guo F, et al. Induction of Foxp3 demethylation increases regulatory CD4+ CD25+ T cells and prevents the occurrence of diabetes in mice. Journal of Molecular Medicine. 2009;**87**(12):1191

[77] HODGE DR, CHO E, COPELAND TD, GUSZCZYNSKI T, YANG E, SETH AK, et al. IL-6 enhances the nuclear translocation of DNA cytosine-5-methyltransferase 1 (DNMT1) via phosphorylation of the nuclear localization sequence by the AKT kinase. Cancer Genomics-Proteomics. 2007;**4**(6):387-398

[78] Wang L, Liu Y, Han R, Beier UH, Thomas RM, Wells AD, et al. Mbd2 promotes Foxp3 demethylation and T-regulatory-cell function. Molecular and Cellular Biology. 2013; **33**(20):4106-4115

[79] Piqué M, López JM, Foissac S, Guigó R, Méndez R. A combinatorial code for CPE-mediated translational control. Cell. 2008;**132**(3):434-448

[80] Anderson P. Post-transcriptional regulons coordinate the initiation and resolution of inflammation. Nature Reviews Immunology. 2010;**10**(1):24-35

[81] Cai Y, Yu X, Hu S, Yu J. A brief review on the mechanisms of miRNA regulation. Genomics, Proteomics & Bioinformatics. 2009;**7**(4):147-154

[82] Mathieu E-L, Belhocine M, Dao L, Puthier D, Spicuglia S. Functions of lncRNA in development and diseases. Medecine Sciences: M/S. 2014;**30**(8-9):790

[83] Muljo SA, Ansel KM, Kanellopoulou C, Livingston DM, Rao A, Rajewsky K. Aberrant T cell differentiation in the absence of Dicer. Journal of Experimental Medicine. 2005; **202**(2):261-269

[84] Xiao C, Srinivasan L, Calado DP, Patterson HC, Zhang B, Wang J, et al. Lymphoproliferative disease and autoimmunity in mice with elevated miR-17– 92 expression in lymphocytes. Nature immunology. 2008;**9**(4):405

[85] Li Q-J, Chau J, Ebert PJ, Sylvester G, Min H, Liu G, et al. miR-181a is an intrinsic modulator of T cell sensitivity and selection. Cell. 2007;**129**(1):147-161

[86] Pan W, Zhu S, Yuan M, Cui H, Wang L, Luo X, et al. MicroRNA-21 and microRNA-148a contribute to DNA hypomethylation in lupus CD4+ T cells by directly and indirectly targeting DNA methyltransferase 1. The Journal of Immunology. 2010;**184**(12):6773-6781

[87] Xue Q, Guo Z-Y, Li W, Wen W-H, Meng Y-L, Jia L-T, et al. Human activated CD4+ T lymphocytes increase IL-2 expression by downregulating microRNA-181c. Molecular Immunology. 2011;**48**(4):592-599

[88] Rossi RL, Rossetti G, Wenandy L, Curti S, Ripamonti A, Bonnal RJ, et al. Distinct microRNA signatures in human lymphocyte subsets and enforcement of the naive state in CD4+ T cells by the microRNA miR-125b. Nature Immunology. 2011;**12**(8):796-803

[89] Sandberg R, Neilson JR, Sarma A, Sharp PA, Burge CB. Proliferating cells express mRNAs with shortened 39 untranslated regions and fewer microRNA target sites. Science. 2008;**320**(5883):1643-1647

[90] Glascock J, Techasintana P, Magee J, Atasoy U. RNA-binding protein HuR controls IL-2 homeostasis in activated T cells by regulating CD25 expression (CCR3P.202). The Journal of Immunology. 2015;**194**(1 Supplement):49.3-.3

[91] Rodriguez A, Vigorito E, Clare S, Warren MV, Couttet P, Soond DR, et al. Requirement of bic/microRNA-155 for normal immune function. Science. 2007;**316**(5824):608-611

[92] Fedeli M, Riba M, Garcia Manteiga JM, Tian L, Viganò V, Rossetti G, et al. miR-17 ~ 92 family clusters control iNKT cell ontogenesis via modulation of TGF-β signaling. Proceedings of the National Academy of Sciences. 2016;**113**(51):E8286-E8E95

[93] Dews M, Fox JL, Hultine S, Sundaram P, Wang W, Liu YY, et al. Myc - miR-17~92 axis blunts TGFβ signaling and production of multiple TGFβ-dependent anti-angiogenic factors. Cancer Research. 2010;**70**(20):8233-8246

[94] Fu D, Yu W, Li M, Wang H, Liu D, Song X, et al. MicroRNA-138 regulates the balance of Th1/Th2 via targeting RUNX3 in psoriasis. Immunology Letters. 2015;**166**(1):55-62

[95] Steiner DF, Thomas MF, Hu JK, Yang Z, Babiarz JE, Allen CD, et al. MicroRNA-29 regulates T-box transcription factors and interferon-γ production in helper T cells. Immunity. 2011;**35**(2):169-181

[96] Ogilvie RL, SternJohn JR, Rattenbacher B, Vlasova IA, Williams DA, Hau HH, et al. Tristetraprolin mediates interferon-γ mRNA decay. Journal of Biological Chemistry. 2009;**284**(17):11,216-11,223

[97] Yarovinsky TO, Butler NS, Monick MM, Hunninghake GW. Early Exposure to IL-4 stabilizes IL-4 mRNA in CD4+ T cells via RNA-binding protein HuR. The Journal of Immunology. 2006;**177**(7):4426-4435

[98] Hosokawa H, Kimura MY, Shinnakasu R, Suzuki A, Miki T, Koseki H, et al. Regulation of Th2 cell development by polycomb group gene bmi-1 through the stabilization of GATA3. The Journal of Immunology. 2006;**177**(11):7656-7664

[99] Casolaro V, Fang X, Tancowny B, Fan J, Wu F, Srikantan S, et al. Posttranscriptional regulation of IL-13 in T cells: Role of the RNA-binding protein HuR. The Journal of Allergy And Clinical Immunology. 2008;**121**(4):853-859.e4

[100] Simpson LJ, Patel S, Bhakta NR, Choy DF, Brightbill HD, Ren X, et al. A microRNA upregulated in asthma airway T cells promotes TH2 cytokine production. Nature Immunology. 2014;**15**(12):1162-1170

[101] Okoye IS, Czieso S, Ktistaki E, Roderick K, Coomes SM, Pelly VS, et al. Transcriptomics identified a critical role for Th2 cell-intrinsic miR-155 in mediating allergy and antihelminth immunity. Proceedings of the National Academy of Sciences of the United States of America. 2014;**111**(30):E3081-E3090

[102] Mattes J, Collison A, Plank M, Phipps S, Foster PS. Antagonism of microRNA-126 suppresses the effector function of TH2 cells and the development of allergic airways disease. Proceedings of the National Academy of Sciences. 2009;**106**(44):18,704-118709

[103] Guerau-de-Arellano M, Smith KM, Godlewski J, Liu Y, Winger R, Lawler SE, et al. Micro-RNA dysregulation in multiple sclerosis favors pro-inflammatory T-cell-mediated autoimmunity. Brain. 2011;**134**(12):3575-3586

[104] Murugaiyan G, da Cunha AP, Ajay AK, Joller N, Garo LP, Kumaradevan S, et al. MicroRNA-21 promotes Th17 differentiation and mediates experimental autoimmune encephalomyelitis. The Journal of Clinical Investigation. 2015;**125**(3):1069

[105] Lu L-F, Thai T-H, Calado DP, Chaudhry A, Kubo M, Tanaka K, et al. Foxp3-dependent microRNA155 confers competitive fitness to regulatory T cells by targeting SOCS1 protein. Immunity. 2009;**30**(1):80-91

[106] Oertli M, Engler DB, Kohler E, Koch M, Meyer TF, Müller A. MicroRNA-155 is essential for the T cell-mediated control of Helicobacter pylori infection and for the induction of chronic gastritis and colitis. The Journal of Immunology. 2011;**187**(7):3578-3586

[107] Escobar Thelma M, Kanellopoulou C, Kugler David G, Kilaru G, Nguyen Cuong K, Nagarajan V, et al. miR-155 activates cytokine gene expression in Th17 cells by regulating the DNA-binding protein Jarid2 to relieve polycomb-mediated repression. Immunity. 2014;**40**(6):865-879

[108] Du C, Liu C, Kang J, Zhao G, Ye Z, Huang S, et al. MicroRNA miR-326 regulates TH-17 differentiation and is associated with the pathogenesis of multiple sclerosis. Nature Immunology. 2009;**10**(12):1252-1259

[109] Takahashi H, Kanno T, Nakayamada S, Hirahara K, Sciumè G, Muljo SA, et al. TGF-[beta] and retinoic acid induce the microRNA miR-10a, which targets Bcl-6 and constrains the plasticity of helper T cells. Nature Immunology. 2012;**13**(6):587-595

[110] Ma F, Liu X, Li D, Wang P, Li N, Lu L, et al. MicroRNA-466 l upregulates IL-10 expression in TLR-triggered macrophages by antagonizing RNA-binding protein tristetraprolin-mediated IL-10 mRNA degradation. The Journal of Immunology. 2010; **184**(11):6053-6059

[111] de Kouchkovsky D, Esensten JH, Rosenthal WL, Morar MM, Bluestone JA, Jeker LT. microRNA-17–92 regulates IL-10 production by regulatory T cells and control of experimental autoimmune encephalomyelitis. Journal of Immunology (Baltimore, Md: 1950). 2013;**191**(4):1594-1605

[112] Fayyad-Kazan H, Rouas R, Fayyad-Kazan M, Badran R, El Zein N, Lewalle P, et al. MicroRNA profile of circulating CD4-positive regulatory T cells in human adults and impact of differentially expressed microRNAs on expression of two genes essential to their function. Journal of Biological Chemistry. 2012;**287**(13):9910-9922

[113] Huang B, Zhao J, Lei Z, Shen S, Li D, Shen G-X, et al. miR-142-3p restricts cAMP production in CD4(+)CD25(−) T cells and CD4(+)CD25(+) T(REG) cells by targeting AC9 mRNA. EMBO Reports. 2009;**10**(2):180-185

[114] Rouas R, Fayyad-Kazan H, El Zein N, Lewalle P, Rothé F, Simion A, et al. Human natural Treg microRNA signature: Role of microRNA-31 and microRNA-21 in FOXP3 expression. European Journal of Immunology. 2009;**39**(6):1608-1618

[115] Kristensen AR, Gsponer J, Foster LJ. Protein synthesis rate is the predominant regulator of protein expression during differentiation. Molecular Systems Biology. 2013;**9**(1):689

[116] Schwanhäusser B, Busse D, Li N, Dittmar G, Schuchhardt J, Wolf J, et al. Global quantification of mammalian gene expression control. Nature. 2011;**473**(7347):337-342

[117] Garcia-Sanz JA, Lenig D. Translational control of interleukin 2 messenger RNA as a molecular mechanism of T cell anergy. The Journal of Experimental Medicine. 1996; **184**(1):159-164

[118] Buxadé M, Parra JL, Rousseau S, Shpiro N, Marquez R, Morrice N, et al. The Mnks are novel components in the control of TNFα biosynthesis and phosphorylate and regulate hnRNP A1. Immunity. 2005;**23**(2):177-189

[119] Cook KD, Miller J. TCR-dependent translational control of GATA-3 enhances Th2 differentiation. The Journal of Immunology. 2010;**185**(6):3209-3216

[120] Bjur E, Larsson O, Yurchenko E, Zheng L, Gandin V, Topisirovic I, et al. Distinct translational control in CD4+ T cell subsets. PLoS Genetics. 2013;**9**(5) e1003494

[121] Mamane Y, Petroulakis E, Rong L, Yoshida K, Lian Wee Ler K, Sonenberg N. eIF4E-from translation to transformation. Oncogene. 2004;**23**(18):3172-3179

[122] Delgoffe GM, Kole TP, Zheng Y, Zarek PE, Matthews KL, Xiao B, et al. The mTOR kinase differentially regulates effector and regulatory T cell lineage commitment. Immunity. 2009;**30**(6):832-844

Section 5

Transcription Controlling Signals that Could Lead to Cancer Generation

Chapter 12

Phosphorylation of PRH/HHEX by Protein Kinase CK2 Regulates Cell Proliferation and Cell Migration in Diverse Cell Types

Padma-Sheela Jayaraman, Kerry S. Wadey,
Sarah J. George and Kevin Gaston

Additional information is available at the end of the chapter

http://dx.doi.org/10.5772/intechopen.72902

Abstract

Disruption of the regulatory mechanisms that control cell proliferation and cell migration results in multiple disease states including cancer and leukaemia. The proline-rich homeodomain protein (PRH)/haematopoietically expressed homeobox protein (HHEX) is a transcription factor that controls cell proliferation and cell migration in a variety of tissues in the adult and in the embryo. Phosphorylation of PRH by Protein Kinase CK2 (Casein Kinase II) stops PRH from binding to DNA and regulating the transcription of its direct target genes. In leukaemic cells, phosphorylation also results in the production of a transdominant-negative truncated PRH phosphoprotein by the proteasome. Phosphorylation of PRH is increased in breast and prostate cancer cells and the consequent loss of PRH activity increases cell proliferation and migration. PRH also regulates the proliferation of vascular smooth muscle cells and CK2-dependent phosphorylation of PRH in these cells accompanies increased cell proliferation during intimal thickening. Thus the ability of PRH to regulate cell behaviour and the control of PRH by CK2 is not limited to a specific cell type or tissue. This raises the possibility that the PRH-CK2 axis could be targeted in a variety of disease states ranging from multiple cancers to the intimal thickening that occurs in vein bypass graft failure and restenosis.

Keywords: cell proliferation, cell migration, cell invasion, tumourigenesis, tumour growth, restenosis, intimal thickening

1. Introduction

The proline-rich homeodomain (PRH) or haematopoietically expressed homeobox (HHEX) protein, is a highly conserved transcription factor belonging to the homeodomain family (reviewed by Soufi et al. [1]). Originally characterised in the haematopoietic compartment

[2–4], PRH has since been found in a wide variety of tissues [1]. PRH is critically important in embryonic development where it regulates anteroposterior axis formation and the development of multiple organ systems including the liver, thyroid, lung, thymus, gallbladder and pancreas [5–8]. In the adult, PRH is expressed in a variety of tissues including the thyroid, lungs, liver and haematopoietic compartment [4, 9]. In these tissues PRH acts as a master regulator of genes important in cell proliferation, cell migration and invasion, and cell differentiation [1]. Changes in PRH activity therefore have profound effects on cell behaviour. This review focuses on the regulation of PRH activity by Protein Kinase CK2 and the role that this plays in tumourigenesis and in the control of vascular smooth muscle cell (VSMC) proliferation during intimal thickening.

2. The regulation of gene expression by PRH

2.1. The PRH protein

The PRH protein has three functional domains; a central homeodomain that mediates DNA binding, with N-terminal and C-terminal domains that regulate transcription (**Figure 1**). The PRH homeodomain is a 60 amino acid sequence that forms three α helices. The second and third helices make up a helix-turn-helix motif and together with amino acids in an N-terminal arm of this domain, this mediates sequence-specific DNA binding. The mutation of asparagine to alanine at position 187 within the PRH homeodomain dramatically reduces DNA binding and prevents PRH from repressing the transcription of its direct target genes [10, 11]. The PRH homeodomain also mediates binding to transcription factor AP1 [12]. The PRH N-terminal domain can repress transcription when attached to a heterologous DNA binding domain [10, 13]. Additionally, the N-terminal domain interacts with a variety of proteins including the promyelocytic leukaemic (PML) protein, eukaryotic initiation factor 4E (eIF-4E), proteasome subunit C8, and the regulatory subunit of Protein Kinase CK2

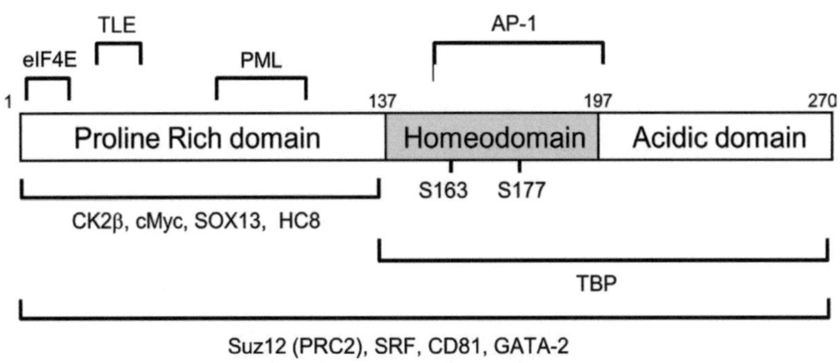

Figure 1. PRH and PRH-interacting proteins. A schematic representation of the PRH protein. The homeodomain and the N- and C-terminal domains are indicated along with the serine residues known to be phosphorylated by CK2 (S163 and S177). PRH-interacting proteins are listed and their binding sites on PRH are indicated by brackets. Some of the protein-protein interactions have not been mapped to defined regions of PRH.

[14–17]. The C-terminal domain is rich in acidic residues and it also functions in transcriptional regulation since its loss prevents PRH from activating transcription of the sodium-dependent bile acid co-transporter (NTCP) gene [18, 19].

The PRH protein forms oligomeric complexes *in vitro* and in cells [20]. The PRH N-terminal domain is resistant to SDS (sodium dodecyl sulphate)-induced denaturation and does not have extensive α-helical or β-sheet secondary structures. However, this domain forms dimers that interact with the PRH homeodomain [20]. *In vitro* studies suggest that octameric PRH oligomers form via the association four PRH dimers [20]. This has implications for DNA binding since although the isolated PRH homeodomain binds to a single DNA site, the full length PRH protein binds to linear arrays of homeodomain binding sites with high affinity [21]. Several genes that are directly regulated by PRH including Goosecoid (GSC), TLE4, VEGFA, VEGFR-1 (FLT1), and endothelial cell-specific molecule-1 (ESM-1) contain multiple, putative PRH-binding sequences [8, 21–23]. This suggests that PRH oligomers bind to these linear arrays to regulate gene expression. However, it is possible that a single PRH binding site may be sufficient to confer gene regulation by PRH.

2.2. The regulation of gene expression

Like many transcription factors PRH can either repress or activate transcription depending on its target gene (see Soufi et al. [1] and Gaston et al. [40] for lists of PRH target genes) and its partner proteins (shown in **Figure 1**). For example, PRH represses the Goosecoid, ESM-1, VEGFA, VEGFR-1, VEGFR-2, and thyroglobulin promoters [8, 21, 23, 24]. An Eh1 motif in PRH N-terminal domain allows PRH to recruit members the Groucho/transducin-like enhancer of split (TLE) family of co-repressor proteins which in turn recruit histone deacetylases [25]. Similarly, PRH can repress transcription by recruiting the polycomb-repressive complex 2 (PRC2) to target genes to bring about histone methylation [26]. These co-repressor interactions can bring about short- and long-range transcriptional repression through histone modification and consequent chromatin condensation. PRH can also repress transcription by interfering with other transcription factors. Binding of PRH to GATA-2 suppresses GATA-2-mediated activation of vascular endothelial growth factor receptor 2 (VEGFR-2) transcription [27]. Similarly, PRH binds to Jun and cMyc inhibiting Jun- and cMyc-dependent transcription activation, respectively [12, 28]. PRH also activates transcription through multiple mechanisms including direct binding to target promoters as in the case of the NTCP promoter [19]. Moreover, PRH binding to hepatocyte nuclear factor 1α (HNF-1α) and serum-response factor (SRF) increases HNF-1α- and SRF-activated transcription [29, 30]. In addition, PRH can regulate gene expression post-transcriptionally through binding to eIF-4E. PRH binding to eIF-4E in PML nuclear bodies disrupts these structures and blocks eIF-4E-dependent transport of cyclin D1 mRNA down-regulating cyclin D1 protein expression [15].

2.3. PRH activity in tumourigenesis

Inappropriate expression and/or aberrant subcellular localization of PRH has been observed in a variety of disease states including acute myelogenous leukaemia (AML) [31, 32], chronic myelogenous leukaemia (CML) [32], breast, thyroid, and prostate cancer [33–36], liver disease, and cardiovascular disease [37, 38]. In normal haematopoietic cells PRH protein is clearly discernable in distinct foci within the nucleus, co-localising with PML and translation factor eIF-4E [14, 25], whereas in AML and CML PRH appears to be mislocalised to the cytoplasm [32]. Comparably, in thyroid cancer and breast cancer cells, PRH appears to be mislocalised from the nuclear compartment to the cytoplasm and often shows down-regulation in expression [33–35]. In breast and prostate cells loss of PRH activity results in increase cell proliferation and increased cell migration and invasion [35, 36]. Moreover, PRH over-expression in mouse mammary tumour cells inhibits tumour growth *in vivo* [36]. Similarly, PRH over-expression in liver cancer cells inhibits tumour growth in a xenograft mouse model [39] and PRH directly interacts with c-Myc to inhibit hepatocyte proliferation [28]. These studies are consistent with PRH playing a tumour suppressive role in these cell types.

In contrast, PRH has been shown to function as an oncoprotein in T-cell lineages and in AML subtypes (reviewed by Gaston et al. [40]). In retroviral insertion experiments in mice (Lvis1)-elevated PRH expression is associated with B-cell- and T-cell-derived leukaemias and lymphomas [41, 42]. Transgenic mice with ectopic PRH expression in T cell progenitors showed increased numbers of progenitors but this did not result in leukaemia [43]. However mice transplanted with bone marrow cells transduced with a retrovirus expressing PRH exhibit aggressive neoplastic transformation within T-cell populations [44] and in mouse models of early T-cell precursor-like acute lymphoblastic leukaemia (ETP-ALL), PRH is important in Lmo2-driven T-cell self-renewal [45, 46]. Furthermore, in a mouse model of AML elevated PRH is essential for the initiation and maintenance of the leukaemia [26]. Interestingly a human AML has been identified where alteration of the Nup98 and PRH genes to form a fusion gene is the only identified cytogenetic abnormality [31].

2.4. PRH in vascular compartments

PRH is expressed in the developing vascular system in haematopoietic and endothelial progenitor cells [9]. PRH over-expression inhibits haematopoietic and vascular development in embryoid bodies [47] while PRH loss leads to abnormal vasculogenesis and cardiac morphogenesis [5]. PRH can inhibit the proliferation of leukaemic cells by repressing the transcription of VEGFA and other genes involved in VEGF signalling and haematopoietic and vascular biology [48]. PRH is also important in neo-angiogenesis; in endothelial cells PRH represses transcription of multiple genes that control blood vessel formation including VEGFR-1, VEGFR-2, tyrosine kinase with Ig and EGF homology domains (TIE)-1, TIE-2, and neuropilin-1 [27, 49]. PRH is also targeted by urokinase-type plasminogen activator (uPA). uPA regulates angiogenesis and vascular permeability by proteolytic degradation of the extracellular matrix and through intracellular signalling. Single chain uPA is transported from the cell surface receptors to the nucleus where it modulates gene transcription by binding to transcription factors including PRH. The binding of uPA to PRH derepresses VEGFR-1 and VEGFR-2 thereby promoting their expression [50].

Importantly, PRH is up-regulated in VSMCs after balloon injury of the rat aorta [37]. During the period of cell dedifferentiation and cell proliferation following injury, PRH activates transcription of SMemb/NMHC-B, a marker for dedifferentiated cells [37]. Moreover, over-expression of PRH in embryonic fibroblasts results in the expression of early, but not late, markers of VSMC differentiation [29]. It has also been reported that in VSMCs infected with Human Cytomegalovirus (HCMV) PRH up-regulation promotes cell proliferation and inhibits apoptosis [51]. Our recent work has shown that PRH inhibits the proliferation of human and rat VSMCs (see Section 6.2 [38]). This suggests that HCMV infection may switch PRH from being an inhibitor of VSMC proliferation to an activator.

3. Protein kinase CK2

3.1. CK2 structure

Protein Kinase CK2 (formerly known as Casein Kinase II) is a ubiquitously expressed enzyme important in a range of cellular functions and processes including cell cycle progression and cell migration and invasion [52]. CK2 is a Ser/Thr kinase with the minimal consensus target sequence Ser/Thr– X – X – Asp/Glu/pSer (where X indicates any non-basic amino acid). However, CK2 can phosphorylate wide variety of target sequences. CK2 exists as a hetero-tetrameric enzyme consisting of two catalytic α subunits and two regulatory β subunits. In humans, two isoenzymic forms of the catalytic subunit, designated α and α', are well-characterised while a more recently discovered α'' subunit is less well understood [53–55].

3.2. CK2 function

CK2 is important in the control of cell migration and cell proliferation and in many other cell functions. To this end CK2 is pleiotropic, in that it has multiple effects via the phosphorylation of numerous cytoplasmic and nuclear proteins. For example, phosphorylation of inhibitor of kappa B (IκB) by CK2 causes disassembly of the nuclear factor kappa-light-chain-enhancer of activated B cells (NF-κB)-IκB complex [56]. This allows NF-κB to regulate the transcription of genes involved in cell cycle progression and cell survival. CK2 is also important in the control of extracellular proteins. For example, phosphorylation of the extracellular matrix protein vitronectin by CK2 is important for the adhesion of VSMCs [57]. CK2 itself is regulated by multiple signalling cascades and can cross talk to co-ordinate cell survival and cell proliferation. The ABL, Src and ERK kinase families all act as upstream regulators of CK2 and inhibitors that target these kinases can be used to inhibit CK2 indirectly [58–60].

3.3. CK2 in tumourigenesis

Aberrant CK2 activity has been demonstrated to be oncogenic and elevated CK2 expression is seen in multiple cancers including breast [61], prostate [62], lung [63], head and neck [64], and kidney cancers [65]. CK2-mediated abrogation of tumour suppressor activity or stimulation of oncogenic proteins has been demonstrated to play a significant role in tumourigenesis. The tumour suppressors promyelocytic leukaemia protein (PML), connexin, and phosphatase and tensin homology protein (PTEN) are all CK2 substrates that are inactivated by phosphorylation [66]. CK2 has additionally been shown to potentiate aberrant activation of oncoproteins including NF-κB [56], and AKT [67]. Drugs that inhibit CK2 have proven to be well-tolerated in a number of clinical trials and systemic or local delivery of these inhibitors is therefore a potential treatment for multiple disease states [68, 69].

4. The regulation of PRH by CK2

4.1. CK2 binds to PRH and phosphorylates the homeodomain

To identify PRH binding proteins we performed a yeast two hybrid screen using PRH as bait. This showed that the regulatory β subunit of CK2 can bind to the PRH N terminal domain [17]. The interaction was confirmed in human chronic myeloid leukaemia K562 cells using pull-down experiments and co-immunoprecipitation [17]. Importantly, PRH is a phosphoprotein in these cells and pharmacological inhibition of CK2 with DMAT (2-dimethylamino-4,5,6,7-tetrabromo-1H-benzimidazole) or TBB (4,5,6,7-tetrabromo-1H-benzotriazole) significantly reduces the amount of phosphorylated PRH (pPRH) indicating that PRH is also a CK2 substrate [17]. CK2β controls substrate specificity and therefore the interaction with PRH is potentially of importance for the control of CK2 activity on other specific substrates as well as in the phosphorylation of PRH.

To map CK2 phosphorylation sites within PRH, purified, human PRH protein was incubated with CK2 and ATP and subjected to surface-enhancer laser desorption/ionisation time-of-flight mass spectrophotometry (SELDI-TOF-MS) analysis. This showed that S163 and S177 located within the PRH homeodomain can be phosphorylated by CK2 [17]. S163 is located within a CK2 target consensus site while S177 is within a non-consensus site. Subsequently further phosphorylation sites have been identified within PRH but these sites have not been associated with a specific kinase.

4.2. Phosphorylation of PRH blocks DNA binding

Phosphorylation of the PRH homeodomain by CK2 abrogates PRH DNA-binding activity *in vitro* [17]. Interestingly DNA binding activity is restored by a subsequent incubation of pPRH with calf intestinal alkaline phosphatase. Thus, CK2-mediated phosphorylation of PRH functions as a reversible switch for DNA binding [17]. CK2 has also been shown to inhibit the binding of PRH to DNA in cells. Ectopic over-expression of PRH in K562 cells represses transcription of the PRH target gene VEGFR-1 but this repression is lost on co-transfection with CK2α and β transgenes [48]. However, the repression of VEGFR-1 transcription by a PRH mutant in which phosphorylation of serine 163 and serine 177 is prevented by the replacement of these residues by cysteine residues is not inhibited by CK2 over-expression [48]. Quantitative chromatin immunoprecipitation (ChIP) showed that CK2 over-expression does not prevent the binding of PRH S163C,S177C to the VEGFR-1 promoter as it does with wild-type PRH [48].

4.3. Phosphorylation of PRH induces protein processing

Hypo-phosphorylated PRH is stable in K562 cells treated with the translation inhibitor anisomycin [48]. However, pPRH is rapidly degraded in these cells. The half-life of pPRH is extended by treatment with proteasome inhibitors showing that phosphorylation targets PRH for proteasome-mediated protein cleavage. Interestingly, pPRH is cleaved to produce is a stable truncated protein that lacks the C-terminal domain (PRHδC). Over-expression of

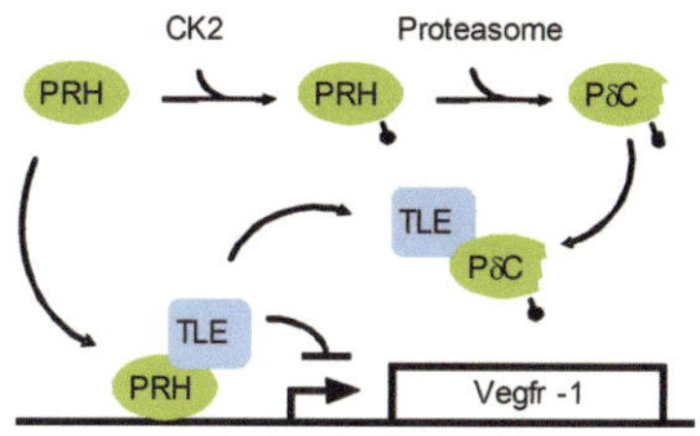

Figure 2. Phosphorylation of PRH by CK2 induces protein cleavage. PRH recruits co-repressor proteins including TLE to target genes such as VEGFR-1 in order to repress transcription. Phosphorylation of PRH by CK2 (shown as a filled lollipop) prevents PRH from binding to DNA and targets the protein for processing by the proteasome. The PRHδC protein cannot bind to DNA but it can sequester TLE proteins (and possibly other PRH interacting proteins) and thereby block transcriptional repression by PRH.

CK2 increases the production of this cleavage product and the truncated protein can act as transdominant negative regulator of full-length PRH by sequestering TLE co-repressor proteins and possibly other PRH interacting proteins [48]. This suggests that phosphorylation of PRH not only blocks DNA binding but also acts to prevent unphosphorylated PRH from regulating transcription (**Figure 2**). As might be expected, PRH S163C,S177C cannot be phosphorylated at these residues and this protein is not processed by the proteasome. In contrast, the phosphomimetic PRH S163E,S177E is more readily processed to produce PRHδC than wild type PRH [48].

4.4. pPRH in tumourigenesis

Pre-clinical studies have shown that pPRH is elevated in benign prostatic hyperplasias and in breast ductal carcinoma *in situ* compared to normal tissues [35, 36]. PRH localization is also altered in prostate and breast tumours compared to normal tissue. Both increased pPRH and increased PRH cytoplasmic localization are indicative of PRH inactivation and it is likely that this contributes to increased cell proliferation in these diseases. Interestingly, pPRH is less highly elevated in aggressive prostate adenocarcinomas and invasive breast carcinomas [35]. This could be due to decreased total PRH expression in these cancers. Thus high levels of pPRH appear to correlate more with hyperproliferative disease in these tissues rather than with advanced cancer.

5. PRH and CK2 in tumourigenesis

5.1. pPRH and PRH as potential biomarkers

The identification of protein modifications that contribute to increased cancer cell proliferation and increased cell migration and invasion is likely to result in new therapeutic approaches that could be of great benefit to patients. Moreover such cancer biomarkers could be useful as prognostic indicators and as indicators of pharmacologic responses to a therapeutic intervention. Prognostic biomarkers that can flag a tumour as potentially benign or requiring further treatment are urgently required. Many breast and prostate tumours for example do not need intervention and are currently over-treated by surgery because of a lack of biomarkers for prognosis. In pre-clinical studies the levels and localization of pPRH and PRH appear to be altered in breast and prostate tumours compared to controls [35, 36]. However, additional studies with large numbers of patients will be required to determine whether pPRH and PRH or the pPRH/PRH ratio is a good prognostic indicator.

5.2. The restoration of PRH function

Since PRH appears to be inactivated in breast and prostate cancer cells by CK2-dependent phosphorylation resulting in increased cell proliferation and cell migration, the inhibition of CK2 in these tissues would be expected to restore PRH function. This would be expected to inhibit cell proliferation and it could inhibit tumour growth. CK2 inhibitors have been proposed as novel treatments for multiple cancers including prostate cancer. In normal immortalised prostate epithelial cells the inhibition of proliferation brought about by the inhibition of CK2 requires the presence of PRH [35]. It is likely that CK2 inhibitors will have similar effects in other cancer cell types through the prevention of PRH phosphorylation and the restoration of PRH function. Indirect inhibition of CK2 activity can also restore PRH function and re-establish the control of cell proliferation. Our previous work showed that in chronic myeloid leukaemia cells Dasatinib decreases CK2 activity and decreases the phosphorylation of PRH [58]. Dasatinib inhibits membrane bound tyrosine kinases and Src family kinases and is an efficacious therapeutic for leukaemias expressing BCR-ABL fusion proteins and those with activated Src [70]. Importantly, Src-kinases are known to stimulate CK2 activity [59]. It is possible that other Abl/Src kinase inhibitors will also restore PRH activity via the indirect inhibition of CK2. However, since PRH can act as oncoprotein in some cell types it is possible that the reduction of PRH phosphorylation in these cell types might be counterproductive.

6. Saphenous vein graft failure

6.1. Intimal thickening in saphenous vein grafts

Atherosclerotic plaque development within coronary arteries is a major precursor for myocardial infarction (commonly known as heart attack). Coronary artery bypass graft (CABG) surgery is an effective treatment for occlusive or ruptured coronary artery atherosclerotic plaques; surgery most often involves harvesting and grafting of healthy, autologous saphenous vein to bypass the occluded artery and facilitate revascularisation of the cardiac tissue [71, 72]. Arteriovenous grafts are however predisposed to reblocking (restenosis), and despite extensive research, 10–15% of CABG patients suffer early vein graft failure within the first year after surgery, and as many as 50% suffer graft failure within 10 years [71–73]. Thrombosis, intimal thickening, and accelerated atherosclerosis are the underlying causes of saphenous vein graft failure. Intimal thickening, which serves as a foundation for superimposed atherosclerosis, is often the cause of late vein graft failure (**Figure 3**), while thrombosis is the cause of early graft failure. Intimal thickening is a product of aberrant VSMC migration into the intima where they proliferate and deposit extracellular matrix.

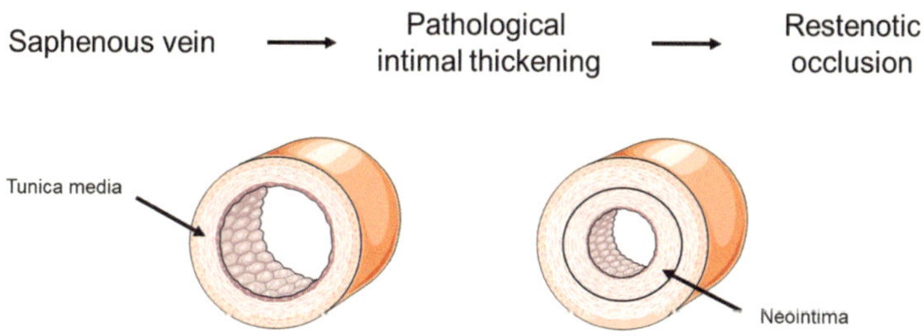

Figure 3. Intimal hyperplasia in saphenous vein grafts. Intimal hyperplasia in saphenous vein grafts is a consequence of the migration of medial VSMCs to the intima and their subsequent proliferation and deposition of extracellular matrix. Neointima formation results in narrowing of the lumen and a consequent restriction of blood flow.

6.2. PRH is up-regulated in neointimal cells

PRH expression is up-regulated in the intimal compartment of rat thoracic aortas injured with a balloon embolectomy catheter – a robust model for neointimal hyperplasia [37]. However, PRH mRNA and protein expression is absent in healthy aorta. Moreover PRH activates transcription of SMemb/NMHC-B, a marker of dedifferentiated VSMCs with a synthetic, proliferative phenotype, and not of differentiated VSMCs with a quiescent, contractile phenotype [37]. Together these findings could indicate that PRH promotes VSMC de-differentiation and accumulation in the intima, thereby accelerating disease progression. However, ectopic overexpression of wild-type PRH in primary cultures of rat aortic VSMCs inhibits cell cycle progression, whereas siRNA-mediated knockdown of PRH promotes cell proliferation [38]. These data clearly indicate an anti-proliferative role for PRH in VSMCs. Transfection of isolated rat aortic VSMCs with a vector expressing PRH F32E, a mutant that does not bind TLE, did not block cell proliferation suggesting that in these cells, PRH inhibits cell cycle progression in a TLE-independent manner (KSW unpublished observations). Interestingly, PRH S163C,S177C exhibited a prolonged anti-mitotic effect with respect to wild-type PRH [38]. This indicates that phosphorylation of PRH at Ser163 and Ser177 prevents PRH from inhibiting VSMC proliferation. Moreover, adenovirus-mediated gene transfer of PRH S163C,S177C retarded intimal thickening in an *ex vivo* human saphenous vein organ culture model [38]. It is hence likely that PRH is up-regulated during neointima formation in dedifferentiated, proliferating VSMCs as a negative feedback mechanism to prevent further rounds of mitosis.

6.3. CK2 activity during intimal thickening

Multiple studies have implicated the involvement of CK2 in the regulation of VSMC proliferation and pathophysiological intimal thickening. For example, treatment of cultured human aortic smooth muscle cells with emodin (1,3,8-trihydroxy-6-methylanthraquinone) – a naturally occurring CK2 inhibitor used in traditional Chinese medicine – blocked platelet-derived growth factor (PDGF)- and tumour necrosis factor α (TNF-α)-induced cell proliferation in a dose-dependent manner [74]. Also, in the rat aortic VSMC line A10, inhibition of CK2 with the synthetic compounds DDZ (daidzein) and DRB (5,6-dichlorobenzimidazole riboside) antagonised lysophosphatidic acid-induced cell division [75]. However, emodin, DDZ and DRB show high promiscuity as inhibitors [76]. PDGF, basic fibroblast growth factor (bFGF), and Wnt proteins are well-recognised atherogenic mitogens that are up-regulated in atherosclerotic and restenotic lesions ([38] and references therein). Interestingly, pharmacological inhibition of CK2 with the highly selective compounds TBB and K66 suppresses PDGF-, bFGF- and Wnt-4-induced cell replication in primary cultures of rat aortic VSMCs [38]. Silencing of CK2 using exogenous siRNAs also inhibited VSMC proliferation further suggesting that CK2 promotes the proliferation of these cells. Furthermore, treatment of human saphenous vein organ cultures with the CK2 inhibitor K66 disrupted neointima formation [38].

6.4. CK2 acts via PRH to modulate VSMC proliferation

One mechanism through which CK2 may facilitate VSMC proliferation could be via blocking PRH activity. Treatment with the K66 failed to arrest PDGF- and bFGF-stimulated cell cycle progression in VSMCs with depleted levels of PRH [38]. Thus CK2-dependent mitogenic signal transduction at least in part requires the presence of PRH (**Figure 4**). Similarly, treatment of human immortalised myelogenous K562 cells with the CK2 inhibitor DMAT inhibits cell proliferation but has no significant effect on the proliferation of K562 cells in which PRH has been knocked down using shRNA [58]. In K562 cells PRH controls cell proliferation via the inhibition of VEGF signalling [24, 58]. Further work is required to determine whether PRH controls VSMC proliferation via the inhibition of VEGF signalling or whether other signalling pathways targeted by PRH are important in this context. For instance, another potential mechanism by which PRH might control VSMC proliferation involves urokinase-type plasminogen activator (uPA)-mediated signalling [77]. uPA is a serine protease that is up-regulated in atheromas and restenotic lesions of human arteries [77–79]. In uPA deficient mice, subsequent to either electrical or mechanical arterial injury, intimal thickening and cell accumulation is significantly reduced compared to wild-type mice [80]. In human umbilical vein VSMCs, endogenous uPA has been shown to be involved in the induction of a mitogenic response by either PDGF or bFGF [77]. Furthermore, in PDGF- or bFGF-stimulated cells, pharmacological inhibition of uPA and CK2 with p-aminobenzamidine and 4 μM TBB, respectively, markedly enhances the anti-proliferative effects of 4 μM TBB alone in an additive manner [77]. Intracellular uPA has recently been shown to bind to PRH in endothelial

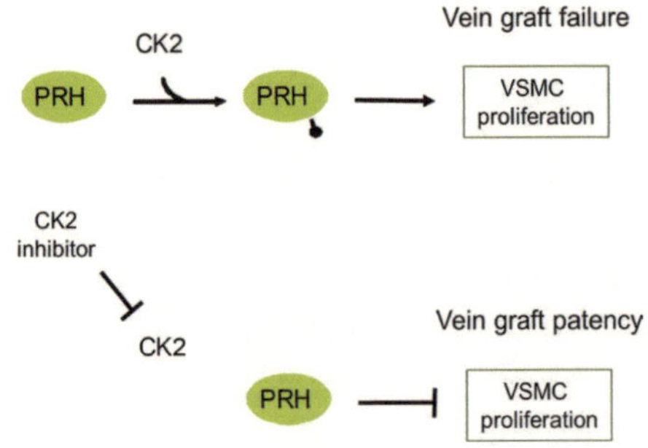

Figure 4. The inhibition of CK2 prevents intimal thickening. Top – phosphorylation of PRH by CK2 prevents PRH from inhibiting VSMC proliferation and this contributes to vein graft failure. Bottom – pharmacological inhibition of CK2 allows PRH to suppress VSMC proliferation and thereby prevent neointima formation. Other CK2 target proteins are also likely to play a role in the prevention of intimal thickening following CK2 inhibition.

cells and to prevent PRH from repressing VEGF signalling genes [50]. Therefore it is possible that the effects of uPA inhibition on endothelial proliferation and CK2 inhibition on VSMC proliferation during intimal thickening are both mediated by PRH.

6.5. Implications for saphenous vein grafts

As protein kinase CK2 is ubiquitously expressed, systemic delivery of a CK2 inhibitor for the treatment of saphenous vein graft degeneration may cause unwanted side effects. However, perivascular drug delivery systems could be employed for localised, sustained release of a CK2 inhibitor to a grafted vein. Such a system has been used to deliver sunitinib in a biocompatible hyaluronic acid-based hydrogel within a polyactide-co-glycolide perivascular wrap [81]. Other approaches for delivery include drug-eluting nanoparticles and drug-linked antibodies [82].

Gene therapy also has therapeutic potential in alleviating saphenous vein graft stenosis, and could be used for the introduction of PRH, particularly PRH S163C,S177C, to grafted vein. Genetic manipulation of a venous graft must however occur peri-operatively, meaning there is only a single opportunity to complete gene transfer. Therefore, helper-dependent adenovirus technology may be necessary to provide prolonged expression of PRH or PRH S163C,S177C within the grafted conduit [83, 84]. In a similar instance, delivery of tissue inhibitor of metalloproteinase 3 (TIMP-3) has been shown to block neointima formation in autologous porcine arteriovenous interposition grafts for up to 3 months [85].

7. Conclusion

The regulation of cell proliferation and cell migration/invasion by PRH is not limited to a particular cell type. Similarly, the control of PRH by CK2-dependent phosphorylation is also seen in multiple cell types. The PRH-CK2 axis is likely to be important for the regulation of cell proliferation and cell behaviour across a broad spectrum of cell types and in a variety of disease states. Further work in this area is therefore likely to be of great clinical relevance.

Acknowledgements

We are grateful to the British Heart Foundation (FS/10/58/28515) and the Medical Research Council for supporting this work. We apologise to the many authors whose papers we have not cited here due to space constraints.

Abbreviations

ATP	adenosine triphosphate
bFGF	basic fibroblast growth factor
CABG	coronary artery bypass graft

CK2	protein kinase CK2 (Casein Kinase II)
DDZ	daidzein
DMAT	2-dimethylamino-4,5,6,7-tetrabromo-1H-benzimidazole)
DRB	5,6-dichlorobenzimidazole riboside
K66	1-carboxymethyl-2-dimethylamino-4,5,6,7-tetrabromo-benzimidazole
PDGF	platelet-derived growth factor
SDS	sodium dodecyl sulphate
SELDI-TOF-MS	surface-enhancer laser desorption/ionisation time-of-flight mass spectrophotometry
TBB	4,5,6,7-tetrabromo-1H-benzotriazole
VSMC	vascular smooth muscle cell

Author details

Padma-Sheela Jayaraman[1], Kerry S. Wadey[2], Sarah J. George[2] and Kevin Gaston[3*]

*Address all correspondence to: kevin.gaston@bristol.ac.uk

1 Institute of Cancer and Genome Biology, College of Medical and Dental Sciences, University of Birmingham, Birmingham, UK

2 Bristol Medical School, University of Bristol, Bristol Royal Infirmary, Bristol, UK

3 School of Biochemistry, University of Bristol, Bristol, UK

References

[1] Soufi A, Jayaraman PS. PRH/Hex: An oligomeric transcription factor and multifunctional regulator of cell fate. Biochemical Journal. 2008;**412**(3):399-413

[2] Crompton MR, Bartlett TJ, MacGregor AD, Manfioletti G, Buratti E, Giancotti V, Goodwin GH. Identification of a novel vertebrate homeobox gene expressed in haematopoietic cells. Nucleic Acids Research. 1992;**20**(21):5661-5667

[3] Hromas R, Radich J, Collins S. PCR cloning of an orphan homeobox gene (PRH) preferentially expressed in myeloid and liver cells 30. Biochemical and Biophysical Research Communications. 1993;**195**(2):976-983

[4] Bedford FK, Ashworth A, Enver T, Wiedemann LM. HEX: A novel homeobox gene expressed during haematopoiesis and conserved between mouse and human. Nucleic Acids Research. 1993;**21**(5):1245-1249

[5] Hallaq H, Pinter E, Enciso J, McGrath J, Zeiss C, Brueckner M, Madri J, Jacobs HC, Wilson CM, Vasavada H, et al. A null mutation of Hhex results in abnormal cardiac development, defective vasculogenesis and elevated Vegfa levels. Development. 2004; **131**(20):5197-5209

[6] Martinez Barbera JP, Clements M, Thomas P, Rodriguez T, Meloy D, Kioussis D, Beddington RS. The homeobox gene Hex is required in definitive endodermal tissues for normal forebrain, liver and thyroid formation. Development. 2000;**127**(11):2433-2445

[7] Keng VW, Yagi H, Ikawa M, Nagano T, Myint Z, Yamada K, Tanaka T, Sato A, Muramatsu I, Okabe M, et al. Homeobox gene Hex is essential for onset of mouse embryonic liver development and differentiation of the monocyte lineage. Biochemical and Biophysical Research Communications. 2000;**276**(3):1155-1161

[8] Brickman JM, Jones CM, Clements M, Smith JC, Beddington RS. Hex is a transcriptional repressor that contributes to anterior identity and suppresses Spemann organiser function. Development. 2000;**127**(11):2303-2315

[9] Manfioletti G, Gattei V, Buratti E, Rustighi A, De IA, Aldinucci D, Goodwin GH, Pinto A. Differential expression of a novel proline-rich homeobox gene (Prh) in human hematolymphopoietic cells. Blood. 1995;**85**(5):1237-1245

[10] Guiral M, Bess K, Goodwin G, Jayaraman PS. PRH represses transcription in hematopoietic cells by at least two independent mechanisms. The Journal of Biological Chemistry. 2001;**276**(4):2961-2970

[11] Desjobert C, Noy P, Swingler T, Williams H, Gaston K, Jayaraman PS. The PRH/Hex repressor protein causes nuclear retention of Groucho/TLE co-repressors. Biochemical Journal. 2009;**417**(1):121-132

[12] Schaefer LK, Shuguang W, Schaefer TS. Functional interaction of Jun and homeodomain proteins. The Journal of Biological Chemistry. 2001;**276**:43074-43082

[13] Tanaka T, Inazu T, Yamada K, Myint Z, Keng VW, Inoue Y, Taniguchi N, Noguchi T. cDNA cloning and expression of rat homeobox gene, Hex, and functional characterization of the protein. Biochemical Journal. 1999;**339**(1):111-117

[14] Topcu Z, Mack DL, Hromas RA, Borden KL. The promyelocytic leukemia protein PML interacts with the proline-rich homeodomain protein PRH: A RING may link hematopoiesis and growth control. Oncogene. 1999;**18**(50):7091-7100

[15] Topisirovic I, Culjkovic B, Cohen N, Perez JM, Skrabanek L, Borden KL. The proline-rich homeodomain protein, PRH, is a tissue-specific inhibitor of eIF4E-dependent cyclin D1 mRNA transport and growth. The EMBO Journal. 2003;**22**(3):689-703

[16] Bess KL, Swingler TE, Rivett AJ, Gaston K, Jayaraman PS. The transcriptional repressor protein PRH interacts with the proteasome. Biochemical Journal. 2003;**374**(3):667-675

[17] Soufi A, Noy P, Buckle M, Sawasdichai A, Gaston K, Jayaraman PS. CK2 phosphorylation of the PRH/Hex homeodomain functions as a reversible switch for DNA binding. Nucleic Acids Research. 2009;**37**:3288-3300

[18] Kasamatsu S, Sato A, Yamamoto T, Keng VW, Yoshida H, Yamazaki Y, Shimoda M, Miyazaki J, Noguchi T. Identification of the transactivating region of the homeodomain protein, hex. Journal of Biochemistry (Tokyo). 2004;**135**(2):217-223

[19] Denson LA, Karpen SJ, Bogue CW, Jacobs HC. Divergent homeobox gene hex regulates promoter of the Na(+)-dependent bile acid cotransporter 5. American Journal of Physiology-Gastrointestinal and Liver Physiology. 2000;**279**(2):G347-G355

[20] Soufi A, Smith C, Clarke AR, Gaston K, Jayaraman PS. Oligomerisation of the developmental regulator proline rich homeodomain (PRH/Hex) is mediated by a novel proline-rich dimerisation domain. Journal of Molecular Biology. 2006;**358**(4):943-962

[21] Williams H, Jayaraman PS, Gaston K. DNA wrapping and distortion by an oligomeric homeodomain protein. Journal of Molecular Biology. 2008;**383**(1):10-23

[22] Cong R, Jiang X, Wilson CM, Hunter MP, Vasavada H, Bogue CW. Hhex is a direct repressor of endothelial cell-specific molecule 1 (ESM-1). Biochemical and Biophysical Research Communications. 2006;**346**(2):535-545

[23] Zamparini AL, Watts T, Gardner CE, Tomlinson SR, Johnston GI, Brickman JM. Hex acts with beta-catenin to regulate anteroposterior patterning via a Groucho-related co-repressor and nodal. Development. 2006;**133**(18):3709-3722

[24] Noy P, Williams H, Sawasdichai A, Gaston K, Jayaraman P-S. PRH/Hhex controls cell survival through coordinate transcriptional regulation of vascular endothelial growth factor signaling. Molecular and Cellular Biology. 2010;**30**(9):2120-2134

[25] Swingler TE, Bess KL, Yao J, Stifani S, Jayaraman PS. The proline-rich homeodomain protein recruits members of the Groucho/Transducin-like enhancer of split protein family to co-repress transcription in hematopoietic cells. Journal of Biological Chemistry. 2004;**279**(33):34938-34947

[26] Shields BJ, Jackson JT, Metcalf D, Shi W, Huang Q, Garnham AL, Glaser SP, Beck D, Pimanda JE, Bogue CW, et al. Acute myeloid leukemia requires Hhex to enable PRC2-mediated epigenetic repression of Cdkn2a. Genes & Development. 2016;**30**(1):78-91

[27] Minami T, Murakami T, Horiuchi K, Miura M, Noguchi T, Miyazaki J, Hamakubo T, Aird WC, Kodama T. Interaction between hex and GATA transcription factors in vascular endothelial cells inhibits flk-1/KDR-mediated vascular endothelial growth factor signaling. Journal of Biological Chemistry. 2004;**279**(20):20626-20635

[28] Marfil V, Blazquez M, Serrano F, Castell JV, Bort R. Growth-promoting and tumourigenic activity of c-Myc is suppressed by Hhex. Oncogene. 2014;**34**(23):3011-3022

[29] Oyama Y, Kawai-Kowase K, Sekiguchi K, Sato M, Sato H, Yamazaki M, Ohyama Y, Aihara Y, Iso T, Okamaoto E, et al. Homeobox protein Hex facilitates serum responsive factor-mediated activation of the SM22alpha gene transcription in embryonic fibroblasts. Arteriosclerosis, Thrombosis, and Vascular Biology. 2004;**24**(9):1602-1607

[30] Tanaka H, Yamamoto T, Ban T, Satoh S, Tanaka T, Shimoda M, Miyazaki J, Noguchi T. Hex stimulates the hepatocyte nuclear factor 1alpha-mediated activation of transcription. Archives of Biochemistry and Biophysics. 2005;**442**(1):117-124

[31] Jankovic D, Gorello P, Liu T, Ehret S, La SR, Desjobert C, Baty F, Brutsche M, Jayaraman PS, Santoro A, et al. Leukemogenic mechanisms and targets of a NUP98/HHEX fusion in acute myeloid leukemia. Blood. 2008;**111**(12):5672-5682

[32] Topisirovic I, Guzman ML, McConnell MJ, Licht JD, Culjkovic B, Neering SJ, Jordan CT, Borden KL. Aberrant eukaryotic translation initiation factor 4E-dependent mRNA transport impedes hematopoietic differentiation and contributes to leukemogenesis. Molecular and Cellular Biology. 2003;**23**(24):8992-9002

[33] D'Elia AV, Tell G, Russo D, Arturi F, Puglisi F, Manfioletti G, Gattei V, Mack DL, Cataldi P, Filetti S, et al. Expression and localization of the homeodomain-containing protein HEX in human thyroid tumors. The Journal of Clinical Endocrinology and Metabolism. 2002;**87**(3):1376-1383

[34] Puppin C, Puglisi F, Pellizzari L, Manfioletti G, Pestrin M, Pandolfi M, Piga A, Di LC, Damante G. HEX expression and localization in normal mammary gland and breast carcinoma. BMC Cancer. 2006;**6**:e192

[35] Siddiqui YH, Kershaw RM, Humphreys EH, Assis Junior EM, Chaudhri S, Jayaraman PS, Gaston K. CK2 abrogates the inhibitory effects of PRH/HHEX on prostate cancer cell migration and invasion and acts through PRH to control cell proliferation. Oncogene. 2017;**6**(1):e293

[36] Kershaw RM, Roberts D, Wragg J, Shaaban AM, Humphreys E, Halsall J, Price L, Bicknell R, Gaston K, Jayaraman PS. Proline-rich homeodomain protein (PRH/HHEX) is a suppressor of breast tumour growth. Oncogene. 2017;**6**(6):e346

[37] Sekiguchi K, Kurabayashi M, Oyama Y, Aihara Y, Tanaka T, Sakamoto H, Hoshino Y, Kanda T, Yokoyama T, Shimomura Y, et al. Homeobox protein hex induces SMemb/nonmuscle myosin heavy chain-B gene expression through the cAMP-responsive element. Circulation Research. 2001;**88**(1):52-58

[38] Wadey KS, Brown BA, Sala-Newby GB, Jayaraman PS, Gaston K, George SJ. Protein kinase CK2 inhibition suppresses neointima formation via a proline-rich homeodomain-dependent mechanism. Vascular Pharmacology. 2017;**99**:34-44

[39] Su J, You P, Zhao JP, Zhang SL, Song SH, ZR F, Ye LW, Zi XY, Xie DF, Zhu MH, et al. A potential role for the homeoprotein Hhex in hepatocellular carcinoma progression. Medical Oncology. 2012;**29**(2):1059-1067

[40] Gaston K, Tsitsilianos MA, Wadey K, Jayaraman PS. Misregulation of the proline rich homeodomain (PRH/HHEX) protein in cancer cells and its consequences for tumour growth and invasion. Cell & Bioscience. 2016;**6**:e12

[41] Hansen GM, Justice MJ. Activation of Hex and mEg5 by retroviral insertion may contribute to mouse B-cell leukemia. Oncogene. 1999;**18**(47):6531-6539

[42] Li J, Shen H, Himmel KL, Dupuy AJ, Largaespada DA, Nakamura T, Shaughnessy JD Jr, Jenkins NA, Copeland NG. Leukaemia disease genes: Large-scale cloning and pathway predictions. Nature Genetics. 1999;**23**(3):348-353

[43] Mack DL, Leibowitz DS, Cooper S, Ramsey H, Broxmeyer HE, Hromas R. Down-regulation of the myeloid homeobox protein Hex is essential for normal T-cell development. Immunology. 2002;**107**(4):444-451

[44] George A, Morse HC III, Justice MJ. The homeobox gene Hex induces T-cell-derived lymphomas when overexpressed in hematopoietic precursor cells. Oncogene. 2003;**22**(43): 6764-6773

[45] McCormack MP, Young LF, Vasudevan S, de Graaf CA, Codrington R, Rabbitts TH, Jane SM, Curtis DJ. The Lmo2 oncogene initiates leukemia in mice by inducing thymocyte self-renewal. Science. 2010;**327**(5967):879-883

[46] Smith S, Tripathi R, Goodings C, Cleveland S, Mathias E, Hardaway JA, Elliott N, Yi Y, Chen X, Downing J, et al. LIM domain only-2 (LMO2) induces T-cell leukemia by two distinct pathways. PLoS One. 2014;**9**(1):e85883

[47] Kubo A, Chen V, Kennedy M, Zahradka E, Daley GQ, Keller G. The homeobox gene HEX regulates proliferation and differentiation of hemangioblasts and endothelial cells during ES cell differentiation. Blood. 2005;**105**(12):4590-4597

[48] Noy P, Sawasdichai A, Jayaraman PS, Gaston K. Protein kinase CK2 inactivates PRH/Hhex using multiple mechanisms to de-repress VEGF-signalling genes and promote cell survival. Nucleic Acids Research. 2012;**40**(18):9008-9020

[49] Nakagawa T, Abe M, Yamazaki T, Miyashita H, Niwa H, Kokubun S, Sato Y. HEX acts as a negative regulator of angiogenesis by modulating the expression of angiogenesis-related gene in endothelial cells in vitro. Arteriosclerosis, Thrombosis, and Vascular Biology. 2003;**23**(2):231-237

[50] Stepanova V, Jayaraman PS, Zaitsev SV, Lebedeva T, Bdeir K, Kershaw R, Holman KR, Parfyonova YV, Semina EV, Beloglazova IB, et al. Urokinase-type plasminogen activator (uPA) promotes angiogenesis by attenuating proline-rich homeodomain protein (PRH) transcription factor activity and de-repressing vascular endothelial growth factor (VEGF) receptor expression. The Journal of Biological Chemistry. 2016;**291**(29):15029-15045

[51] Li L, Liu M, Kang L, Li Y, Dai Z, Wang B, Liu S, Chen L, Tan Y, Wu G. HHEX: A cross-talker between HCMV infection and proliferation of VSMCs. Frontiers in Cellular and Infection Microbiology. 2016;**6**:e169

[52] Litchfield DW. Protein kinase CK2: Structure, regulation and role in cellular decisions of life and death. Biochemical Journal. 2003;**369**(1):1-15

[53] Wirkner U, Voss H, Lichter P, Ansorge W, Pyerin W. The human gene (CSNK2A1) coding for the casein kinase II subunit alpha is located on chromosome 20 and contains tandemly arranged Alu repeats. Genomics. 1994;**19**(2):257-265

[54] Bodenbach L, Fauss J, Robitzki A, Krehan A, Lorenz P, Lozeman FJ, Pyerin W. Recombinant human casein kinase II. A study with the complete set of subunits (alpha, alpha' and beta), site-directed autophosphorylation mutants and a bicistronically expressed holoenzyme. European Journal of Biochemistry. 1994;**220**(1):263-273

[55] Yang-Feng TL, Naiman T, Kopatz I, Eli D, Dafni N, Canaani D. Assignment of the human casein kinase II alpha' subunit gene (CSNK2A1) to chromosome 16p13.2-p13.3. Genomics. 1994;**19**(1):173

[56] Wang D, Westerheide SD, Hanson JL, Baldwin AS Jr. Tumor necrosis factor alpha-induced phosphorylation of RelA/p65 on Ser529 is controlled by casein kinase II. The Journal of Biological Chemistry. 2000;**275**(42):32592-32597

[57] Stepanova V, Jerke U, Sagach V, Lindschau C, Dietz R, Haller H, Dumler I. Urokinase-dependent human vascular smooth muscle cell adhesion requires selective vitronectin phosphorylation by ectoprotein kinase CK2. The Journal of Biological Chemistry. 2002;**277**(12):10265-10272

[58] Noy P, Gaston K, Jayaraman PS. Dasatinib inhibits leukaemic cell survival by decreasing PRH/Hhex phosphorylation resulting in increased repression of VEGF signalling genes. Leukemia Research. 2012;**36**(11):1434-1437

[59] Donella-Deana A, Cesaro L, Sarno S, Ruzzene M, Brunati AM, Marin O, Vilk G, Doherty-Kirby A, Lajoie G, Litchfield DW, et al. Tyrosine phosphorylation of protein kinase CK2 by Src-related tyrosine kinases correlates with increased catalytic activity. Biochemical Journal. 2003;**372**(3):841-849

[60] Mishra S, Reichert A, Cunnick J, Senadheera D, Hemmeryckx B, Heisterkamp N, Groffen J. Protein kinase CKIIalpha interacts with the Bcr moiety of Bcr/Abl and mediates proliferation of Bcr/Abl-expressing cells. Oncogene. 2003;**22**(51):8255-8262

[61] Landesman-Bollag E, Song DH, Romieu-Mourez R, Sussman DJ, Cardiff RD, Sonenshein GE, Seldin DC. Protein kinase CK2: Signaling and tumorigenesis in the mammary gland. Molecular and Cellular Biochemistry. 2001;**227**(1-2):153-165

[62] Yenice S, Davis AT, Goueli SA, Akdas A, Limas C, Ahmed K. Nuclear casein kinase 2 (CK-2) activity in human normal, benign hyperplastic, and cancerous prostate. Prostate. 1994;**24**(1):11-16

[63] Daya-Makin M, Sanghera JS, Mogentale TL, Lipp M, Parchomchuk J, Hogg JC, Pelech SL. Activation of a tumor-associated protein kinase (p40TAK) and casein kinase 2 in human squamous cell carcinomas and adenocarcinomas of the lung. Cancer Research. 1994;**54**(8):2262-2268

[64] Faust RA, Gapany M, Tristani P, Davis A, Adams GL, Ahmed K. Elevated protein kinase CK2 activity in chromatin of head and neck tumors: Association with malignant transformation. Cancer Letters. 1996;**101**(1):31-35

[65] Stalter G, Siemer S, Becht E, Ziegler M, Remberger K, Issinger OG. Asymmetric expression of protein kinase CK2 subunits in human kidney tumors. Biochemical and Biophysical Research Communications. 1994;**202**(1):141-147

[66] Scaglioni PP, Yung TM, Cai LF, Erdjument-Bromage H, Kaufman AJ, Singh B, Teruya-Feldstein J, Tempst P, Pandolfi PP. A CK2-dependent mechanism for degradation of the PML tumor suppressor. Cell. 2006;**126**(2):269-283

[67] Di Maira G, Salvi M, Arrigoni G, Marin O, Sarno S, Brustolon F, Pinna LA, Ruzzene M. Protein kinase CK2 phosphorylates and upregulates Akt/PKB. Cell Death and Differentiation. 2005;**12**(6):668-677

[68] Battistutta R, Cozza G, Pierre F, Papinutto E, Lolli G, Sarno S, O'Brien SE, Siddiqui-Jain A, Haddach M, Anderes K, et al. Unprecedented selectivity and structural determinants of a new class of protein kinase CK2 inhibitors in clinical trials for the treatment of cancer. Biochemistry. 2011;**50**(39):8478-8488

[69] Martins LR, Lucio P, Melao A, Antunes I, Cardoso BA, Stansfield R, Bertilaccio MT, Ghia P, Drygin D, Silva MG, et al. Activity of the clinical-stage CK2-specific inhibitor CX-4945 against chronic lymphocytic leukemia. Leukemia. 2014;**28**(1):179-182

[70] Steinberg M. Dasatinib: A tyrosine kinase inhibitor for the treatment of chronic myelogenous leukemia and philadelphia chromosome-positive acute lymphoblastic leukemia. Clinical Therapeutics. 2007;**29**(11):2289-2308

[71] Yusuf S, Zucker D, Peduzzi P, Fisher LD, Takaro T, Kennedy JW, Davis K, Killip T, Passamani E, Norris R, et al. Effect of coronary artery bypass graft surgery on survival: Overview of 10-year results from randomised trials by the coronary artery bypass graft surgery trialists collaboration. Lancet. 1994;**344**(8922):563-570

[72] Eagle KA, Guyton RA, Davidoff R, Edwards FH, Ewy GA, Gardner TJ, Hart JC, Herrmann HC, Hillis LD, Hutter AM Jr, et al. ACC/AHA 2004 guideline update for coronary artery bypass graft surgery: A report of the American College of Cardiology/American Heart Association task force on practice guidelines (committee to update the 1999 guidelines for coronary artery bypass graft surgery). Circulation. 2004;**110**(14):e340-e437

[73] Harskamp RE, Lopes RD, Baisden CE, de Winter RJ, Alexander JH. Saphenous vein graft failure after coronary artery bypass surgery: Pathophysiology, management, and future directions. Annals of Surgery. 2013;**257**(5):824-833

[74] Heo SK, Yun HJ, Park WH, Park SD. Emodin inhibits TNF-alpha-induced human aortic smooth-muscle cell proliferation via caspase- and mitochondrial-dependent apoptosis. Journal of Cellular Biochemistry. 2008;**105**(1):70-80

[75] YJ X, Rathi SS, Chapman DC, Arneja AS, Dhalla NS. Mechanisms of lysophosphatidic acid-induced DNA synthesis in vascular smooth muscle cells. Journal of Cardiovascular Pharmacology. 2003;**41**(3):381-387

[76] Pagano MA, Bain J, Kazimierczuk Z, Sarno S, Ruzzene M, Di Maira G, Elliott M, Orzeszko A, Cozza G, Meggio F, et al. The selectivity of inhibitors of protein kinase CK2: An update. The Biochemical Journal. 2008;**415**(3):353-365

[77] Padro T, Mesters RM, Dankbar B, Hintelmann H, Bieker R, Kiehl M, Berdel WE, Kienast J. The catalytic domain of endogenous urokinase-type plasminogen activator is required for the mitogenic activity of platelet-derived and basic fibroblast growth factors in human vascular smooth muscle cells. Journal of Cell Science. 2002;**115**(9):1961-1971

[78] Lupu F, Heim DA, Bachmann F, Hurni M, Kakkar VV, Kruithof EKO. Plasminogen activator expression in human atherosclerotic lesions. Arteriosclerosis, Thrombosis, and Vascular Biology. 1995;**15**(9):1444-1455

[79] Raghunath PN, Tomaszewski JE, Brady ST, Caron RJ, Okada SS, Barnathan ES. Plasminogen activator system in human coronary atherosclerosis. Arteriosclerosis, Thrombosis, and Vascular Biology. 1995;**15**(9):1432-1443

[80] Carmeliet P, Moons L, Herbert J-M, Crawley J, Lupu F, Lijnen R, Collen D. Urokinase but not tissue plasminogen activator mediates arterial neointima formation in mice. Circulation Research. 1997;**81**(5):829-839

[81] Sanders WG, Hogrebe PC, Grainger DW, Cheung AK, Terry CM. A biodegradable perivascular wrap for controlled, local and directed drug delivery. Journal of Controlled Release: Official Journal of the Controlled Release Society. 2012;**161**(1):81-89

[82] Thomas AC. Targeted treatments for restenosis and vein graft disease. ISRN Vascular Medicine. 2012;**2012**:23

[83] Oka K, Pastore L, Kim IH, Merched A, Nomura S, Lee HJ, Merched-Sauvage M, Arden-Riley C, Lee B, Finegold M, et al. Long-term stable correction of low-density lipoprotein receptor-deficient mice with a helper-dependent adenoviral vector expressing the very low-density lipoprotein receptor. Circulation. 2001;**103**(9):1274-1281

[84] Belalcazar LM, Merched A, Carr B, Oka K, Chen KH, Pastore L, Beaudet A, Chan L. Long-term stable expression of human apolipoprotein A-I mediated by helper-dependent adenovirus gene transfer inhibits atherosclerosis progression and remodels atherosclerotic plaques in a mouse model of familial hypercholesterolemia. Circulation. 2003;**107**(21):2726-2732

[85] George SJ, Wan S, Hu J, MacDonald R, Johnson JL, Baker AH. Sustained reduction of vein graft neointima formation by ex vivo TIMP-3 gene therapy. Circulation. 2011;**124**(11 Suppl):S135-S142

Chapter 13

Dual Role of METCAM/MUC18 Expression in the Progression of Cancer Cells

Guang-Jer Wu

Additional information is available at the end of the chapter

http://dx.doi.org/10.5772/intechopen.72742

Abstract

The altered expression of cell adhesion molecules (CAMs) correlates with the malignant progression of many epithelial tumors. MUC18/CD146/A32/MelCAM/S-endo 1, a CAM in the immunoglobulin gene superfamily, is an integral membrane glycoprotein. MUC18 is not a mucin, resulting from its misleading nomenclature by the original discoverer. We re-named it as METCAM (metastasis-regulating CAM), based on its very interesting biological roles in tumor formation and metastasis of many epithelial tumors. Initial findings show that METCAM/MUC18 expression has a positive effect (as a tumor and metastasis promoter) on the progression of breast cancer, most melanoma cell lines, nasopharyngeal carcinoma (NPC) type II, and prostate cancer. Later research results show that METCAM/MUC18 expression has a negative effect (as a tumor suppressor and metastasis suppressor) on the progression of ovarian cancer, one mouse melanoma cell line, and nasopharyngeal carcinoma type I, and perhaps hemangioma. Since the above dual function of METCAM/MUC18 occurs only in different cell lines from the same cancer type or in those from different cancer types, we suggest that the different effect of METCAM/MUC18 on tumor formation and metastasis of different cancer cell line may be due to different intrinsic properties (co-factors) in each cancer cell line that modify the biological functions of METCAM/MUC18 in the intrinsic properties of tumor cells and their interactions with the tumor microenvironment. This chapter will review the published work and present some possible mechanisms for the METCAM/MUC18-mediated cancer progression for future studies.

Keywords: METCAM/MUC18, breast cancer, melanoma, nasopharyngeal carcinoma, ovarian cancer, prostate cancer, tumors

1. Introduction

Cancer progression is very complex because many genes are directly or indirectly involved in the process. The accumulation of the multiple intrinsic changes leading to aberrant alterations of gene expression can contribute to tumorigenesis and its progression to the malignant phenotype. This is because the genome of malignant tumor cells has greater instability than non-malignant tumor cells and renders malignant tumor cells more prone to acquiring multiple mutations [1]. Tumorigenesis involves expression of many oncogenes and tumor suppressor genes [2, 3], which will not be elaborated here. Likewise, metastasis also involves many metastasis enhancer genes and metastasis suppressor genes [2, 3] ever since the successful conversion of a non-metastatic Ha-ras-transformed NIH 3 T3 fibroblast cells to metastatic tumor cells by transfecting the cells with the DNA fragments isolated from a human metastatic tumor [4]. This also suggests that many alternative pathways are possible for metastasis, similar to multiple alternative pathways leading to tumorigenesis [2, 3]. This includes the genes encoding cell adhesion molecules (CAMs), such as E-cadherin [5], integrins $\alpha2\beta1$ [6] and $\alpha V\beta3$ [7], CD44 [8], EPCAM [9, 10], ALCAM [11], and METCAM/MUC18 [12, 13]. The list of these genes has been rapidly lengthened because of the advent of modern state-of-the-art technologies, such as SAGE analysis [14, 15], DNA chip microarray analysis [16–19], and proteomics [20–22]. Some of these genes may be commonly used by metastatic tumors derived from different tissues, if these genes render tumor cells with a metastatic advantage over other tumor cells, regardless of their origins. Some oncogenes or tumor suppressor genes may also play direct or indirect roles in tumor metastasis, if they directly or indirectly alter cytoskeleton structure, cellular motility, invasiveness, and render them having growth advantages in target organs.

Tumor metastases fortunately are a rare event due to metastatic inefficiency. It was originally thought that only a very small population of the metastatic cells could reach and establish the growth in the distant target organs after they successfully intravasate or extravasate the vasculatures or lymphatics, and then survive the assaults in the circulatory system, which includes the attacks from the immune system and the destructive hydrodynamic shearing [23]. However, recent results of observing the process with *in vivo* video microscopy appear to support the notion that metastatic inefficiency is more likely due to that only a small percentage of tumor cells are able to dock and establish secondary growths in distant organs after survival from the attacks from the immune system and the assault from the mechanical shearing, since both highly metastatic cells and non-metastatic cells have similar migratory and invasive abilities to intravasate or extravasate the circulatory systems [24]. The successful establishment of secondary growth by metastatic cells may result from a complex interaction of tumor cells with the extracellular matrix in the favorable microenvironment of the target organs. This interaction may also be due to the altered expressions of many cell adhesion molecules (CAMs) in metastatic cells that alter their ability to interact with the extracellular matrix.

CAMs govern the social behaviors of the cells. The altered expression of CAMs affects cell-cell interactions and cell-extracellular matrix interactions, which results in changing the cellular motility and invasiveness [25]. Altered expression of CAMs also can affect survival and growth of tumor cells and alter angiogenesis [26]. As such, CAMs may promote or suppress the metastatic potential of tumor cells [26]. The metastatic potential of a tumor cell could be the consequence of a complex participation of many over- or under-expressed CAMs, as documented in many carcinomas [27]. For example, integrins αV, $\alpha 4$, and $\beta 3$, I-CAM, METCAM/MUC18, and HLA-DR are over-expressed, whereas E-cadherin, α-catenin, and VCAM are under-expressed in metastatic melanomas [28]. On the other hand, the metastatic potential of a tumor cell could be due to the altered expression of a single CAM. For example, over-expression of integrin α2β1 decreases the metastasis of breast carcinoma cells [6], whereas over-expression of integrin αVβ3 increases the metastatic potential of human prostate carcinoma cells [7].

Effects of altered expression of I-CAM, V-CAM, some integrins (αV, α4, and ß3), L1CAM, METCAM/MUC18 [28], and E-cadherin [29] on the metastasis of melanoma have been demonstrated. Studies of the altered expression of CAMs on the metastasis of prostate cancers are E-cadherin [5], CD44 [8, 30], CEA-CAM [31, 32], and some integrins [7, 33, 34]. Increased expression of E-cadherin [35] and the standard form of CD44 [8] suppresses metastasis of prostate carcinoma. On the contrary, increased expression of a splicing variant form of CD44, CD44v7-v10, correlates with the progression of prostate carcinoma and enhances *in vitro* invasiveness of human prostate cancer cell lines [30]. Increased expression of CEA-CAM1 suppresses tumorigenesis [32]; however, the effect on metastasis has not been tested. The effect of a single integrin mostly is not obvious except αVβ3, α6β1, and α3β1 integrins in prostate cancer, perhaps many members of the integrin family are functionally compensatory to each other [33–36]. Aberrant expression of CAMs has been associated with nasopharyngeal carcinoma (NPC). For examples, up-regulation of ICAM [37] and down-regulation of E-cadherin [38, 39] and connexin 43 [40] correlate with the progression of NPC; however, the expression of CD44 does not [38]. Aberrant expression of various CAMs associated with the malignant progression of ovarian cancer are mucins [41], integrins [42], CD44 [43], L1CAM [44], E-cadherin [45], claudin-3 [46], EpCAM [9, 10], and METCAM/MUC18 [47, 48].

For the past two decades, we have focused our research on the role of METCAM/MUC18 in the progression of several epithelial tumors: first, we tried to correlate the expression level of METCAM/MUC18, which was determined by using the methods of immunohistochemistry and/or RT-PCR, with the pathological state of the tumor tissues and from the results to propose a hypothesis to predict the possible positive or negative role played by METCAM/MUC18 in the progression of each cancer. Then we tested the hypothesis by investigating effects of METCAM/MUC18 over-expression or under-expression on *in vitro* cellular behaviors and tumorigenesis and on *in vivo* tumorigenesis in athymic nude mice, or if possible, in syngeneic mice. We studied the effect of the expression of METCAM/MUC18 on the progression of melanoma cell lines [49, 50] and prostate cancer cell lines [51–55], and then extended our research to breast cancer cell lines [56–58], ovarian cancer cell lines [48, 59, 60], and nasopharyngeal carcinoma cell lines [61] Possible mechanisms played by METCAM/MUC18 were preliminarily determined by analyzing the expression levels of several downstream effectors in the tumor tissues excised from these mice. In this chapter, I will summarize the findings of the above research activities and review the dual role of METCAM/MUC18 in the progression of breast cancer, melanoma, nasopharyngeal carcinoma, ovarian cancer, and prostate cancer [48–62]. I will also propose some possible mechanisms of METCAM/MUC18-mediated tumorigenesis and metastasis for future studies.

2. METCAM/MUC18

Human METCAM/MUC18 (huMETCAM/MUC18), a CAM in the immunoglobulin gene superfamily, is an integral membrane glycoprotein [63]. The name "MUC18", which was originally coined by Judy Johnson [63], has often been mistaken as a new member in the mucin family. Other names, such as CD146, A32, and S-endo 1, were not used because they did not reflect its biological functions [63–68]. The names MCAM and MELCAM with an over-emphasis on its role in melanoma [28] are discarded because MUC18 is involved in the metastasis of many cancers besides melanoma ([69] and this review). To eliminate confusion and to reflect its biochemical properties and key role in the progression of epithelial tumors, we have created a new name for MUC18: METCAM (metastasis CAM), an immunoglobulin-like CAM that regulates metastasis [69]. MUC18 is included in our nomenclature to commemorate its original discovery [63].

Judy Johnson's group was the first group to clone and characterize the sequence of a huMETCAM/MUC18 cDNA from human melanoma [63]. Later my group cloned the huMETCAM/MUC18 cDNA from several human melanoma cell lines and human prostate cancer cell lines [70]. The DNA sequences of our huMETCAM/MUC18 cDNA clones from three human melanoma cell lines, three human prostate cancer cell lines, and several human nasopharyngeal tissues are similar; therefore, we conclude that our huMETCAM/MUC18 cDNA gene is the major common form in comparison to that of Judy Johnson. The amino acid sequences deduced from the DNA sequence of our huMETCAM/MUC18 cDNA differ from that of Johnson's group in seven amino acids [63, 70]. Regardless of minor differences in amino acid sequences, all huMETCAM/MUC18 cDNAs encode 646 amino acids that include a N-terminal extracellular domain of 558 amino acids, of which at the N-terminus it has 28 amino acids characteristic of a signal peptide sequence, a transmembrane domain of 24 amino acids (amino acid #559–583), and an intracellular cytoplasmic domain of 64 amino acids at the C-terminus (**Figure 1**). The molecular weight of the un-glycosylated form of huMETCAM/MUC18 protein is estimated to be about 72 kDa [63, 69, 70]. Since huMETCAM/MUC18 has eight putative N-glycosylation sites (Asn-X-Ser/Thr), it is often heavily glycosylated and sialylated resulting with an apparent molecular weight between 113,000 and 150,000, dependent upon the tissue origin. The extracellular domain of the protein contains five immunoglobulin-like domains (V-V-C2-C2-C2) [63, 70] and an X domain [69, 70]. The cytoplasmic domain contains peptide sequences that are potentially be phosphorylated by protein kinase A (PKA), protein kinase C (PKC), and casein kinase 2 (CK 2) [63, 64, 69, 70]. My lab has also cloned the mouse METCAM/MUC18 (moMETCAM/MUC18) cDNA, which contains 648 amino acids with 76.2% identity with huMETCAM/MUC18 [71]. The structure of the huMETCAM/MUC18 protein is illustrated in **Figure 1**.

Similar to other CAMs, the functions of huMETCAM/MUC18 has been studied in relation to cell-cell and cell-extracellular matrix interactions, which trigger a cascade of signals that affect cytoskeleton structure and cellular motility and invasiveness. **Figure 1** shows the six conserved

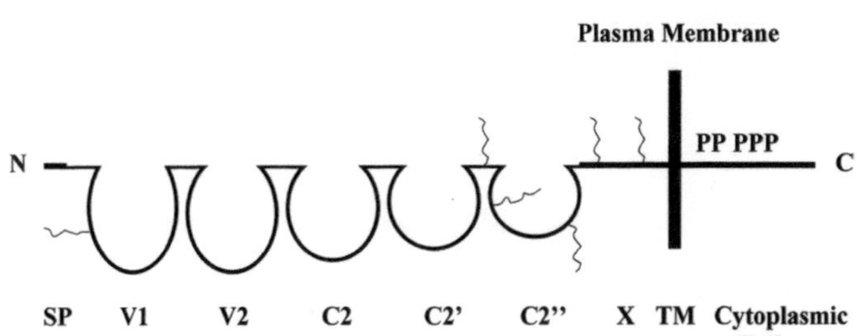

Figure 1. The protein structure of human METCAM/MUC18.

N-glycosylation sites, which are located in the V1, the region between the C2′ and the C2″, the C2″, and the X domains in the extracellular domain, and five potential phosphorylation sites in the intracellular cytoplasmic tail. From the protein structure, we predicted that METCAM/MUC18 may have additional functions, which may include synergistic interactions with growth factor receptors (as a co-receptor) to modulate cell functions and to trigger on intracellular signaling pathways, activation of matrix metalloproteinases (MMPs), serving as a co-activator for other cell functions, and serving as a co-transporter for extracellular small molecules (for example, calcium ion influx) [69], as summarized in **Figure 2**.

HuMETCAM/MUC18 is expressed in several normal tissues/cells, such as endothelial cells, hair follicular cells, smooth muscle cells, normal breast epithelial cells, basal cells in bronchial epithelium, the cerebellum, intermediate trophoblasts, some activated T cells [66], ovarian epithelial cells [48], and normal nasopharynx epithelial cells [61]. In addition, huMETCAM/MUC18 is expressed in several cancers, such as melanoma, gestational trophoblastic tumors, leiomyosarcoma, angiosarcoma, hemangioma, Kaposi's sarcoma, schwannoma, some lung squamous and small cell carcinomas, some breast cancer, and some neuroblastoma [66]. For the past two decades, we have also found that huMETCAM/MUC18 is also expressed in prostate cancer [72], ovarian cancer [48], and nasopharyngeal carcinoma [61].

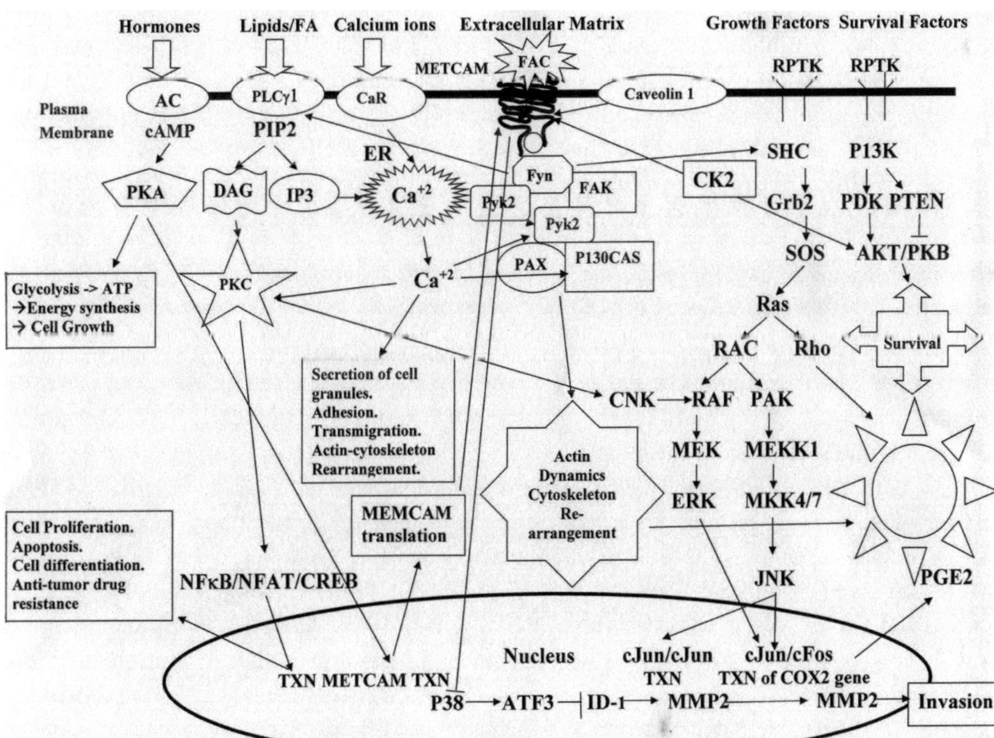

Figure 2. A proposed model for the outside-in and inside-out signaling of METCAM/MUC18 and its possible crosstalk with signal transduction pathways.

3. Role of METCM/MUC18 in the tumorigenesis and metastasis of different human cancers

3.1. METCAM/MUC18 plays a positive role in the progression of breast cancer

METCAM/MUC18 was suggested by two groups to play a tumor suppressor role [73, 74], but by the two other groups as a tumor promoter in the progression of human breast cancer [75, 76]. To resolve the controversial role of METCAM/MUC18 in the progression of human breast cancer, we set out independent studies to investigate the actual role played by METCAM/MUC18 in the progression of human breast cancer. We found that enforced expression of METCAM/MUC18 in both MCF-7 and SK-BR-3 cell lines increased their *in vitro* motility, invasiveness, and colony formation in soft agar (*in vitro* tumorigenesis). Furthermore, enforced expression of METCAM/MUC18 in both cell lines increased tumor-take and tumorigenesis in athymic nude mice [56–58].

Moreover, anti-METCAM/MUC18 antibody decreased the motility and invasiveness of the two basal-like cell lines, MDA-MB-231 and MDA-MB-468 [57]. Enforced expression of METCAM/MUC18 increases the metastasis of both basal-like cell lines in athymic nude mice [77]. Taken together, METCAM/MUC18 plays a positive role in the progression of four human breast cancer cell lines. Therefore, METCAM/MUC18 is a novel oncogene for mammary carcinoma cells and may be useful as a therapeutic target for the treatment of breast cancer. From further preliminary mechanical studies we suggest that METCAM/MUC18 promotes the progression of human breast cancer cells by increasing proliferation, angiogenesis, switching to aerobic glycolysis, and epithelial-to-mesenchymal transition (EMT) [56–58], thus its downstream signaling molecules may also be used as therapeutic targets for the treatment of breast cancer.

3.2. METCAM/MUC18 plays a dual role in the progression of melanoma

HuMETCAM/MUC18 was highly expressed on the cellular surface of most malignant human melanomas and has been suggested to play a positive role in the progression of human melanoma [63, 64]. Three groups demonstrate that the stably ectopic expression of the huMETCAM/MUC18 cDNA gene in three non-metastatic human cutaneous melanoma cell lines increases the metastatic ability of these cell lines in immune-deficient mouse models [12, 67]. Our group focused our studies on mouse melanomas, we show that stable, ectopic expression of moMETCAM/MUC18 in two low-metastatic mouse melanoma cell lines, K1735-3 and K1735-10, increases their metastatic abilities in immune-competent syngeneic mice [49]. METCAM/MUC18 enables melanoma cells to establish pulmonary metastasis only when the cells are injected into the tail vein (experimental metastasis) [12, 13, 49, 50], thus bypassing the initial stages of metastasis. In contrast, no metastasis was found when METCAM/MUC18-expressing melanoma cells were injected subcutaneously (spontaneous metastasis) either in immune-deficient mouse models [12, 67] or in immune-competent syngeneic mouse models [13, 49]. We concluded that moMETCAM/MUC18 may promote melanoma metastasis only in the later stages of metastasis. This result is consistent with the observation of one of the three original groups that huMETCAM/MUC18 does not initiate the conversion (transformation) of melanocytes into melanoma [78].

In contrast to the role of moMETCAM/MUC18 in promoting metastasis in the two mouse melanoma cell lines K1735 clone 3 and clone 10, surprisingly we found that over-expression of moMETCAM/MUC18 in one mouse melanoma cell line K1735 clone 9 decreased subcutaneous tumorigenesis and decreased pulmonary lung nodule formation when cells were injected into the tail vein in an isogenic mouse model [50]. Thus MCAM/MUC18 acts as a tumor and metastasis suppressor for the K1735-9 subline, different from its role in other K1735 sublines, K1735-3 and K1735-10. We suggest that ectopic expression of MCAM/MUC18 in different sublines may interact with different intrinsic co-factors/ligands, which may contribute to these intrinsic properties, such as adhesion-associated signaling cascades and cytoskeleton rearrangement, leading to different epithelial-to-mesenchymal transition of these cells and hence the intrinsic tumorigenic and metastatic potential of these cells. Different intrinsic co-factors in different K1735 sublines, which may modulate the functions of MCAM/MUC18 in the cells, leading to interact differently with the tumor microenvironment, may render sublines manifest differently in tumorigenicity and metastasis *in vivo*. Moreover, interactions of METCAM/MUC18 with these co-factors/ligands may render different sublines/cell lines being regulated by other physiological factors *in vivo*, which may enhance or inhibit *in vivo* growth of the tumor cells by altering metabolic switch, by altering apoptosis, or by up-regulating or down-regulating angiogenesis, as well as by boosting up or suppressing immune system in the tumor microenvironment and in the lung [50].

These syngeneic mouse systems are more useful models than the immune-deficient mouse systems for better understanding mechanisms of the complex role played by MCAM/MUC18 in the progression of melanoma cells. Furthermore, since these syngeneic mouse models more closely mimic the clinical melanoma cases in comparison to xenograft models, the knowledge gained from using these systems may also be useful for designing efficacious clinical therapies. Therefore, when therapeutic means are developed, we should keep in mind the dual role played by MCAM/MUC18. We should also be aware of the response of immunotherapy by using anti-METCAM/MUC18 monoclonal antibodies [79] and therapy by using MCAM/MUC18-specifc siRNAs [80] may be different in different patients.

3.3. METCAM/MUC18 plays a dual role in the progression of nasopharyngeal carcinoma

Nasopharyngeal carcinoma (NPC) is a malignant head and neck cancer; 90% of that develops in the non-lymphomatous, squamous epithelial lining of posterior nasopharynx [81]. NPC is heterogeneous: it manifests one of the three subtypes (or three patterns): keratinizing squamous cell carcinomas (WHO type I), non-keratinizing squamous cell carcinomas (WHO type II), and undifferentiated carcinomas (WHO type III) [61, 81]. Epidemiological studies suggest that three major etiological factors, such as genetic susceptibility, environmental factors, and infection with Epstein Barr virus (EBV), contribute to the extraordinary incidence in endemic areas [61]. However, how these major etiological factors contribute to the initiation and development and final progression is not known. Nevertheless, these etiological factors may induce aberrant expression of cell adhesion molecules (CAMs) in NPC and leading to tumorigenesis and malignant progression. Aberrant expression of CAMs has been associated with the progression of NPC [37–40]. However, the possible aberrant expression of METCAM/MUC18 in nasopharyngeal carcinoma has not been studied.

We initiated the study of the possible roles of METCAM/MUC18 in the malignant progression of NPC by using immunohistochemistry to determine the expression of the protein in the tissues of normal nasopharynx and NPC and two established NPC cell lines [61]. We found that METCAM/MUC18 was expressed in all of the normal nasopharynx, but weakly expressed in only 27% of the NPC tissues, suggesting that METCAM/MUC18 may function as a tumor suppressor in the development of NPC during the progression of the disease [61]. To test the hypothesis, we investigated the effect of METCAM/MUC18 over-expression on *in vitro* cellular behavior and *in vivo* tumorigenesis of two NPC cell lines in athymic nude mice. Indeed, METCAM/MUC18 over-expression suppressed the tumor growth of NPC-TW01 cells, which were established from type I NPC [81], as shown in [82, 83]. We suggested that METCAM/MUC18 plays a tumor suppressor role in the type I NPC [82, 83]. On the contrary, over-expression promoted the tumor growth of NPC-TW04 cells, which were established from type II NPC [81], as shown in [82, 84]. We suggest that METCAM/MUC18 plays a tumor promoter role in the type II NPC [82, 84].

We suggest that the dual role played by METCAM/MUC18 in the progression of two different types of NPC's may be modulated by different intrinsic factors and also in different stromal microenvironment. These two NPC cell lines may serve as models for understanding the contribution of three etiological factors to trigger the malignant progression of NPC and for translational applications. Radiotherapy has been used for the treatment of NPC; however, NPC has been notoriously resistant to radiotherapy. Thus, we sought the possibility of altering the radiosensitivity of NPC by ectopically increased expression of METCAM/MUC18 in NPC cell lines. Our preliminary studies show that radio-sensitivity of the tumors induced from both cell lines in athymic nude mice was increased by increased expression of METCAM/MUC18. Thus, ectopically increased expression of this protein may be used for clinical treatment [data not shown].

3.4. METCAM/MUC18 plays a negative role in the progression of ovarian cancer

METCAM/MUC18 expression has been recently to correlate with the progression of ovarian cancer [47, 48], and perhaps affect the *in vitro* behaviors of ovarian cancer cells [85]; however, the role of METCAM/MUC18 in the progression of epithelial ovarian cancer has not been directly studied in animal models. For this purpose, we initiated the studies by directly testing the effect of over-expression of METCAM/MUC18 on the ability of SK-OV-3 cells in *in vitro* motility and invasiveness, and *in vivo* tumor formation in nude mice after subcutaneous (SC) injection and *in vivo* progression in nude mice after intraperitoneal (IP) injection. Over-expression of METCAM/MUC18 inhibited *in vitro* motility and invasiveness [59] and suppressed *in vivo* tumorigenesis and malignant progression of the human ovarian cancer cell line SK-OV-3 [59]. Similar results were shown in another human ovarian cancer cell line, BG-1 (data not shown).

Taken together, we provided *in vitro* and *in vivo* evidence to support the notion that METCAM/MUC18 plays a suppressing role in tumorigenesis and malignant progression of two human ovarian cancer cell lines [59, 60]. We strongly suggested that METCAM/MUC18 is a novel tumor and metastasis suppressor for the progression of human ovarian cancer cells.

3.5. METCAM/MUC18 plays a positive role in the progression of prostate cancer

Over-expression of METCAM/MUC18 is not limited to melanoma as previously thought and also later research carried out by one of the original three groups proved that MelCAM/MCAM/MUC18 did not play an important role in converting normal melanocyte into melanoma [78]. With this in mind, we have initiated the study of trying to correlate the huMETCAM/MUC18 expression with prostate cancer at different pathological stages. Molecular biological and immunological methods were used to study the expression of huMETCAM/MUC18 in two prostate cancer cell lines (DU145 and PC-3) and in human tissues of normal prostates, BPH, PIN, and prostate cancer, and immunohistochemistry was used for its expression in tissue sections of paraffin-embedded human prostate cancer [70, 72]. From the results, we suggested a possibility that huMETCAM/MUC18 may be used as a novel early diagnostic marker for the metastatic potential of human prostate cancer. These notions are further strengthened by the results of our studies in a transgenic mouse model, *tr*ansgenic *a*denocarcinoma *m*ouse *p*rostate (TRAMP) [52]. Furthermore, we have suggested a hypothesis that huMETCAM/MUC18 very likely plays an important role in tumorigenesis and metastasis of human prostate cancer cells [72]. Then we carried out systematic studies of huMETCAM/MUC18-mediated prostate cancer metastasis in animal models to test the above hypothesis. We have tested the effect of ectopic expression of huMETCAM/MUC18 in human prostate LNCaP cells on their ability to form tumor in the non-orthotopic subcutaneous sites [53] and in the orthotopic prostate glands and to initiate metastasis in nude mice [51]. In contrast to melanoma cells, we have obtained evidence to prove that huMETCAM/MUC18 is a key determinant in initiating the metastasis of prostate cancer [51]. The detailed evidence is briefly described as follows:

3.5.1. Over-expression of huMETCAM/MUC18 correlates with the development and malignant progression of human prostate cancer

Two groups initiated the studies by testing possible huMETCAM/MUC18 expression in prostate cancer cell lines and prostate cancer tissues; however, they were unable to obtain positive results because the monoclonal antibodies used were incapable of recognizing the huMETCAM/MUC18 epitopes in prostate cancer cell lines and tissues [65, 86]. But we were able to use our chicken polyclonal antibodies for Western blot analysis and immunohistochemistry to detect the expression of huMETCAM/MUC18 antigens in prostate cancer cell lines and human prostate cancer tissues. We confirmed these results by using the RT-PCR analysis to show the presence of huMETCAM/MUC18 mRNA [70, 72]. We found that huMETCAM/MUC18 was neither expressed in most (90%) of the normal epithelial cells in the prostatic ducts/acini nor in any (100%) of these cells in BPH, but it was detectable in the majority (greater than 80%) of the neoplastic prostate epithelial cells (high-grade PIN), high-grade prostate adenocarcinomas, and metastatic lesions. HuMETCAM/MUC18 was expressed in two metastatic human prostate cancer cell lines, DU145 and PC-3, and one bladder cancer cell line, Tsu-Pr1, but not in one non-metastatic prostate cancer cell line, LNCaP [70, 72]. Thus, we conclude that huMETCAM/MUC18 is not expressed in normal and benign hyperplastic human prostate tissues, but its expression increases during prostate cancer initiation (high-grade PIN), progression to carcinoma, and in metastatic cell lines and metastatic lesions. Taken together, over-expression of METCAM/MUC18 correlates with the initiation of malignant progression of human prostate cancer [70, 72], suggesting that huMETCAM/MUC18 may be a useful marker for monitoring the metastatic potential of prostate cancer cells [70, 72]. Furthermore, the extent of *in vitro* motility and invasiveness is directly proportional to the extent of huMETCAM/MUC18 expression in four human cancer cell lines [70]. Our anti-huMETCAM/MUC18 antibody was able to significantly block the *in vitro* motility and invasiveness of various human prostate cancer cell lines [70]. Therefore, we propose the hypothesis that huMETCAM/MUC18 may directly mediate the increased epithelial-to-mesenchymal transition and initiate the progression of prostate cancers.

3.5.2. Correlation of over-expression of mouse METCAM/MUC18 with the malignant progression of prostate cancer in a transgenic mouse model (TRAMP)

If the above hypothesis is correct, we should be able to correlate moMETCAM/MUC18 expression with the development and progression of prostate cancer in a transgenic mouse model. To test this possibility, we have used the autochthonous TRAMP (*tr*ansgenic *a*denocarcinoma *m*ouse *p*rostate) model for the experiment by collaborating with Dr Norman Greenberg's group. The TRAMP model established by Dr Norman Greenberg [87] is one of two transgenic mouse models that have been established for studying the tumorigenesis and metastasis of prostate cancer [87, 88]. This model was created by transfecting the germ line of the C57BL/6 inbred strain of mice with fusion gene of the rat probasin (PB) gene promoter and the SV40 T antigen (Tag) gene. The expression of the PB-Tag transgene is regulated by androgens and only localized to the prostatic epithelial cells in the dorsolateral and ventral lobes. When the mice reach an age of 12–20 weeks, TRAMP mice histologically show mild to severe hyperplasia with cribriform structures. By an age of 26 weeks, severe hyperplasia and adenocarcinoma is manifested. By an age of 26–33 weeks, all TRAMP males show primary tumors and metastasis in the lymph nodes and lungs and less frequently in the bones, kidney, and adrenal glands. In this transgenic model, the epithelial origin of the tumors and metastatic deposits has been successfully shown [87] in prostates.

MoMETCAM/MUC18 expression was determined by Western blot analysis and/or immunohistochemistry by using our chicken anti-moMETCAM/MUC18 antibodies [71] during the progression of mouse prostate adenocarcinoma in this transgenic mouse model. When these mice reached 12–20 weeks of age, they began to show PIN in the prostate glands. When they reached 178–181 days of age (25.7–25.9 weeks), they had primary tumors in the prostate glands and the expression of moMETCAM/MUC18 mRNA and protein was detectable. Tumors continued to grow beyond an age of 32.4 weeks, when some mice were found dead. Interestingly, metastasis was found even when tumors were small (less than 0.5 g) and the level of moMETCAM/MUC18 expression was much lower. MoMETCAM/MUC18 was not detectable in the prostates of the control group (presumably having the normal organ). The tumor metastasizes to peri-aortic lymph nodes in all the mice that had primary tumors. Metastatic lesions were also observed in seminal vesicles, abdomen cavity, livers, and lungs in some mice. The expression of MoMETCAM/MUC18 was detectable in all PINs, prostate adenocarcinomas, and metastatic lesions. We concluded that the moMETCAM/MUC18 expression was increased during the progression of the mouse prostate cancer in this transgenic mouse model [52]. Bone metastasis has been observed, though we have not analyzed the bone samples of these transgenic mice [89].

3.5.3. Over-expression of huMETCAM/MUC18 increases the tumor-take and metastasis of human prostate cancer cells

To test the hypothesis that huMETCAM/MUC18 may increase the metastatic potential of human prostate cancer cells, we successfully obtained G418-resistant clones that express a high level of huMETCAM/MUC18 after transfecting the huMETCAM/MUC18 cDNA gene into a human prostate cancer LNCaP cell line that did not previously express huMETCAM/MUC18 and had a minimal ability to metastasize. We then injected these clones orthotopically into one of the dorsolateral lobes of the prostate. We found that ectopically enforced huMETCAM/MUC18 expression increases the tumor-take and initiates the metastasis of LNCaP cells to various organs, such as the seminal vesicles, the ureter, the kidney, and the peri-aortic lymph nodes, in athymic nude mice [51]. Since metastatic lesions were only observed in the mice with tumors, we also concluded that metastasis is closely associated with the tumorigenesis, as suggested by Weiss [23], but tumor formation without the expression of huMETCAM/MUC18 did not lead to metastasis.

Alternatively, we have also established a xenograft mouse model to further study how the expression of huMETCAM/MUC18 mediates tumorigenesis of LNCaP cells. We subcutaneously injected the huMETCAM/MUC18-expressing LNCaP cells together with Matrigel and observed the appearance of tumors at different times in a nude mouse model [53]. We found that ectopic (or enforced) expression of huMETCAM/MUC18 increased the early on-set of tumorigenesis of LNCaP cells in this mouse model [53]. Ectopic (or enforced) expression of huMETCAM/MUC18 increases the tumor formation of LNCaP cells [53]. We concluded that the enforced expression of huMETCAM/MUC18 in human prostate cancer LNCaP cells increased the tumor growth more than the control cells.

These results confirming that huMETCAM/MUC18 plays an important role in increasing tumorigenesis and initiating metastasis of LNCaP cells, consistent with our earlier findings that huMETCAM/MUC18 is frequently expressed in the pre-malignant high-grade PIN and in human prostate cancer tissues [72]. Taken together, the hypothesis that METCAM/MUC18 plays an important role in initiating prostate cancer progression is well-supported by evidence.

Recently, we further shown that huMETCAM/MUC18 also played a positive role in the progression of another prostate cancer cell line, DU145, by showing that the tumorigenesis of DU145 in an athymic nude mouse model was decreased when the endogenously expressed METCAM/MUC18 was decreased by knock-down with SiRNAs [54, 55].

3.6. METCAM/MUC18 plays a dual role in other tumors

In addition to melanoma, prostate cancer, breast cancer, ovarian cancer, and NPC, METCAM/MUC18 is also expressed in other cancers, such as gestational trophoblastic tumors, leiomyosarcoma, angiosarcoma, Kaposi's sarcoma, some lung squamous and small cell carcinomas, and some neuroblastoma; however, the role of METCAM/MUC18 in the development of most of these cancers has not been investigated [65, 66]. In our preliminary tests, we observed that moMETCAM/MUC18 was expressed at a higher level in one angiosarcoma clone, SVR, which was transfected with H-Ras, than in an immortalized normal endothelial cell line control, MS-1 [62]. The higher expression level of moMETCAM/MUC18 was correlated with the higher tumorigenicity of the SVR cell line [69, 90], suggesting that METCAM/MUC18 promoted the development of angiosarcoma [62, 69, 90]. Recent findings from other groups also suggest that METCAM/MUC18 also plays a positive role in the progression of osteosarcoma [91], hepatocellular carcinoma [92, 93], gastric cancer [94], non-small cell lung adenocarcinoma [95], small cell lung cancer [96], and pancreatic cancer [98].

On the other hand, the possible tumor and metastasis suppressor role of METCAM/MUC18 has also been extended from melanoma, ovarian cancer, and NPC, to colorectal cancer [97], pancreatic cancer [99], and perhaps, hemangioma [100]. **Table 1** summarizes the role of METCAM/MUC18 in the tumor formation and/or cancer metastasis of various tumors/cancers.

Tumor/cancers	Tumorigenesis	Metastasis	References
Clinical prostate cancer and human prostate cancer cell lines	Increasing	Increasing and affecting initiation in the early stage (PIN)	[51, 53–55, 70, 72]
Prostate adenocarcinoma in TRAMP mice	Increasing	Increasing and affecting initiation in the early stage	[52]
Clinical melanoma and human melanoma cell lines	No effect	Increasing and affecting at the late stage	[12, 67]
Mouse melanoma cells (K1735-3 and 10)	No effect or suppression	Increasing and affecting at the late stage	[13, 49, 71]
Mouse melanoma cells (K1735-9)	Suppression	Suppression	[13, 50, 71]
Angiosarcoma	Increasing	Possible promotion, by not determined	[62, 69, 90]
Human breast cancer cell line MCF-7	Promotion	Not determined	[56]
Human breast cancer cell line SK-BR-3	Promotion	Not determined	[57–58]
Human breast cancer cell lines MDA-MB-231 and 468	Promotion	Promotion	[57, 77]
Hemangioma	Possible suppression, but bot determined	Not determined	[100]
Nasopharyngeal carcinoma type I	Suppression	Possible suppression, but not determined	[82, 83]
Nasopharyngeal carcinoma type II	Promotion	Possible augmentation, but not determined	[82, 84]
Ovarian cancer	Suppression	Suppression	[48, 59, 60]
Colorectal cancer	Suppression	Suppression	[97]
Gastric cancer	Promotion	Not determined	[94]
Non-small cell lung carcinoma	Promotion	Not determined	[95]
Small cell lung carcinoma	Promotion	Not determined	[96]
Hepatocellular carcinoma	Promotion	Promotion	[92, 93]
Osteosarcoma	Promotion	Not determined	[91]
Pancreatic cancer	Promotion or suppression	Not determined	[98, 99]

Table 1. The possible role of METCAM/MUC18 in tumor formation and/or cancer metastasis of various tumors/cancers.

Taken together, the dual role of METCAM/MUC18 may be explained by that the intrinsic properties of each cancer cell line may provide co-factors that either positively or negatively regulate METCAM/MUC18-mediated tumorigenesis and metastasis. To understand further the role of METCAM/MUC18 in these processes, it is essential to identify these intrinsic co-factors in the future studies.

4. Possible molecular mechanisms of the huMETCAM/MUC18-mediated progression of cancer

Since the discovery of huMETCAM/MUC18 in the 1980s, about three groups have worked on the role of huMETCAM/MUC18 in melanoma metastasis [12, 63, 64, 67], another group on the role of huMETCAM/MUC18 in the biology of endothelial cells [68], and our group joined in the effort to study the role of huMETCAM/MUC18 in the progression of melanoma and prostate cancer, and later breast cancer, ovarian cancer, and NPC, as described above. Though we are beginning to understand the biology of METCAM/MUC18-mediated cancer progression, however, many questions of linking the regulation of the expression of this gene to its role in cancer progression are remained to be answered. For examples, the contribution of the protein structure and the glycosylation of the protein to the function of huMETCAM/MUC18 in the progression of cancer have not been systematically studied. How the protein mediates the interaction of tumor cells with the tumor microenvironment is not well studied. Though only limited information is available for huMETCAM/MUC18's outside-in and inside-out signaling in endothelial cells, and the signaling information for the METCAM/MUC18-mediated progression of various cancer cells are not much known. How the expression of METCAM/MUC18 is regulated at the level of transcription is minimally studied. We will try to address these questions by taking advantage of the currently known information from various sources to propose possibilities for much needed studies in the future.

4.1. The presentation of huMETCAM/MUC18 on the surface of cancer tissues may be different from cancer to cancer

Our unique contribution to the biology of METCAM/MUC18 was mainly attributed to the high specificity of our chicken antibodies [70, 71], to reconcile the different, sometimes controversial, findings [73, 86], we suggest that the presentation of huMETCAM/MUC18 on the cellular surface in normal and carcinoma tissues may be different from cancer to cancer [70, 72]. HuMETCAM/MUC18 may be presented differently in various cancer cell lines because of different carbohydrate composition, differential distribution of huMETCAM/MUC18 in the cholesterol-enriched lipid raft membrane fraction of the plasma membrane, different interactions of huMETCAM/MUC18 with other membrane proteins, and different lipid modification of the protein. There appears to have some correlation of the predominant cytoplasmic expression of huMETCAM/MUC18 antigens with the malignant progression of human prostate carcinomas, but not in human melanoma. To test the above possibilities, it is necessary to express the whole or a fragment of the protein in a large scale in human cancer cells lines in order to purify the protein for biochemical characterization and for crystallization and physical structure studies. Alternatively, to probe the functions of different parts of the molecule and for translational research, a complete set of monoclonal antibodies can be induced from the purified whole protein or its fragments. In line with these, a repertoire of mouse monoclonal antibodies has been successfully constructed by Yen's group [101]. We also intend to make a repertoire of rabbit monoclonal antibodies for the above purpose.

4.2. Which domains of huMETCAM/MUC18 are required for tumorigenesis and metastasis?

The relation of the protein structure of huMETCAM/MUC18 to its functions in tumorigenesis and metastasis has not been systematically defined. For this purpose, the partial known information of the functional domain(s) of the two huMETCAM/MUC18-related cell adhesion molecules in the Ig-like gene superfamily, such as CEA-CAM [31, 32] and ALCAM [102–104], might be used as a guide for designing tests to probe the functional domains in the external domain of huMETCAM/MUC18. The known functions of the cytoplasmic tail of several cell adhesion molecules may also provide clues to understand the function of the cytoplasmic tail of huMETCAM/MUC18 in crosstalk with signal pathways leading to tumorigenesis and metastasis [105–107]. For example, the domain of CEACAM1 required for tumorigenesis seems to reside in the intracellular cytoplasmic tail, but not in the extracellular domain [31, 32]. The N-terminal most Ig-like domain of the extracellular portion of ALCAM seems to be responsible for homophilic and heterophilic interactions [103, 104]. However, the domain(s) of these two molecules required for metastasis have not yet been studied. Since the information from these related proteins is very limited, we cannot logically predict the role of both the extracellular domain and the intracellular tail of the Ig-like CAMs in tumorigenesis and metastasis. To begin addressing this question, in the past, we have generated mutants deleted different domains of huMETCAM/MUC18 by using a special PCR method [108] and used them to determine their contribution to tumorigenesis. The ecto-domain of huMETCAM/MUC18 was similar to the whole wild type cDNA to be able to induce tumorigenesis of LNCaP cells in nude mice, suggesting that the ecto-domain alone was sufficient to induce tumor of human prostate cancer cells *in vivo*, implying that the cytoplasmic domain was not essential for this process [data not shown].

However, similar tests of using only the cytoplasmic domain have not been performed for LNCaP cells. Rather, the function of the cytoplasmic domain of huMETCAM/MUC18 was tested for the human ovarian cancer cell line BG-1 that the cytoplasmic domain alone was able to induce tumors in nude mice [data not shown].

In conclusion, we are not clear if this is true only for BG-1 cells or this is generally true for all cancer cell lines, which requires further studies.

4.3. The possible role of glycosylation in the huMETCAM/MUC18-mediated cancer metastasis

Glycosylation of a protein has been shown to affect the proper folding, stability, and/or activity of a protein [109]. Furthermore, the glycosylation of a cell adhesion molecule may affect its ability to induce metastasis of cancer cells [110–113].

Both huMETCAM/MUC18 and moMETCAM/MUC18 have an apparent molecular weight of about 150 kDa [114], because they are heavily glycosylated, sialylated, and post-translationally modified. We have shown that the apparent molecular weight of huMETCAM/MUC18 expressed in different human cancer cell lines was decreased after digestion with N-glycosidase F and neuraminidase (sialidase), but not with O-glycosidase or endoglycosidase H [62, 69], suggesting that huMETCAM/MUC18 has both sialic acid and N-glycans as carbohydrate side chains. Glycosylation in different cancer may be different that has been shown by using the anti-HNK-1 monoclonal antibody Leu 7 to probe the expression of HNK-1 epitope, a sulfated-glycan with the structure of sulfo → 3GlcAβ1 → 3Galβ1 → 4GlcNA-cβ1→ R, in melanomas and prostate cancer tissues [115–120]. The expression level of the HNK-1 epitope is proportional to that of human METCAM/MUC18 in human melanoma, and both are predominantly expressed on the plasma membrane of melanoma cells. In contrast, the HNK-1 epitope is found to be predominantly present in the cytoplasm of human prostate epithelial cells. In addition, different from the increased expression level of huMETCAM/MUC18 in prostate cancer, the expression of the HNK-1 epitope is decreased in the more advanced grades of human prostate cancer [120]. We suggest that the sugar moieties in the N-glycans of huMETCAM/MUC18 in human prostate cancer cells are different from that in melanoma cells; this may be related to its more profound effect on promoting the tumorigenesis and metastasis of human prostate cancer LNCaP cells than that of melanoma cells [12, 51, 69, 70]. Thus, we hypothesize that the N-glycans at the N-glycosylation sites of huMETCAM/MUC18 should have a significant effect on their *in vitro* motility and invasiveness and other *in vitro* cellular behaviors (for example, cell-cell adhesion and cell-extracellular matrix interaction) as well as tumorigenesis and metastasis of human prostate cancer and melanoma cells and very likely also in other human cancer cells that express METCAM/MUC18, since glycosylation of huMETCAM/MUC18 may affect its ability to mediate cell-cell adhesion and cell-extracellular matrix interaction. This notion is supported by a recent publication that GCNT3 is an upstream regulator of METCAM and it glycosylates METCAM/MUC18 and extends its half-life, leading to further elevation of S100A8/A9-mediated cellular motility in melanoma cells [121].

The human huMETCAM/MUC18 protein has nine potential N-glycosylation sites (Asn-X-Ser/Thr or N-X-S/T sites) [63, 64, 70] and the mouse METCAM/MUC18 has seven [71]. Their locations on huMETCAM/MUC18 are depicted in **Figure 1**. Six N-glycosylation sites are conserved between the two proteins: 56/58 NL/FS, 418/420NRT, 449/451NLS, 467NCT/469NCS, 507NTS/509NTT, and 544/546NST [69]. Since the apparent molecular weight of huMETCAM/MUC18 and moMETCAM/MUC18 in the SDS gel are similar, we suggest that only these six conserved N-glycosylation sites are actually glycosylated. All these N-glycosylation sites are located in the external domains of V1, C′, C″, and X. The effect of N-glycosylation on the function of huMETCAM/MUC18 can be tested by using genetic means to alter the N-glycosylation sites. First, we should test the effect of mutations in the six conserved sites of the huMETCAM/MUC18 on *in vitro* cell-cell aggregation and cell-extracellular matrix adhesion and on *in vivo* tumorigenesis and metastasis of human cancer cells. The N-glycosylation site can be point mutated from Asn to Ala or Gln [122, 123] or may be linker-scanning mutated by replacing the three codons (the nine nucleotide sequence) with a nine bp oligonucleotide containing a unique restriction site sequence [124]. Both kinds of mutation are better than deletion mutations, since they do not change the relative physical location of the mutated sequences and thus the phenotype of the mutant is directly related to the substituted sequence without the complicated influence of the added sequences from the surrounding region of interest. The linker-scanning mutations from our experience are superior to the point mutations because they usually manifest a more dramatic phenotype [124].

4.4. The heterophilic ligands of METCAM/MUC18 may play an important role in the cell-cell and cell-extracellular matrix interactions and cancer metastasis

To further understand how huMETCAM/MUC18 mediates metastasis of cancer cells to certain target organs, it is important to identify the heterophilic ligand(s) of huMETCAM/MUC18 and to know how it regulates cellular behaviors, and how it interacts with members of the signal transduction pathways. Previous studies suggest that huMETCAM/MUC18 prefers to interact with heterophilic ligand(s) [125, 126], which, however, has not been identified. But at least we know that some components of proteoglycans such as, glycosaminoglycan, hyaluronic acid, dermatan sulfate, keratan sulfate, heparin, heparan sulfate, chondroitin-6-sulfate, and heparan sulfate proteoglycan, have been excluded [125, 126]. The heterophilic ligands of huMETCAM/MUC18 are highly likely to be proteins. The proteins possessing SH3 domain [127] may be the possible candidates; however, the proteins containing the SH3 domain may not be the real ligands since they interact with MUC18 with a low affinity. The neurite outgrowth factor (a member of the laminin family) [128] may be another possible candidate; however, the cDNA gene of the neurite outgrowth factor has not been cloned for further characterization. To identify the authentic heterophilic ligands of huMETCAM/MUC18, stringent biochemical criteria should be employed.

To search for the ligand(s), many methods may be employed, such as immunoaffinity pull-down method [129], METCAM/MUC18-GST fusion protein pull-down method [69], METCAM/MUC18-AP fusion method to screen an expression library [130, 131], or METCAM/MUC18 used for screening counter-acting peptides in a phage library expressing random peptides [132, 133]. So far, we have attempted to use an immunoaffinity pull-down method to identify the heterophilic ligands of huMETCAM/MUC18. From our preliminary results, we found that a protein of 72 kDa may be a potential ligand, which is expressed on the cellular surface of two human prostate cancer cell lines and one human melanoma cell line [69]. This putative ligand protein appeared to be present in the extract of the human prostate cancer cell line, PC-3, more than that in DU145. We excluded the possibility that this protein may be the breakdown product of huMETCAM/MUC18 because of its discrete size. We are in the process of preparing a sufficient quantity of the protein for further characterization with mass spectrometry. In addition, we have successfully expressed a huMETCAM/MUC18-ectodoamin-GST fusion protein in LNCaP cells. The fusion protein will be purified and also used for pulling down ligands. Alternatively, we have used a huMETCAM/MUC18-AP fusion protein to screen a human brain cDNA expression library; preliminary trials indicated that this methodology appears to be promising.

4.5. METCAM/MUC18-mediated signal transduction and cancer metastasis

The intracellular cytoplasmic tail of huMETCAM/MUC18 contains three consensus sequences to be recognized by PKC, one by PKA, and one by CK2 [63, 69, 70]. Though not biochemically proven, the cytoplasmic tail presumably is phosphorylated by these kinases. It probably has a capacity to crosstalk and network different signal pathways, similar to the cytoplasmic tails of other CAMs [106, 107, 134, 135]. Thus METCAM/MUC18, as an integral membrane protein and a cell adhesion molecule, should mediate inside-out and outside-in signals, which may be participating in cell-cell communication, cell-extracellular matrix interaction, and affecting the cellular motility and invasiveness [134, 135]. Furthermore, its interaction with cognate heterophilic ligand(s) may affect how it promotes angiogenesis and how it mediates targeting to specific organs and facilitates metastasis. Moreover, it may interact with androgen/androgen receptor, growth factors/receptors, chemokines/receptors, and Ca^{2+}-mediated signaling members. **Figure 2** summarizes the possible crosstalk of huMETCAM/MUC18 with many members of signal transduction pathways, which are supported by the following:

The downstream signal transduction of this protein has been studied in endothelial cells. Anfosso et al. [68] showed that antibody cross-linked huMETCAM/MUC18 (which mimics cell adhesion on the cell surface) induces phosphorylation of both FAK and PyK2 (a member of the FAK family) and association of FAK with paxillin in the endothelial cells, which leads to the activation of focal adhesion complexes, similar to the outside-in signaling triggered by the engagement of integrins with the extracellular matrix. In addition, the engagement of huMETCAM/MUC18 also triggers direct association with Fyn, a member of the c-Src family, which activates adhesion-associated signaling cascades and cytoskeleton rearrangement, leading to increasing motility, and invasiveness. Since FAK and PyK2 do not directly associate with huMETCAM/MUC18 and the molecules that link the huMETCAM/MUC18 with FAK or PYK2 have not been identified, but huMETCAM/MUC18, similar to integrins, may use Fyn (and talin) for this purpose. We suggest that it is likely that focal adhesion complexes and signaling cascades may also be present in the prostate cancer and melanoma cells, since the over-expression of huMETCAM/MUC18 increases motility and invasiveness of human prostate cancer cells and melanoma cells.

Anfosso et al. further found that huMETCAM/MUC18 engagement also induces a Ca^{2+} influx, indicating that it is also able to initiate a store-operated calcium mobilization [136]. Ca^{2+} inside the cell may play a very important role—more so than other secondary messengers—in focal adhesion-induced actin cytoskeleton rearrangement and cellular motility, which is supported by the fact that locally elevated Ca^{2+} inside the cell triggers focal adhesion disassembly and enhances residency of focal adhesion kinase at focal adhesions [137, 138]. The link between the cell adhesion role of huMETCAM/MUC18 with Ca^{2+} influx is supported by the evidence that human METCAM/MUC18 is coupled to a Fyn-dependent pathway that triggers activation of phospholipase C-γ1 via tyrosine phosphorylation, which leads to increased Ca^{2+} influx that is in turn required for the tyrosine phosphorylation of PyK2 and $p130^{Cas}$ and formation of a complex between PyK2, $p130^{Cas}$, and paxillin, which in turn leads to cell adhesion and cell motility. Taken together, huMETCAM/MUC18 is a signaling molecule involved in the dynamics of actin cytoskeleton rearrangement. The elevation of Ca^{2+} influx also has other effects: it is linked to Ras-Raf1-MAP kinase via PyK2 and involved in cell proliferation by activating phospholipase C-γ1, which in turn activates PKCs that affects cell proliferation, differentiation, and transcriptional control of other genes (for example, c-Myc target genes); and it may directly activate transcription factors, such as NF-kB, NF-AT, and CREB, which regulate transcription of genes in proliferation, survival, and/or apoptosis [139].

AKT (or PKB), the cellular homolog of the retroviral oncogene v-AKT, is a serine/threonine kinase. AKT is a key member in the AKT/PI3K/PTEN signaling pathway [140]. AKT is activated by phosphorylation at Thr 308 and Ser473 by its upstream factor, PI3 kinase, and is inactivated by de-phosphorylation by PTEN, a tumor suppressor. Upon activation, AKT promotes cell survival by interfering with the cell apoptosis (when cells are exposed to pro-apoptotic signals, such as growth factor withdraw, irradiation, DNA damage, detachment, and the administration of apoptosis-inducing reagents) [140] and also promotes motility, proliferation, growth, angiogenesis, and the activation of mTOR (mammalian target of rapamycin) [141]. AKT also can be activated by Ras, which in turn is activated by a growth factor receptor or by RTK and survival factors, IGF1. In melanoma cells, when AKT activation is inhibited, huMETCAM/MUC18 expression is reduced. When AKT is super-activated, huMETCAM/MUC18 expression is increased. On the other hand, the over-expression of huMETCAM/MUC18 in melanoma cells led to further activation of AKT, resulting in cell survival under stress conditions [142]. It is not clear how the expression of AKT is directly or indirectly affecting the expression of huMETCAM/MUC18 and which isoforms is involved, since there are three isoforms of AKT: AKT-1, AKT-2, and AKT-3. One possible crosstalk between METCAM/MUC18 and AKT may be linked by casein kinase 2, as described further.

Casein kinase 2 (CK2) was discovered in the 1950s. The history of CK2 is full of paradoxes and unexpected findings [143]. The α-subunits and the β-subunits of CK2 are found to be un-coordinately distributed in different cellular compartments, suggesting that the interaction partners of the α-subunits and the β-subunits may be different and much more complex than we have previously thought. CK2 is constitutively active, and no oncogenic CK2 mutant is known; but high CK2 activity correlates to neoplasia. It was thought to be one of the most pleiotropic protein kinases. However, a phospho-proteomics analysis of these CK2 null cells suggests that CK2 pleiotropy may be less pronounced than expected, supporting the idea that the phospho-proteome generated by this kinase is flexible and not rigidly pre-determined. Furthermore, CK2 is dispensable, since it can be replaced by other kinases to perform the phosphorylation of critical sites whenever CK2 activity is nullified. CK2 may also be involved in cell survival by directly affecting AKT activity or indirectly interacting with members of the AKT survival pathway. We suggest that a potential sequence present in the huMETCAM/MUC18 cytoplasmic tail may be recognized by CK2 as its substrate and may link the reciprocal mutual effect between huMETCAM/MUC18 and AKT.

PKC is the most extensively studied among all protein kinases. A huge number of members are involved in the family of PKC. PKCs are encoded by nine different genes. It has a large family including three major families of isozymes with distinct regulation: cPKC (PKCα, PKCβI, PKCβII, and PKCγ), nPKC (PKCδ, PKCε, PKCη, and PKCθ), and aPKC (PKCλ, PKCζ, and PKCι) [144]. In addition, there are the PKC-related kinases, PRK ½ [145] and PKC-binding partners [146]. The classical PKCs (cPKCs) are activated by PS, calcium, and DAG or PMA; the novel PKCs (nPKCs) are activated by PS and DAG or PMA; the atypical PKCs (aPKCs) are independent of PS, calcium, and DAG. PKC isozymes are key regulators of cellular function, such as growth, differentiation, cell survival, neurotransmission, carcinogenesis, and cancer progression [144]. PKCs control multiple functions associated with cancer progression, in many cases in opposite manners. Depending on the context, PKCs can act either as promoters or suppressors of the cancer phenotype [147]. The PKC-related kinases, PRK ½ and PKC-binding partners may regulate and expand the functions of PKCs by positioning individual PKCs in the appropriate location to respond to specific receptor-mediated activating signals, bringing them in close contact with substrate proteins, directing them in vesicle trafficking between compartments, or integrating PKC-mediated signaling with other signaling pathways [145, 146]. Increased regulation of PKCα has been associated with the malignant progression of melanoma and that of PKCβII with the progression of colon/rectal cancer [144]. Up-regulation of PKCα, PKCε, and PKCζ, and down-regulation of PKCβ was associated with the progression of prostate cancer [144]. Over-expression of PKCε was sufficient to transform androgen-sensitive LNCaP cells into an androgen-independent variant [144]. The contribution of PKCs to METCAM/MUC18-mediated tumor growth and metastasis has not been studied. At least, it is highly possible that PKCs may phosphorylate the cytoplasmic tail of METCAM/MUC18 at the three potential PKC phosphorylation sites; however, it is not clear which isoform of PKC is responsible it. Furthermore, some inside-out signals may turn on some of the PKC members, which in turn may interact with the cytoplasmic tail of huMETCAM/MUC18, leading to tumor cell survival, tumor vascularization, cytoskeleton re-organization, focal adhesion, migration, and invasiveness [147].

PKA is involved in cAMP-mediated signal transduction. The huMETCAM/MUC18 promoter may be regulated by PKA [148], since it contains a consensus CREB-binding site, as shown in **Figure 3**. Thus, the expression of huMETCAM/MUC18 may be regulated by PKA. Furthermore, the activity/function of huMETCAM/MUC18 may be regulated by PKA-mediated signals, perhaps after the phosphorylation of the cytoplasmic tail. Since PKA has been shown to regulate the Ca^{2+} channels and pumps, the Ca^{2+} influx induced by the huMETCAM/MUC18 engagement may also be regulated by PKA [139]. The effect of PKA on *in vitro* tumor growth and *in vitro* motility and invasiveness may be investigated after augmentation of the PKA activity by treatment of cells with forskolin. The effect of PKA on these processes may be reversed by treatment with specific inhibitors to reduce the PKA activity.

4.6. Transcriptional regulation of huMETCAM/MUC18 gene

Only a few studies have been done to understand the mechanism of transcriptional control of METCAM/MUC18 gene. The sequence of 900 bp in the core promoter region of huMETCAM/MUC18 has been characterized [64]. This promoter does not have a TATA box, but is GC-rich, which contains putative binding sites for SP-1, CREB [148], AP-2 [149, 150], c-Myb [151], N-Oct2 (Brn2) [152], Ets [153], CArG [154], and Egr-1 [155] and three insulin responsive elements (one Ets and two E-box motifs) [156], suggesting that huMETCAM/MUC18 expression may be regulated by growth-related signals [62, 69] (**Figure 3**).

AP-2 is a transcription repressor for the huMETCAM/MUC18 gene and it is also a suppressor for the huMETCAM/MUC18-mediated metastasis [149, 150]. This is supported by the evidence that transfection of highly metastatic melanoma cells (AP-2$^-$/MUC18$^+$) with the AP-2 gene resulted in a down-regulation of huMETCAM/MUC18 gene and inhibited their tumor growth and metastasis in nude mice [149]. Similar down-regulation of huMETCAM/MUC18 probably occurs in human prostate cancer cells [150]. Since the loss of AP-2 expression is at the early stage of prostate cancer development, this is consistent with our notion that MEMCAM/MUC18 plays an important role in initiating the development of prostate cancer. The loss of AP-2 expression at the late stage of melanoma is also consistent with our hypothesis that MEM/MUC18 plays a key role only in the late stage of the development of melanoma. ZBTB7A has

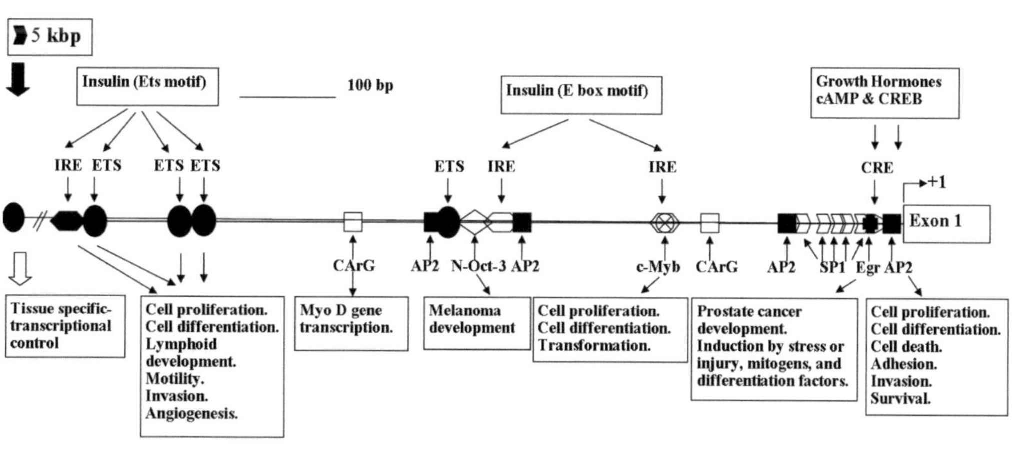

Figure 3. Putative transcription factor-recognized motifs in the 900 bp core promoter and 5–10 kbp upstream region of the huMETCAM/MUC18 gene.

been shown to repress transcription of METCAM/MUC18 gene in melanoma [157]. METCAM/MUC18 gene in osteosarcoma has been partly controlled by the transcription factor YY1 [158].

In addition to the sequence in the core promoter region, some upstream sequences should be required for the tissue-specific regulation of huMETCAM/MUC18 gene, since this 900 bp promoter region did not contain the necessary sequences to confer tissue specificity of the huMETCAM/MUC18 expression [159]. A recent finding appears to support this notion that Ets sequence in the 10 kbp upstream region is involved in the regulation of the expression of huMETCAM.MUC18 gene [160]. The sequence of the upstream region of the huMETCAM/MUC18 promoter may be obtained by searching in the Celera or other web sites. We have obtained several clones that contain at least 4 kbp of the gene for future studies.

Furthermore, epigenetic control of the huMETCAM/MUC18 gene has not been extensively studied. Nevertheless, the epigenetic control of the expression of huMETCAM/MUC18 gene has been demonstrated in NPC [161] and prostate cancer [162]. HuMETCAM/MUC18 gene is located on human chromosome 11q23.3 [127] which has been shown to be methylated in NPC, suggesting that the expression of this gene may be regulated by epigenetic controls. METCAM/MUC18 has been shown to be methylated in most of the early stage of prostate cancer [162].

5. Conclusions and clinical applications

METCAM/MUC18 may play a key positive function in the progression of prostate cancer, melanoma, breast cancer, gastric cancer, hepatocellular carcinoma, lung cancer, pancreatic cancer, and NPC type II. On the other hand, it may also have a key function in suppressing the progression of one mouse melanoma cell line, ovarian cancer, NPC type I, colorectal cancer, hemangioma, and perhaps other cancers. To further understand its role in these processes, it is essential to further define its functional domains, identify its cognate ligands and regulators, and study its crosstalk with members of various signal transduction pathways and the regulation of its expression at the level of transcription. The knowledge obtained from our studies should be useful for designing effective means to arrest, or even better, to block the metastatic potential of these cancers. For example, a preclinical trial of using doxazosin, a α1-adrenergic antagonist, which has been used to treat the BPH patients, has been shown to reduce prostate cancer metastasis in the TRAMP mouse model [163]. Furthermore, the success of preclinical trials has been demonstrated in using a fully humanized anti-METCAM/MUC18 antibody against melanoma growth and metastasis [164] and in using a mouse anti-METCAM/MUC18 monoclonal antibody against angiogenesis and tumor growth (hepatocellular carcinoma, leiomyosarcoma, and pancreatic cancer) [165]. However, the dual role of METCAM/MUC18 in cancer progression warns us an important point in clinical applications that we should not be hasty in using monoclonal antibodies or siRNA for clinical trials, rather we should spend more effort on tailoring a personalized treatment in the future.

Acknowledgements

I thank Mr Jonathan C.-Y. Wu and Mrs Mei-Whey Wu for critical reading the manuscript and for proofreading English. I thank the support of grants from National Research Council, Taiwan.

Author details

Guang-Jer Wu[1,2*]

*Address all correspondence to: guangj.wu@gmail.com

1 Department of Bioscience Technology, Center for Biomedical Technology, Chung Yuan Christian University, Taoyuan, Taiwan

2 The Winship Cancer Institute, Department of Microbiology and Immunology, Emory University School of Medicine, Atlanta, GA, USA

References

[1] Lengauer C, Kinzler KW, Vogelstein B. Genetic instabilities in human cancers. Nature. 1998;**396**:643-649

[2] Ruddon RW. Chapter 11: Biology of tumor metastasis. In: Ruddon RW, editor. Cancer Biology. 4th ed. New York, Oxford: Oxford University Press; 2007. pp. 402-427

[3] Hanahan D, Weinberg RA. Hallmarks of cancer: The next generation. Cell. 2011;**144**:646-674. DOI: 10.1016/j.cell.2011.02.013

[4] Bernstein SC, Weinberg RA. Expression of the metastatic phenotype of cells transfected with human metastatic tumor DNA. Proceedings of the National Academy of Sciences of the United States of America. 1985;**82**:1726-1730

[5] Umbas R, Schalken JA, Aalders TW, Carter BS, Karthaus HFM, Schaafsma HE, Debruyne FMJ, Isaacs WB. Expression of the cellular adhesion molecule E-cadherin is reduced or absent in high-grade prostate cancer. Cancer Research. 1992;**52**:5104-5109

[6] Zutter MM, Santoro SA, Staatz WD, Tsung YL, et al. Re expression of the α2β1 integrin abrogates the malignant phenotype of breast carcinoma cells. Proceedings of the National Academy of Sciences of the United States of America. 1995;**92**:7411-7415

[7] Zheng DQ, Wooddard AS, Fornaro M, Tallini G, Languino LR. Prostatic carcinoma cell migration via αVβ3 integrin is modulated by a focal adhesion kinase pathway. Cancer Research. 1999;**59**:1655-1664

[8] Gao AC, Lou W, Dong JT, Isaacs JT. CD44 is a metastasis suppressor gene for prostate cancer located on human chromosome 11p13. Cancer Research. 1997;**57**:846-849

[9] Pietzner K, Woopen H, Richter R, Joens T, Braicu EI, Dimitrova D, et al. Expression of EpCAM in paired tumor samples of patients with primary and recurrent serous ovarian cancer. International Journal of Gynecological Cancer. 2013;**23**(5):797-802

[10] Schneck H, Gierke B, Uppenkamp F, Behrens B, Niederacher D, Stoecklein NH, Templin MF, Pawlak M, Fehm T, Neubauer H, Disseminated Cancer Cell Network (DCC Net) Duesseldorf. EpCAM-independent enrichment of circulating tumor cells in metastatic breast cancer. PLoS One. 2015 Dec 22;**10**(12):e0144535. DOI: 10.1371/journal.pone.0144535 eCollection 2015. Erratum in: PLoS One. 2016;**11**(2):e0149315

[11] Weidle UH, Eggle D, Klostermann S, Swart GW. ALCAM/CD166: Cancer-related issues. Cancer Genomics & Proteomics. 2010;**7**(5):231-243

[12] Xie S, Luca M, Huang S, Gutman M, Reich R, Johnson JP, Bar-Eli M. Expression of MCAM/MCU18 by human melanoma cells leads to increased tumor growth and metastasis. Cancer Research. 1997;**57**:2295-2303

[13] Wu GJ, Peng Q, Fu P, Wang SWC, Wu MWH. Effect of MUC18 expression on in vitro invasiveness, and in vivo tumorigenesis and metastasis of murine melanoma cell lines in a syngeneic mouse model. In: The Proceedings of the 92nd Annual Meeting of American Association for the Cancer Research. April 2001. Vol. 42. Philadelphia: AACR; 2001. p. 516. Abstract # 2776

[14] Velculescu VE, Zhang L, Volgelstein B, Kinzler KW. Serial analysis of gene expression. Science. 1995;**270**:484-487

[15] Zhang L, Zhou W, Velculescu VE, Kern SE, Hruban RH, Hamilton SR, Volgelstein B, Kinzler KW. Gene expression profiles in normal and cancer cells. Science. 1997;**276**: 1268-1272

[16] Clark EA, Golub TR, Lander ES, Hynes RO. Genomic analysis of metastasis reveals an essential role for RhoC. Nature. 2000;**406**:532-535

[17] Morin PJ. Functional genomics approaches in cancer research. Current Genomics. 2002; **3**:425-436

[18] LaTulipope E, Satagopan J, Smith A, Scher H, Scardino P, Reuter V, Gerald WL. Comprehensive gene expression analysis of prostate cancer reveals distinct transcriptional programs associated with metastatic disease. Cancer Research. 2002;**62**:4499-4506

[19] Leung YF, Cavalieri D. Fundamentals of cDNA microarray data analysis. Trends in Biotechnology. 2003;**19**:649-659

[20] YatesIII JR. Mass spectrometry from genomics to proteomics. Trend in Genetics. 2000; **16**:5-8

[21] Lee KH. Proteomics: A technology-driven and technology-limited discovery science. Trends in Biotechnology. 2001;**19**:217-222

[22] Martin DB, Gifford DR, Wright ME, Keler A, Yi E, Goodlett DR, Aebersold R, Nelson PS. Quantitative proteomic analysis of proteins released by neoplastic prostate epithelium. Cancer Research. 2004;**64**:347-355

[23] Weiss L. Metastatic inefficiency. Advances in Cancer Research. 1990;**54**:159-211

[24] Chambers AF, MacDonald IC, Schmidt EE, Koop S, Morris VL, Khokha R, Groom AC. Step in tumor metastasis: New concepts from intravital videomicroscopy. Cancer & Metastasis Reviews. 1995;**14**:279-301

[25] Mohler JL. Cellular motility and prostate carcinoma metastases. Cancer & Metastasis Reviews. 1993;**12**:53-67

[26] Cavallaro U, Christofori G. Cell adhesion and signaling by cadherins and Ig-CAMs in cancer. Nature Reviews/Cancer. 2005;**4**:118-132

[27] Bellone S, Siegel ER, Cocco E, Cargnelutti M, Silasi DA, Azodi M, et al. Over-expression of epithelial cell adhesion molecule in primary, metastatic, and recurrent/chemotherapy-resistant epithelial ovarian cancer: Implications for epithelial cell adhesion molecule-specific immunotherapy. International Journal of Gynecological Cancer. 2009;**19**(5):860-866

[28] Herlyn M. Molecular and cellular biology of melanoma. Austin, TX: RG Landes Co. 1993. pp 1-97

[29] Hsu MY, Wheelock MJ, Johnson KR, Herlyn M. Shifts in cadherin profiles between human normal melanocytes and melanomas. Journal of Investigative Dermatology Symposium Proceedings. 1996;**1**:188-194

[30] Omara-Opyene AL, Qiu J, Shah GV, Iczkowski KA. Prostate cancer invasion is influenced more by expression of a CD44 isoform including variant 9 than MUC18. Lab Investigation. 2004;**84**:894-907

[31] Cheung PH, Luo W, Qiu Y, Zhang X, Earley K, Millirons P, Lin SH. Structure and function of C-CAM1: The first immunoglobulin domain is required for intercellular adhesion. The Journal of Biological Chemistry. 1993;**268**:24303-24301

[32] Kleinerman DI, Zhang W, Lin S, Van NT, von Eschenbach AC, Hsieh JT. Application of a tumor suppressor (C-CAM1)-expressing recombinant adenovirus in androgen-independent human prostate cancer therapy: A preclinical study. Cancer Research 1995; **55:**2831-2836

[33] Edlund M, Miyamoto T, Sikes RA, Ogle R, Laurie GW, Farach-Carson MC, Otey CA, Zhau HE, Chung LWK. Integrin expression and usage by prostate cancer cell lines on laminin substrata. Cell Growth & Differentiation. 2001;**12**:99-107

[34] Moro L, Perlino E, Marra E, Languino LR, Greco M. Regulation of β1C and β1A integrin expression in prostate carcinoma cells. The Journal of Biological Chemistry. 2004; **279**:1692-1702

[35] Scivolino PJ, Abate-Shen C. Molecular biology of prostate development and prostate cancer. Annals of Medicine. 1998;**30**:357-368

[36] Demetriou MC, Cress AE. Integrin clipping, a novel adhesion switch? Journal of Cellular Biochemistry. 2004;**91**:26-35

[37] Yu Y, Dong W, Zhou X, et al. The significance of soluble intercellular adhesion molecule 1 (ICAM-1) and transformation growth factor alpha in patients with nasopharyngeal carcinomas. Archives of Otolaryngology—Head & Neck Surgery. 2004;**130**:1205-1208

[38] Huang GW, Mo WN, Kuang GQ, et al. Expression of p16, nm-23-H1, E-cadherin, and CD44 gene products and their significance in nasopharyngeal carcinomas. The Laryngoscope. 2001;**111**:1465-1471

[39] Li Z, Ren Y, Lin SX, et al. Association of E-cadherin and β-catenin with metastasis in nasopharyngeal carcinomas. Chinese Medical Journal. 2004;**117**:1232-1239

[40] Yi ZC, Wang H, Zhang GY, et al. Downregulation of connexin 43 in nasopharyngeal carcinoma cells is related to promoter methylation. Oral Oncology. 2006;**11**:004. DOI: 10.1016/j.oraloncology.2006.11.004

[41] Rump A, Morikawa Y, Tanaka M, Minami S, Umesaki N, Takeuchi M, et al. Binding of ovarian cancer antigen CA125/MUC16 to mesothelin mediates cell adhesion. The Journal of Biological Chemistry. 2004;**279**:9190-9198

[42] Strobel T, Cannistra SA. β1-integrins partly mediate binding of ovarian cancer cells to peritoneal mesothelium in vitro. Gynecology Oncology. 2004;**73**:362-367

[43] Bourguignon LYW, Gilad E, Rothman K, Peyrollier K. Hyaluronan-CD44 interaction with IQGAP1 promotes Cdc42 and ERK signaling, leading to actin binding, Elk-1/estrogen receptor transcription activation, and ovarian cancer progression. The Journal of Biological Chemistry. 2005;**280**:11961-11972

[44] Euer NI, Kaul S, Deissler H, Mobus VJ, Zeillinger R, Weidle UH. Identification of L1CAM, Jagged2, and neuromedin U as ovarian cancer-associated antigens. Oncology Reports. 2005;**13**:375-387

[45] Imai T, Horiuchi A, Shiozawa T, Osada R, Kikuchi N, Ohira S. Elevated expression of E-cadherin and alpha-, beta-, and gamma-catenins in metastatic lesions compared with primary epithelial ovarian carcinomas. Human Pathology. 2004;**35**:1469-1476

[46] D'Souza T, Agarwal R, Morin PJ. Phosphorylation of claudin-3 at threonine 192 by cAMP-dependent protein kinase regulates tight junction barrier function in ovarian cancer cells. The Journal of Biological Chemistry. 2005;**280**:26233-26240

[47] Aldovini D, Demichelis F, Doglioni C, Di Vizio D, Galligioni E, Brugnara S, et al. M-CAM expression as marker of poor prognosis in epithelial ovarian cancer. International Journal of Cancer. 2006;**119**(8):1920-1926

[48] Wu GJ, Dickerson EB. Frequent and increased expression of human METCAM/MUC18 in cancer tissues and metastatic lesions associates with the clinical progression of human ovarian carcinoma. Taiwanese Journal of Obstetrics and Gynecology. 2014;**53**:509-517

[49] Wu GJ, Fu P, Wang SW, Wu MWH. Enforced expression of MCAM/MUC18 increases *in vitro* motility and invasiveness and *in vivo* metastasis of two mouse melanoma K1735 sublines in a syngeneic mouse model. Molecular Cancer Research. 2008;**6**(11):1666-1677

[50] Wu GJ. Ectopic expression of MCAM/MUC18 increases in vitro motility and invasiveness, but decreases in vivo tumorigenesis and metastasis of a mouse melanoma K1735-9 subline in a syngeneic mouse model. Clinical & Experimental Metastasis. 2016;**33**(8):817-828. DOI: 10.1007/s10585-016-9812-z

[51] Wu GJ, Peng Q, Fu P, Chiang CF, Wang SWC, Dillehay DL, Wu MWH. Ectopical expression of human MUC18 increases metastasis of human prostate cancer LNCaP cells. Gene. 2004;**327**:201-213

[52] Wu GJ, Chiang CF, Fu P, Hess W, Greenberg N, Wu MWH. Increased expression of MUC18 correlates with the metastatic progression of mouse prostate adenocarcinoma in the (TRAMP) model. Journal of Urology. 2005;**173**:1778-1783

[53] Wu GJ, Wu MWH, Liu Y. Enforced expression of human METCAM/MUC18 increases the tumorigenesis of human prostate cancer cells in nude mice. Journal of Urology. 2011; **185**:1504-1512

[54] Wu GJ. Human METCAM/MUC18 as a novel biomarker to drive and its specific SiRNAs to block the malignant progression of prostate cancer. Journal of Cell Science & Therapy. 2015;**6**:5.1000227

[55] Wu GJ. Human METCAM/MUC18 is a new diagnostic marker of and a driver for promoting and its specific siRNAs, derived oligopeptides and antibodies be used for decreasing the malignant progression of prostate cancer. Journal of Stem Cell Research & Therapeutics. 2016;**1**(5):00035

[56] Zeng GF, Cai SX, Wu GJ. Up-regulation of METCAM/MUC18 promotes motility, invasion, and tumorigenesis of human breast cancer cells. BMC Cancer. 2011;**11**:113. DOI: 10.1186/1471-2407-11-113

[57] Zeng GF, Cai SX, Liu Y, Wu GJ. METCAM/MUC18 augments migration, invasion, and tumorigenicity of human breast cancer SK-BR-3 cells. Gene. 2012;**492**:229-238

[58] Huang CY, Wu GJ. METCAM/MUC18 promoted tumorigenesis of human breast cancer SK-BR-3 cells in a dosage-specific manner. Taiwanese Journal of Obstetrics & Gynecology. 2016;**55**(2):202-212. DOI: 10.1016/j.tjog.2016.02.010

[59] Wu GJ, Zeng GF. METCAM/MUC18 is a novel tumor and metastasis suppressor for the human ovarian cancer SKOV3 cells. BMC Cancer. 2016;**16**:136. DOI: 10.1186/S12885-016-2181-9

[60] Wu GJ. METCAM/MUC18 plays a novel tumor and metastasis suppressor role in the progression of human ovarian cancer cells. Obstetrics & Gynecology International Journal. 2017;**6**(4):00210 pp. 1-8

[61] Lin JC, Chiang CF, Wang SW, Wang WY, Kwuan PC, Wu GJ. Significance and expression of human METCAM/MUC18 in nasopharyngeal carcinoma (NPC) and metastatic lesions. Asian Pacific Journal of Cancer Prevention. 2014;**15**(1):245-252

[62] Wu GJ. Dual role of METCAM in the progression of different cancers. Journal of Oncology. 2012;**2012**:853797. DOI: 10.1155/2012/853797

[63] Lehmann JM, Reithmuller G, Johnson JP. MUC18, a marker of tumor progression in human melanoma. Proceedings of the National Academy of Sciences of the United States of America. 1989;**86**:9891-9895

[64] Sers C, Kirsch K, Rothbacher U, Riethmuller G, Johnson JP. Genomic organization of the melanoma-associated glycoprotein MUC18: Implications for the evolution of the immunoglobulin domains. Proceedings of the National Academy of Sciences of the United States of America. 1993;**90**:8514-8518

[65] Shih IM, Nesbit M, Herlyn M, Kurman RJ. A new Mel-CAM (CD146)-specific monoclonal antibody, MN-4, on paraffin-embedded tissue. Modern Pathology. 1998;**11**:1098-1106

[66] Shih IM. The role of CD146 (Mel-CAM) in biology and pathology. Journal of Pathology. 1999;**189**:4-11

[67] Schlagbauer-Wadl H, Jansen B, Muller M, Polterauer P, Wolff K, Eichler HG, Pehamberger H, Konak E, Johnson JP. Influence of MUC18/MCAM/CD146 expression on human melanoma growth and metastasis in SCID mice. International Journal of Cancer. 1999;**81**:951-955

[68] Anfosso F, Bardin N, Frances V, Vivier E, Camoin-Jau L, Sampol J, Dignat-George F. Activation of human endothelial cells via S-Endo-1 antigen (CD146) stimulates the tyrosine phosphorylation of focal adhesion kinase p125[FAK]. The Journal of Biological Chemistry. 1998;**273**:26852-26858

[69] Wu GJ. METCAM/MUC18 expression and cancer metastasis. Current Genomics. 2005; **6**:333-349

[70] Wu GJ, Wu MWH, Wang SW, Liu Z, Peng Q, Qu P, Yang H, Varma VA, Sun Q, Petros JA, Lim S, Amin MB. Isolation and characterization of the major form of human MUC18 cDNA gene and correlation of MUC18 over-expression in prostate cancer cells and tissues with malignant progression. Gene. 2001;**279**:17-31

[71] Yang H, Wang SWC, Liu Z, Wu MWH, McAlpine B, Ansel J, Armstrong C, Wu GJ. Isolation and characterization of murine MUC18 cDNA gene, and correlation of MUC18 expression in murine melanoma cell lines with metastatic ability. Gene. 2001;**265**:133-145

[72] Wu GJ, Varma VA, Wu MWH, Yang H, Wang SWC, Liu Z, Petros JA, Lim S, Amin M. Expression of a human cell adhesion molecule, MUC18, in prostate cancer cell lines and tissues. The Prostate. 2001;**48**:305-315

[73] Shih IM, Hsu MY, Palazzo JP, Herlyn M. The cell-cell adhesion receptor MEL-CAM acts as a tumor suppressor in breast carcinoma. American Journal of Pathology. 1997; **151**:745-751

[74] Ouhtit A, Gaur RL, Abd Elmageed ZY, Fernando A, Thouta R, Trappey AK, Abdraboh ME, El-Sayyad HI, Rao P, Raj MGH. Towards understanding the mode of action of the multifaceted cell adhesion receptor CD146. Biochimica et Biophysica Acta. 2009; **1795**:130-136

[75] Garcia S, Dales JP, Charafe-Jauffret E, Carpentier-Meunier S, Andrac-Meyer L, Jacquemier J, Andonian C, Lavaut MN, Allasia C, Bonnier P, Charpin C. Poor prognosis in breast carcinomas correlates with increased expression of targetable CD146 and c-Met and with proteomic basal-like phenotype. Human Pathology. 2007;**38**:830-841

[76] Zabouo G, Imbert AM, Jacquemier J, Finetti P, Moreau T, Esterni B, Birnbaum D, Bertucci F, Chabannon C. CD146 expression is associated with a poor prognosis in human breast tumors and with enhanced motility in breast cancer cell lines. Breast Cancer Research. 2009;**11**:R1. DOI: 10.1186/bcr2215

[77] Zeng Q, Li W, Lu D, Wu Z, Duan H, Luo Y, Feng J, Yang D, Fu L, Yan X. CD146, an epithelial-mesenchymal transition inducer, is associated with triple-negative breast cancer. Proceedings of the National Academy of Sciences of the United States of America. 2012;**109**(4):1127-1132

[78] Meier F, Caroli U, Satyamoorthy K, Schittek B, Bauer J, Berking C, Moller H, Maczey E, Rassner G. Herlyn M, Garbe C. Fibroblast growth factor-2 but not Mel-CAM and/or β3 integrin promotes progression of melanocytes to melanoma. Experimental Dermatology. 2003;**12**:296-306

[79] Leslie MC, Zhao YJ, Lachman LB, Hwu P, Wu GJ, Bar-Eli M. Immunization against MUC18/MCAM, a novel antigen that drives melanoma invasion and metastasis. Gene Therapy. 2007;**14**:316-323 382

[80] Takahashi Y, Nishikawa M, Takakura Y. Non-viral vector-mediated RNA interference: Its gene silencing characteristics and important factors to achieve RNAi-based gene therapy. Advance Drug Delivery Reviews. 2009;**61**:760-766

[81] Lin CT, Wong CI, Chan WY, et al. Establishment and characterization of two nasopharyngeal carcinoma cell lines. Laboratory Investigation. 1990;**62**:713-724

[82] Liu YC. Putative roles of huMETCAM in modulating the development and progression of nasopharyngeal arcinoma. Thesis of Master Science degree under the supervision of Dr. Guang-Jer Wu. Taiwan: Department of Bioscience Technology, Chung Yuan Christian University; 2014. http://www.lib.cycu.edu.tw/thesis

[83] Liu YC, Chen, YR, Wu GJ. METCAM/MUC18 plays a tumor suppressor role in the development of nasopharyngeal carcinoma type I. 2017 (submitted)

[84] Liu YC, Ke CC, Chen YR, Wu GJ. METCAM/MUC18 plays a tumor promoter role in the development of nasopharyngeal carcinoma type II. 2017 (submitted)

[85] Wu Z, Wu Z, Li J, Yang X, Wang Y, Yu Y, et al. MCAM is a novel metastasis marker and regulates spreading, apoptosis and invasion of ovarian cancer cells. Tumor Biology. 2012;**33**:1619-1628

[86] Putz E, Witter K, Offner S, Stosiek P, Zippeliux A, Johnson J, Zahn R, Riethmuller G, Pantel K. Phenotypic characteristics of cell lines derived from disseminated cancer cells in bone marrow of patients with solid epithelial tumors: Establishment of working models for human micrometastases. Cancer Research. 1999;**59**:241-248

[87] Greenberg NM, DeMayo F, Finegold MJ, Medina D, Tilley WD, Aspinall JO, Cunha GR, Donjacour AA, Matusik RJ, Rosen JM. Prostate cancer in a transgenic mouse. Proceedings of the National Academy of Sciences of the United States of America. 1995;**92**:3439-3443

[88] Garabedian EM, Humphrey PA, Gordon JI. A transgenic mouse model of metastatic prostate cancer originating from neuroendocrine cells. Proceedings of the National Academy of Sciences of the United States of America. 1998;**95**:15382-15387

[89] Foster B. New paradigms for prostate cancer research-TRAMP bone metastasis cell lines. In: The Proceeding of the AACR Special Conference: New Discoveries in Prostate Cancer Biology and Treatment; The Registry Resort, Naples, FL; 5-9 December 2001

[90] LaMontagne KR Jr, Moses MA, Wiederschain D, Mahajan S, Holden J, Ghazizadeh H, Frank DA, Arbiser J. Inhibition of MAP kinase kinase causes morphological reversion and dissociation between soft agar growth and *in vivo* tumorigenesis in angiosarcoma cells. American Journal of Pathology. 2000;**157**:1937-1945

[91] Westrøm S, Bønsdorff TB, Abbas N, Bruland ØS, Jonasdottir TJ, Mælandsmo GM, Larsen RH. Evaluation of CD146 as target for radioimmunotherapy against osteosarcoma. PLoS One. 2016;**11**(10):e0165382. DOI: 10.1371/journal.pone.0165382 eCollection 2016

[92] Chen K, Ding A, Ding Y, Ghanekar A. High-throughput flow cytometry screening of human hepatocellular carcinoma reveals CD146 to be a novel marker of tumor-initiating cells. Biochemistry and Biophysics Reports. 2016;**8**:107-113

[93] Jiang G, Zhang L, Zhu Q, Bai D, Zhang C, Wang X. CD146 promotes metastasis and predicts poor prognosis of hepatocellular carcinoma. Journal of Experimental & Clinical Cancer Research. 2016;**35**:38. DOI: 10.1186/s13046-016-0313-3

[94] Zeng P, Li H, Lu PH, Zhou LN, Tang M, Liu CY, Chen MB. Prognostic value of CD146 in solid tumor: A systematic review and meta-analysis. Scientific Reports. 2017;**7**(1):4223. DOI: 10.1038/s41598-017-01061-3

[95] Kristiansen G, Yu Y, Schlüns K, Sers C, Dietel M, Petersen I. Expression of the cell adhesion molecule CD146/MCAM in non-small cell lung cancer. Analytical Cellular Pathology. 2003;**25**:77-81

[96] Jiang Y, Huang Y, Du Y, Zhao Y, Ren J, Ma S, Wu C. Identification of prognostic genes and pathways in lung adenocarcinoma using a Bayesian approach. Cancer Informatics. 2017;1-7. DOI: 10.1177/1176935116684825

[97] Liu D, Du L, Chen D, Ye Z, Duan H, Tu T, Feng J, Yang Y, Chen Q, Yan X. Reduced CD146 expression promotes tumorigenesis and cancer stemness in colorectal cancer through activating Wnt/β-catenin signaling. Oncotarget. 2016;**7**(26):40704-40718

[98] von Burstin J, Bachhuber F, Paul M, Schmid RM, Rustgi AK. The TALE homeodomain transcription factor MEIS1 activates the pro-metastatic melanoma cell adhesion molecule MCAM to promote migration of pancreatic cancer cells. Molecular Carcinogenesis. 2017;**56**(3):936-944

[99] Zheng B, Ohuchida K, Chijiiwa Y, Zhao M, Mizuuchi Y, Cui L, Horioka K, Ohtsuka T, Mizumoto K, Oda Y, Hashizume M, Nakamura M, Tanaka M. CD146 attenuation in cancer-associated fibroblasts promotes pancreatic cancer progression. Molecular Carcinogenesis. 2016;**55**(11):1560-1572

[100] Li Q, Yu Y, Bischoff J, Milliken JB, Olsen BR. Differential expression of CD146 in tissues and endothelial cells derived from infantile hemangioma and normal human skin. Journal of Pathology. 2003;**201**:296-302

[101] Zhang Y, Zheng C, Zhang J, Yang D, Feng J, Lu D. Yan X, Generation and characterization of a panel of monoclonal antibodies against distinct epitopes of human CD146. Hybridoma. 2008;**27**(5):345-352. DOI: 10.1089/hyb.2008.0034

[102] Bowen MA, Patel DD, Li X, Modrell B, Malacko AR, Wang WC, Marquardt H, Neubauer M, Pesando JM, Francke U, Haynes BF, Aruffo A. Cloning, mapping, and characterization of ALCAM, a CD6 ligand. The Journal of Experimental Medicine. 1995;**181**:2213-2220

[103] Skonier JE, Bowen MA, Emswiler J, Aruffo A, Bajorath J. Mutational analysis of the CD6 binding site in ALCAM. Biochemistry. 1996;**35**:14743-14748

[104] Van Kempen LCLT, Nelissen JMDT, Degen WGJ, Torensma R, Weidle UH, Bloemers HPJ, Figdor CG, Swart GWM. Molecular basis for the homophilic activated leukocyte

cell adhesion molecule (ALCAM)-ALCAM interaction. The Journal of Biological Chemistry. 2001;**276**:25783-25790

[105] Ozawa M. p120-independent modulation of E-cadherin adhesion activity by the membrane-proximal region of the cytoplasmic domain. The Journal of Biological Chemistry. 2003;**278**:45014-46020

[106] Morgan MR, Thomas GJ, Russell A, Hart IR, Marshall JF. The integrin cytoplasmic-tail motif EKQKVDLSTDC is sufficient to promote tumor cell invasion mediated by matrix metalloproteinase MMP-2 or MMP-9. The Journal of Biological Chemistry. 2004; **279**:26533-26539

[107] Heiz M, Grunberg J, Schubiger PA, Novak-Hofer I. Hepatocyte growth factor-induced ectodomain shedding of cell adhesion molecule L1-role of the cytoplasmic domain. The Journal of Biological Chemistry. 2004;**279**:31149-31156

[108] Geiser M, Cebe R, Drewello D, Schmitz R. Integration of PCR fragments at any specific site within cloning vectors without the use of restriction enzymes and DNA ligase. BioTechniques. 2001;**31**:88-92

[109] Parodi A. Protein glycosylation and its role in protein folding. Annual Review of Biochemistry. 2000;**69**:69-93

[110] Varki A. Glycosylation changes in tumor cells. In: Varki A, Cumming R, Esko J, Freeze H, Hart G, Marth J. editors. Essentials of Glycobiology. NY: Cold Spring Harbor Laboratory Press; 1999. pp. 537-549

[111] Fukuda M. Possible roles of tumor-associated carbohydrate antigens. Cancer Research. 1996;**56**:2237-2244

[112] Hakomori S. Tumor malignancy defined by aberrant glycosylation and sphingo(glyco) lipid metabolism. Cancer Research. 1996;**56**:5309-5318

[113] Yamamoto H, Oviedo A, Sweeley C, Saito T, Moskal JR. α2,6-sialylation of cell-surface N-glycans inhibits glioma formation *in vivo*. Cancer Research. 2001;**61**:6822-6829

[114] Lehmann JM, Holzmann B, Breitbart EW, Schmiegelow P, Riethmuller G, Johnson JP. Discrimination between benign and malignant cells of melanocytic lineage by two novel antigens, a glycoprotein with a molecular weight of 113,000 and a protein with a molecular weight of 76,000. Cancer Research. 1987;**47**:841-845

[115] Lanier LL, Le AM, Phillips JH, Warner NL, Babcock GF. Subpopulations of human NK cells defined by expression of the leu-7 (HNK-1) and Leu-11 (NK-15) antigens. Journal of Immunology. 1983;**131**:1789-1796

[116] Chou DKH, Ilyas AA, Evans JE, Costello C, Quarles RH, Jungalwala FB. Structure of sulfated glucuronyl glycolipids in the nervous systems reacting with HNK-1 antibody and some IgM paraproteins in neuropathy. The Journal of Biological Chemistry. 1986;**261**:11717-11725

[117] Bezouska K, Yuen CT, O'Brien J, Childs RA, Chai W, Lawson AM, Drbal K, Fiserova A, Pospissil M, Feizi T. Oligosaccharide ligands for NKR-P1 protein activate NK cells and cytotoxicity. Nature. 1994;**372**:150-157

[118] Shih IM, Schnaar RL, Gearhart JD, Kurman RJ. Distribution of cells bearing the HNK-1 epitope in the human placenta. Placenta. 1997;**18**:667-674

[119] Ong E, Suzuki M, Belot F, Yeh J, Franceschi I, Angata K, Hindsgaul O, Fukuda M. Biosynthesis of HNK-1 glycans on O-linked oligosaccharides attached to the NCAM. The Journal of Biological Chemistry. 2002;**277**:18182-18190

[120] Liu XH, Yoshiki T, Kokuho M, Okada Y, Tomoyoshi T. The prognostic value of the HNK-1 (leu-7) antigen in prostatic cancer. Acta Urologica. 1993;**39**:439-444

[121] Sumardika W, Youyi C, Kondo E, Inoue Y, Ruma MW, Murata H, Kinoshita R, Yamamoto KI, Tomida S, Shien K, Satoh H, Yamauchi A, Futami J, Putranto EW, Hibino T, Toyooka S, Nishibori M, Sakaguchi M. β-1,3-galactosyl-O-glycosyl-glycoprotein β-1,6-N-acetylglucosaminyltransferase 3 increases MCAM stability, which enhances S100A8/A9-mediated cancer motility. Oncology Research. 2017. DOI: 10.3727/096504017X15031557924123

[122] Dubuisson J, Duvet S, Meunier JC, Op De Beeck A, Cacan R, Wychowski C, Cocquerel L. Glycosylation of the hepatitis C virus envelope protein E1 is dependent on the presence of a downstream sequence on the viral polyprotein. The Journal of Biological Chemistry. 2000;**275**:30605-30609

[123] Wu G, Lai H, Lin Y, Chu Y, Chern Y. N-glycosylation and residues Asn905 and Asn890 are involved in the functional properties of type VI adenyl cyclase. The Journal of Biological Chemistry. 2001;**276**:35450-35457

[124] Railey JF, Wu GJ. Organization of multiple regulatory elements in the control region of the adenovirus type 2 VARNA1 gene: Fine mapping with linker-scanning mutants. Molecular and Cellular Biology. 1988;**8**:1147-1159

[125] Shih IM, Speicher D, Hsu MY, Levine E, Herlyn M. Melanoma cell-ell interactions are mediated through heterophilic Mel-/CAM ligand adhesion. Cancer Research. 1997;**57**:3835-3840

[126] Johnson JP, Bar-Eli M, Jansen B, Markhop E. Melanoma progression-associated glycoprotein MUC18/MCAM mediates homotypic cell adhesion through interaction with a heterophilic ligand. International Journal of Cancer. 1997;**73**:769-774

[127] Wu GJ. MCAM (melanoma cell adhesion molecule). Atlas of Genetics and Cytogenetics in Oncology and Haematology (Open Access Journal). 2012. DOI: 10.4267/2042/47418. ID41314ch11q23. The manually annotated biomax human genome database version 4.0, biomax informatics AG, www.biomax.com, the biomax solutions Inc., Falmouth, MA, USA

[128] Taira E, Takaha N, Taiura H, Kim CH, Miki N. Molecular cloning and functional expression of gicerin, a novel cell adhesion molecule that binds to neurite outgrowth factor. Neuron. 1994;**12**:861-872

[129] Sampath R, Gallagher PJ, Pavalko FM. Cytoskeletal interactions with the leukocyte integrin β2 cytoplasmic tail. The Journal of Biological Chemistry. 1998;**273**:33588-33594

[130] Flanagan JG, Leder P. The kit ligand: A cell surface molecule altered in steel mutant fibroblasts. Cell. 1990;**63**:185-194

[131] Jiang P, Lagenaur CF, Narayanan V. Integrin-associated protein is a ligand for the P84 neural adhesion molecule. The Journal of Biological Chemistry. 1999;**274**:559-562

[132] Yeh RH, Lee TR, Lawrence DS. From consensus sequence peptide to high affinity ligand, a library scan strategy. The Journal of Biological Chemistry. 2001;**276**:12235-12240

[133] Barbas CF III, Burton DR, Scott JK, Silverman GJ. Phage Display—A Laboratory Manual. New York. Cold Spring Harbor Laboratory Press: Cold Spring Harbor; 2001

[134] Sastry SK, Horwitz AF. Integrin cytoplasmic domains: Mediators of cytoskeletal linkages and extra- and intracellular initiated transmembrane signaling. Current Opinion in Cell Biology. 1993;**5**:819-831

[135] Schoenwaelder SM, Burridge K. Bidirectional signaling between the cytoskeleton and integrins. Current Opinion in Cell Biology. 1999;**11**:274-286

[136] Anfosso F, Bardin N, Vivier E, Sabatier F, Sampol J, Dignat-George F. Outside-in signaling pathway linked to CD146 engagement in human endothelial cells. The Journal of Biological Chemistry. 2001;**276**:1564-1569

[137] Giannone G, Ronde P, Gaire M, Beaudouin J, Haiech J, Ellenberg J, Takeda K. Calcium rises locally trigger focal adhesion disassembly and enhance residency of focal adhesion kinase at focal adhesions. The Journal of Biological Chemistry. 2004;**279**:28715-28723

[138] Rahn JJ, Shen Q, Mah BK, Hugh JC. MUC1 initiates a calcium signal after ligation by intercellular adhesion molecule-1. The Journal of Biological Chemistry. 2004;**279**: 29386-29390

[139] Berridge MJ, Lipp P, Bootman MD. The versatility and universality of calcium signaling. Nature Review Molecular Cell Biology. 2000;**1**:11-21

[140] Brazil DP, Yang ZZ, Hemmings BA. Advances in protein kinase B signaling: AKTion on multiple fronts. Trends in Biochemical Sciences. 2004 May;**29**(5):233-242

[141] Cao F, Zhang C, Han W, Gao XJ, Ma J, YW H, Gu X, Ding HZ, Li-Xia Zhu LX, Qin L. P-Akt as a potential poor prognostic factor for gastric cancer: A systematic review and meta-analysis. Oncotarget. 2017;**8**:59878-59888

[142] Li G, Kalabis J, Xu X, Meier F, Oka M, Bogenrieder T, Herlyn M. Reciprocal regulation of MelCAM and AKT in human melanoma. Oncogene. 2003;**22**:6891-6899

[143] Franchin C, Borgo C, Zaramella S, Cesaro L, Arrigoni G, Salvi M, Pinna LA. Exploring the CK2 paradox: Restless, dangerous, dispensable. Pharmaceuticals. 2017;**10**:11. DOI: 10.3390/ph10010011

[144] Hofmann J. Protein kinase C isozymes as potential targets for anticancer therapy. Current Cancer Drug Targets. 2004;**4**:125-146

[145] Mellor H, Parker PJ. The extended protein kinase C superfamily. The Biochemical Journal. 1998;**332**:281-292

[146] Jaken S, Parker PJ. Protein kinase C binding partners. BioEssays. 2000;**22**:245-254

[147] Cooke M, Magimaidas A, Casado-Medrano V, Kazanietz MG. Protein kinase C in cancer: The top five unanswered questions. Molecular Carcinogenesis. 2017;**56**:1531-1542

[148] Rummel MM, Sers C, Johnson JP. Phorbol ester and cyclic AMP-mediated regulation of the melanoma-associated cell adhesion molecule MUC18/MCAM. Cancer Research. 1996;**56**:2218-2223

[149] Jean D, Gershenwald JE, Huang S, Luca M, Hudson MJ, Tainsky MA, Bar-Eli M. Loss of AP-2 results in up-regulation of CAM/MUC18 and an increase in tumor growth and metastasis of human melanoma cells. The Journal of Biological Chemistry. 1998; **273**:16501-16508

[150] Ruiz M, Pettaway C, Song R, Stoeltzing O, Ellis L, Bar-Eli M. Activator protein 2a inhibits tumorigenicity and represses vascular endothelial growth factor transcription in prostate cancer cells. Cancer Research. 2004;**64**:631-638

[151] Ness SA. The Myb oncoprotein: Regulating a regulator. Biochimica et Biophysica Acta. 1996;**1299**:F123-F139

[152] Thomson JAF, Murphy K, Baker E, Sutherland GR, Parsons PG, Sturm RA. The brn-2 gene regulates the melanocytic phenotype and tumorigenic potential of human melanoma cells. Oncogene. 1995;**11**:691-700

[153] Yordy JS, Li R, Sementchenko VI, Pei H, Muise-Helmericks RC, Watson DK. S100 expression modulates ETS1 transcriptional activity and inhibits cell invasion. Oncogene. 2004; **23**:6654-6665

[154] L'honore A, Lamb NJ, Vandromme M, Turowski P, Carnac G, Fernandez A. MyoD distal regulatory region contains an SF binding CArG element required for MyoD expression in skeletal myoblasts and during muscle regeneration. Molecular Biology of the Cell. 2003;**14**:2151-2162

[155] Baron V, Duss S, Rhim J, Mercola D. Antisense to the early growth response-1 gene (Egr-1) inhibits prostate tumor development in TRAMP mice. Annals of the New York Academy of Sciences. 2003;**1002**:197-216

[156] O'Brien RM, Streeper RS, Ayala JE, Stadelmaier BT, Hornbuckle LA. Insulin-regulated gene expression. Biochemical Society Transactions. 2001;**29**:552-558

[157] Liu XS, Genet MD, Haines JE, Mehanna EK, Wu S, Chen HI, et al. ZBTB7A suppresses melanoma metastasis by transcriptionally repressing MCAM. Molecular Cancer Research. 2015;**13**:1206-1217

[158] Schiano C, Grimaldi V, Casamassimi A, Infante T, Esposito A, Giovane A, et al. Different expression of CD146 in human normal and osteosarcoma cell lines. Medical Oncology. 2012;**29**:2998-3002

[159] Johnson JP, Rummel MM, Rothbacher U, Sers C. MUC18: A cell adhesion molecule with a potential role in tumor growth and tumor cell dissemination. Curr Topics Microbiol & Immunol. 1997;**213**:95-106

[160] Sechler M, Parrish JK, Birks DK, Jedlicka P. The histone demethylase KDM3A, and its downstream target MCAM, promote Ewing Sarcoma cell migration and metastasis. Oncogene. 2017;**36**(29):4150-4160

[161] Lung HL, Cheng Y, Kumaran MK, et al. Fine mapping of the 11Q22-23 tumor suppressive region and involvement of TSLC1 in nasopharyngeal carcinoma. International Journal of Cancer. 2004;**112**:628-635

[162] Brait M, Banerjee M, Maldonado L, Ooki A, Loyo M, Guida E, Izumchenko E, Mangold L, Humphreys E, Rosenbaum E, Partin A, Sidransky D, Hoque MO. Promoter methylation of MCAM, ERα and ERβ in serum of early stage prostate cancer patients. Oncotarget. 2017;**8**(9):15431-15440. DOI: 10.18632/oncotarget.14873

[163] Chiang CF, Son EL, Wu GJ. Oral treatment of the TRAMP mice with doxazosin suppresses prostate tumor growth and metastasis. The Prostate. 2005;**64**:408-418

[164] Mills L, Tellez C, Huang S, Baker C, McCarty M, Green L, Gudas JM, Feng X, Bar-Eli M. Fully human antibodies to MCAM/MUC18 inhibit tumor growth and metastasis of human melanoma. Cancer Research. 2002;**62**:5106-5114

[165] Yan X, Lin Y, Yang D, Shen Y, Yuan M, Zhang Z, Li P, Xia H, Li L, Luo D, Liu Q, Mann K, Bader B. A novel anti-CD146 monoclonal antibody, AA98, inhibits angiogenesis and tumor growth. Blood. 2003;**102**:184-191

Chapter 14

Methylation of NF-κB and its Role in Gene Regulation

Han Wei, Lakshmi Prabhu, Antja-Voy Hartley,
Matthew Martin, Emily Sun, Guanglong Jiang,
Yunlong Liu and Tao Lu

Additional information is available at the end of the chapter

http://dx.doi.org/10.5772/intechopen.72552

Abstract

The nuclear factor κB (NF-κB) is one of the most pivotal transcription factors in mammalian cells. In many pathologies NF-κB is activated abnormally. This contributes to the development of various disorders such as cancer, acute kidney injury, lung disease, chronic inflammatory diseases, cardiovascular disease, and diabetes. This book chapter focuses on how methylation of NF-κB regulates its target genes differentially. The knowledge from this chapter will provide scientific strategies for innovative therapeutic intervention of NF-κB in a wide range of diseases.

Keywords: arginine, epigenetic enzymes, gene regulation, lysine, methylation, NF-κb, transcription factor

1. Introduction

The nuclear factor κB (NF-κB) is one of the most pivotal transcription factors in mammalian cells. In many pathologies NF-κB is activated abnormally. This contributes to the development of various disorders such as cancer, acute kidney injury, lung disease, chronic inflammatory diseases, cardiovascular disease, and diabetes [1]. NF-κB family is comprised of five family members: p65 (RelA), RelB, c-Rel, p50/p105 (NF-kB1), and p52/p100 (NF-kB2). Among them, the Rel homology domain (RHD) at their N-termini is a commonly share feature (**Figure 1**). It is necessary for protein dimerization, the inhibition of NF-κB (IκB) interaction, nuclear targeting, and DNA binding [2]. Additionally, a carboxy-terminal transactivation domain (TAD) also exists in the Rel proteins, such as p65 (**Figure 1**), RelB, and c-Rel. Among the NF-κB dimers, the p65:p50 heterodimer is the prototype.

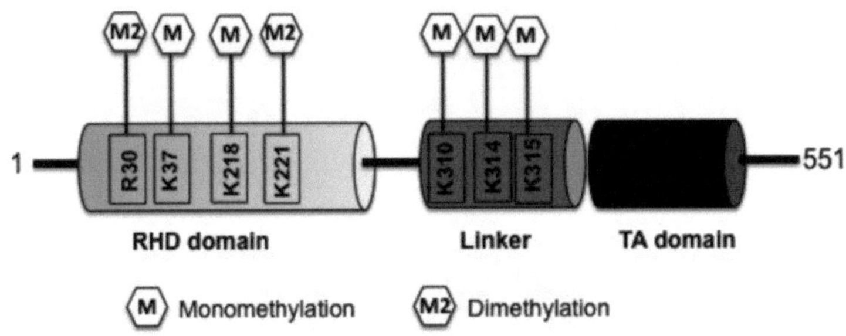

Figure 1. Diagram of the p65 subunit of NF-κB with methylation modifications. In the diagram, the arginine (R) 30 and lysine (K) 37, 218 and 221 are located at the Rel homology domain (RHD) (light gray), other 3 lysine sites K310, 314 and 315 are located in the linker region (gray) between RHD and Transactivation domain (TA) (dark gray).

The activity of NF-κB is frequently regulated by various modifications, namely, post-translational modifications (PTM). Among which, methylation is the newest type of modification that is discovered. The knowledge on NF-κB methylation is still scarce and not popularized among wide range of readers. Thus, in this chapter, we will focus on how methylation of NF-κB regulates its target genes differentially and provide perspectives and future directions in term of the research and application of NF-κB methylation. The knowledge from this chapter will provide scientific strategies for innovative therapeutic intervention of NF-κB in a wide range of diseases.

2. NF-κB signaling pathways

The NF-κB signaling pathways play a very important role in signaling innate and adaptive immune responses and in many cellular processes. NF-κB signaling and subsequent target gene activation can be induced by a variety of factors including cytokines, stress, radiation, and also bacteria and viruses [3]. This signaling can be broken down into two signaling pathways: the canonical and non-canonical branches of the NF-κB pathway (**Figure 2**). In the canonical pathway, activity is regulated by interactions between IκB proteins and the p65:p50 complex. IκB proteins hold NF-κB proteins in inactive conformations by binding in the cytoplasm and preventing nuclear localization. Extracellular signals including cytokines such as interleukin 1 β (IL-1β) and tumor necrosis factor α (TNFα), stress, free radicals, or radiation cause IκB kinase (IKK) activation. IKK is a complex that consists of the IKKα and IKKβ kinases and a third regulatory subunit known as NEMO/IKKγ [4, 5]. In the canonical pathway, IKKβ phosphorylates the N-terminal serine residues 32 and 36 of IκBα, resulting in its polyubiquitination and subsequent rapid proteasomal degradation [3]. This degradation allows the release of p65:p50 into the cytoplasm. The two-unit NF-κB complex then binds to the protein importin and translocates to the nucleus where it further binds to DNA and promotes increased expression of NF-κB target genes [6]. In the noncanonical pathway, the p100 and RelB proteins form an inactive dimer in the cytoplasm. Upon stimulation by a certain group of stimuli, such as B-cell activation factor (BAF) or CD40 ligand (CD40L), IKKα is subsequently activated through NF-κB-inducing kinase (NIK) mediation, leading to the ubiquitin/proteasomal processing of

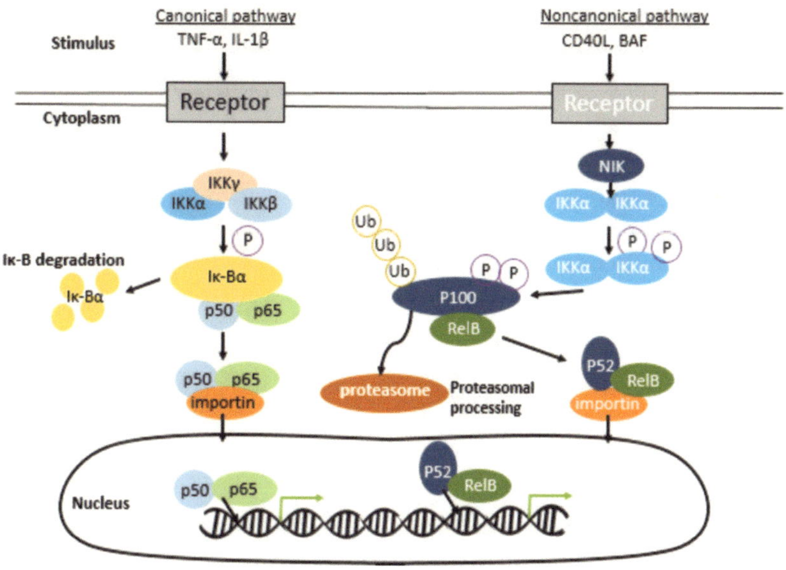

Figure 2. Two important NF-κB pathways. **Left**, in the canonical pathway, NF-κB subunit dimers are bound to inhibitory IκB proteins, which act to hold NF-κB complexes in an inactive state in the cytoplasm. Following stimulus of a receptor, the IκB kinase (IKK) complex becomes phosphorylated. IKK is made of two catalytically active kinases, IKKα and IKKβ, and the regulatory subunit IKKγ (NEMO). IKK then phosphorylates IκB proteins which are subsequently ubiquitinated and proteasomally degraded. This releases the bound subunits of NF-κB p65 and p50 into the cytoplasm. Following cytoplasmic release the subunits bind to importin and translocate to the nucleus where they can bind to the promoter and trigger the transcriptional activation of NF-κB target genes. **Right**, in the noncanonical pathway, the p100/RelB dimer remains in an inactive state until stimulated by a signaling cascade triggered by factors including CD40L or BAFF. Following stimulus and subsequent phosphorylation of IKKα by NIK, IKKα phosphorylates p100 associated with RelB, which leads to its ubiquitination and proteasomal processing to p52. The complexed p52/RelB can then translocate to the nucleus and bind to the target gene promoters and further activate the transcription of the NF-κB target genes.

p100 to p52. Once this processing has occurred, the RelB/p52 complex can translocate to the nucleus and bind to DNA to promote increased expression of NF-κB target genes [7].

3. The state of post-translational modifications (PTM) of NF-κB

Given the role of NF-κB in a wide range of important cellular and physiological processes, the potentially disastrous consequences of dysregulated NF-κB necessitates highly complex and finely regulated mechanisms for controlling NF-κB activity. NF-κB signaling can be influenced at multiple levels, many of which converge on various components of the pathway including the IKK complex and the IκB family of proteins [8]. For instance, the IKK complex remains one of the best-studied central regulators of NF-κB activation, and its phosphorylation of IκBα constitutes an essential event for subsequent signal transduction to both the canonical and non-canonical heterodimeric subunits of NF-κB [8, 9] as described above.

In addition to regulation by the IKK complex and the inhibitory IκB proteins, the NF-κB/Rel dimeric proteins are themselves subject to intricate regulation via a host of critical post-translational modification (PTM) events [10–12]. PTMs on p65, the prototypical subunit of NF-κB, include [13, 14], acetylation [15–19], methylation [20–23], ubiquitination [24], nitrosylation [25], and sumoylation [26]. The consequences of these regulatory modifications are context dependent, and vary based on the nature and abundance of the NF-κB pathway stimulators [11, 22]. Moreover, the sites and/or crosstalk between modifications [16, 27] can yield different outcomes with even the same modifications yielding quite distinct physiological effects [28–31]. Eventually, these PTMs work to dictate the duration and strength of activation and, accordingly, the degree of transcriptional output [10, 32]. Moreover, some of these modifications serve as important means for crosstalk with other signaling pathways [33].

Our laboratory is one of the first few groups to discover that p65 can be methylated on lysine residues upon cytokine stimulation [20]. Subsequently, we pioneered the identification of arginine 30 (R30) methylation of p65 [22]. Below, we will thoroughly discuss the impact of these methylation sites on NF-κB-mediated differential gene regulation.

4. Methylation of the p65 subunit of NF-κB

4.1. Lysine methylation of p65

To date, a total of six lysine methylation sites have been reported: K37, 218, 221, 310, 314, and 315 [18, 20]. By using a novel genetic approach, our lab identified that p65 can be methylated by a lysine methylase, the nuclear receptor-binding SET domain-containing protein 1 (NSD1), and demethylated by a lysine demethylase, the F-box and leucine-rich repeat protein 11 (FBXL11) [20]. This reversible lysine methylation of p65 is targeted at K218/K221 sites and affects NF-κB activity. K218/K221 methylation induces over 80% p65-dependent gene expression in mouse embryonic fibroblast cells (MEFs). The observation indicates that PTMs play an important role in fine-tuning the regulation of NF-κB [20].

Zhang *et al.* provided strong evidence regarding the function of p65 methylation by reporting that in response to TNFα, plant homeodomain finger protein 20 (PHF20) promotes NF-κB transcriptional activity by interacting with methylated p65 at K218/221. The methylation of p65 blocks recruitment of PP2A to p65, thereby leading to the persistent phosphorylation of p65 [34]. By using the immunohistochemistry (IHC) staining method, the authors showed that PHF20 and phosphorylated p65 are localized in the nucleus in glioma tissue specimens. The PHF20 expression levels are also tightly correlated with the clinical tumor grade after univariate analysis with a P value of 0.0018 ($P < 0.05$ is considered to be significant). These findings highlight the interrelated connections between overexpressed PHF20, methylation, and phosphorylation of p65 in human malignant gliomas [34].

In addition to our discovery of the methylation of K218/221, Ea *et al.* revealed that p65 is monomethylated by histone methyltransferase, the Set domain-containing protein 9 (Set9) at K37 in response to both IL-1β and TNFα treatment. The authors showed that TNFα induced p65 monomethylation is essential for the expression of NF-κB regulated genes. Methylated p65 stays in the nucleus, and Set9 might regulate its nuclear function.

Moreover, monomethylation of p65 increases the NF-κB DNA binding ability and recruitment to the promoter of NF-κB target genes [18]. Interestingly, Yang *et al.* described that Set9 may also monomethylate p65 at K314 and K315 in addition to K37, and negatively regulate p65. The authors suggested that methylation of K314/315 inhibits the transcriptional activity of NF-κB through proteasome-mediated degradation, and it downregulates NF-κB target gene expression [19], a phenomenon quite different from that of K37 methylation. Collectively, this evidence suggests the complexity of p65 methylation, and indicates that the same enzyme, such as SET9, may have different functions depending on the lysine residues it modifies. There is also a possibility that K37 modification occurs before K314/K315 methylation. It is likely that K37 methylation is required for gene activation, while K314/315 methylation is required for the termination of NF-κB activity [18].

Besides the methylated lysine residues on p65 discussed above, another SET family member SETD6, was also reported to monomethylate p65 at K310 under basal condition. Levy and colleagues observed that under the unstimulated condition, a proportion of p65 can be monomethylated by SETD6. This methylation event negatively regulates NF-κB target gene expression, including those involved in inflammatory response. The phenotype was proven in various cell lines, such as bone osteosarcoma U2OS, peripheral blood THP-1, and bone marrow-derived macrophages (BMDM), and therefore represents diverse disease models. Interestingly, Levy *et al.* found that K310 monomethylation-mediated NF-κB inhibition is due to the involvement of another protein, the G9A-like protein (GLP). By binding to monomethylated K310, GLP enriches histone H3K9 dimethylation on the p65 target gene promoters, resulting in gene suppression. This SETD6-initiated lysine-methylation repressive pathway can be terminated by p65 phosphorylation at serine 311 (S311) and by the atypical protein kinase PKC-ζ [23]. This study presents a delicate example of how methylation and phosphorylation on p65 may regulate each other and be an integral part of a more sophisticated regulatory system of NF-κB.

An overlook of the biological roles of p65 lysine methylation and their modifying enzymes is shown in **Table 1**. It is evident that under various experimental conditions, p65 lysine methylation may affect NF-κB nucleus localization, transcriptional activity, and NF-κB target gene expression.

4.2. Arginine methylation of p65

Distinct from the methylation of lysine residues, our lab used Mass Spectrometry to discover that p65 can also be symmetrically methylated at arginine 30 residue (R30) [20, 22]. This important modification is carried out by the protein arginine methyltransferase 5 (PRMT5), an enzyme that belongs to the PRMT superfamily, contains 637 amino acids, and catalyzes the formation of symmetrically dimethylated arginine.

We reported that PRMT5 catalyzed p65 dimethylation upon IL-1β treatment. R30 to A mutant (R30A) of p65 decreased NF-κB activity and led to the downregulation of a subgroup of NF-κB inducible genes; among these are cytokine and chemokine genes. Conditional media from cells expressing the R30A mutant of p65 had much less NF-kB-inducing activity than its wild-type cohort. Additionally, through *In Silico* prediction we proposed that dimethylation

Type of methylation	Site modified	Enzymes	Biological function	Reference
Monomethylation	K37	SET9	Stabilizes nuclear localization and enhances p65 binding ability	[18]
Monomethylation	K218	NSD1/FBXL11	Promotes NF-κB transcriptional activity and maintains p65 phosphorylation on S536	[20, 34]
Dimethylation	K221	NSD1/ FBXL11	Promotes NF-κB transcriptional activity and maintains p65 phosphorylation on S536	[20, 34]
Monomethylation	K310	SETD6	Decreases NF-κB target gene expression	[23]
Monomethylation	K314	SET9	Decreases NF-κB activity and target gene expression	[19]
Monomethylation	K315	SET9	Decreases NF-κB activity and target gene expression	[19]
Symmetric dimethylation	R30	PRMT5	Enhances NF-κB DNA binding and transcriptional activities, and increases NF-κB target gene expression	[22, 35]
Asymmetric dimethylation	R30	PRMT1	Reduces NF-κB DNA binding ability and decreases NF-κB target genes expression	[22, 35]

Table 1. Types of NF-κB methylation and its biological roles.

of R30 may mediate *van der Waals* contacts and stabilize domain interactions. The key residues involved are aspartic acid (D) 277, glutamic acid (E) 279, and threonine (T) 191. Since phenylalanine (F) 184 positions closely to R30 and T191, R30 is sandwiched between F184/T191 on one side and D277/E279 on the other. This evidence affirms the importance of R30 methylation in increasing the ability of p65 to bind to DNA, resulting in the changes in its target gene expression [22].

Further demonstrating the complexity of R30 methylation, Reintjes *et al.* reported that PRMT1, another member of the PRMT superfamily, may asymmetrically methylate p65 at the same R30 that is symmetrically methylated by PRMT5 [35]. The information of R30 methylation by both PRMT5 and 1 is also included in **Table 1**. Different from PRMT5, PRMT1 is an enzyme containing 361 amino acids which catalyzes the formation of monomethyl-arginine and asymmetric dimethyl-arginine [36]. Reintjes and colleagues proposed an interesting model suggesting that symmetric dimethylation of R30 by PRMT5 seems to be induced at early time points, however, asymmetric dimethylation of R30 by PRMT1 is enriched at later time points. This idea presents an overall picture of the "meticulously calculated" regulation of NF-κB signaling, through symmetric and/or asymmetric R30 dimethylation that occurs at different stages of NF-κB responses. This model represents a specific on/off switch mechanism for adjusting cytokine-induced NF-κB responses [35].

4.3. Differential gene regulation by lysine and arginine methylation

As we mentioned earlier, a total of six lysine methylation sites can be methylated by different histone lysine methyltransferases in response to activating signals. Among them, K37, K218, and K221 are located in the RHD domain, while K310, K314, and K315 are in the linker region between RHD and the transactivation domain (TA) [36] (**Figure 1**). Using site mutagenesis, we generated the K218/221Q double mutant (DKQ) or the K37Q single mutant of p65. We found that in response to cytokines, such as IL-1β treatment, ~350 genes were rapidly induced within 5 min after treatment, while an additional ~300 genes were significantly upregulated 30 min later. Additionally, 1500 genes were further induced between the time points of 1 and 24 h. We revealed that *early growth response protein 1* (*EGR1*) was upregulated within 30 min and then began to decrease after 2 h. While *C-X-C motif chemokine 10* (*CXCL10*, also known as *IP10*), and *Interleukin 8* (*IL-8*) were upregulated after 1 h or longer treatment. However, their expression is much more stable than the *EGR* gene [21]. To further explore the different effects of DKQ and K37Q on gene expression, we conducted an Illumina array analysis, observing that DKQ is responsible for ~50%, while K37Q is only responsible for ~25% of NF-κB target gene regulation. Among these genes, some were exclusively regulated by either DKQ or K37Q, while others were commonly regulated by both DKQ and K37Q. This is a very interesting phenomenon. Our work showed that a very tiny difference in NF-κB methylation, such as methylation on different lysine residues, could lead to dramatically different gene induction patterns. By using ChIP-seq and bioinformatics approaches, we further uncovered that NF-κB target genes can be classified into multiple subgroups based on the effects of DKQ or K37Q (up- or down-regulation, or lysine site sensitivity) [21]. This data offers a valuable picture of the dynamic complexity of gene regulation by methylation of NF-κB on different lysine residues.

To further determine the difference between K and R methylation of p65 on NF-κB regulation, we conducted similar experiments as described above [21]. R30A and DKA (K218/221 K-A) mutants were generated in HEK293 cells. Illumina microarray experiments were carried out to analyze the gene populations affected by these mutations. We found that ~75% of NF-κB target genes were down-regulated by twofold or more by the R30A mutation, while significantly fewer (~48%) genes were downregulated by the DKA mutation. This data suggests that R30 methylation is in charge of most NF-κB target gene expression, while K218/221 methylation controls a much smaller population of the genes. Not surprisingly, Ingenuity Pathway Analysis **(Figure 3)** revealed that R30A and DKA control different functional networks. For instance, the top network for R30A is regarding the functions of *Cellular Movement, Hematological System Development and Function, Immune Cell Trafficking*, while the top network for DKA is related to *Cell-mediated Immune Response, Cellular Development, Cellular Function and Maintenance*, affirming the quite distinct cellular functions of R30 and K218/221 methylation. **Figure 4** illustrates a representative network from either R30A or DKA regulated genes. Importantly, the NF-κB complex is identified as a critical node in both networks. Two typical NF-κB target genes, IL8 (CXCL8) and IP10 (CXCL10), are also shown as important components in both networks.

Collectively, the evidence described above proves that methylation on different lysine residues or on different types of amino acids (lysine *vs.* arginine) on the p65 subunit of NF-κB,

Rank	Top Networks (Ingenuity Pathway Analysis): Associated Network Functions	
	R30A	DKA
1.	Cellular Movement, Hematological System Development and Function, Immune Cell Trafficking	Cell-mediated Immune Response, Cellular Development, Cellular Function and Maintenance
2.	Cell-To-Cell Signaling and Interaction, Hematological System Development and Function, Inflammatory Response	Cell Cycle, Cell-To-Cell Signaling and Interaction, Hematological System Development and Function
3.	Cardiovascular Disease, Organismal Injury and Abnormalities, Glomerular Injury	Cellular Development, Connective Tissue Development and Function, Tissue Development
4.	Respiratory System Development and Function, Cell Morphology, Embryonic Development	Cancer, Cell Death and Survival, Organismal Injury and Abnormalities
5.	Cellular Function and Maintenance, Humoral Immune Response, Protein Synthesis	Nucleic Acid Metabolism, Small Molecule Biochemistry, Gene Expression

Figure 3. Top networks that are affected by either R30A or DKA mutations. Ingenuity pathway analysis (IPA), showing top five different functional networks that are associated with R30A or DKA mutation.

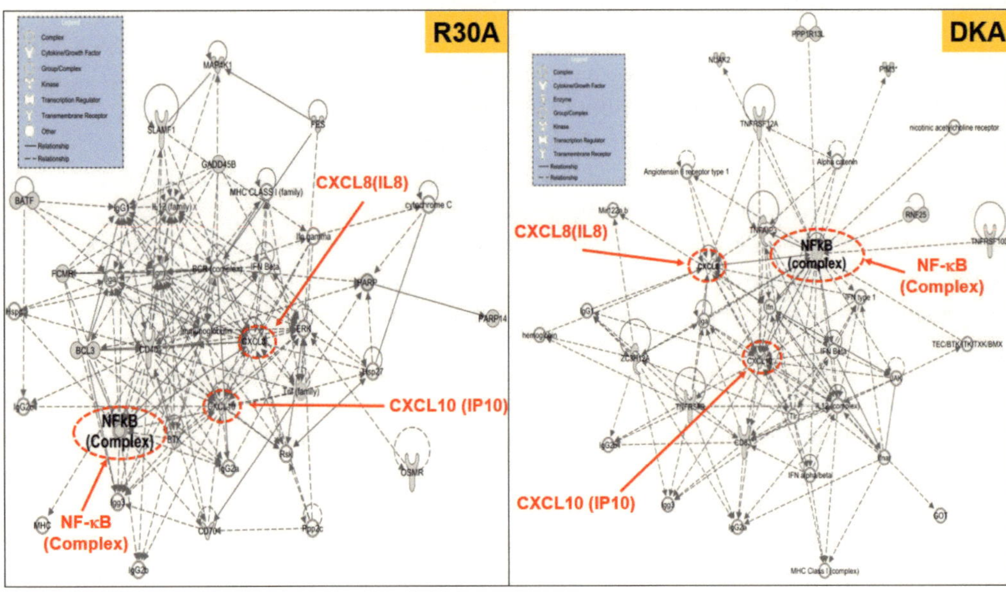

Figure 4. Example networks of R30A and DKA mutations, with NF-κB as a master node. **Left panel,** R30A mutation affects NF-κB orchestrated network. **Right panel,** DKA mutation interferes with NF-κB signaling. However, these two networks show quite distinct topographies and interactions with other signaling components. Note: Both *IL8* and *IP10* are within the networks.

dictates differential gene regulation, leading to complex and distinct outcomes. The work on methylation of NF-κB has offered a unique angle for understanding the mechanisms underlying the extreme plasticity of the biological responses led by the finely tuned regulation of NF-κB. The knowledge gained by this study will enable us to better understand why NF-κB is dysregulated in a variety of disease states, thus providing critical guidance to the design of disease-specific therapeutics.

5. Histone methylases as potential therapeutic targets in cancer

Due to the important role of NF-κB methylation in differential gene regulation, it is logical to recognize the essential roles of the enzymes that catalyze these methylation modifications. These enzymes are frequently histone methylases, and there are quite a few examples. Since the role of histone methylases in cancer has been well reviewed by Albert and Helin [37], below, we will only focus on PRMT5.

PRMT5 has been increasingly recognized as an important tumor promoter. We and others have observed elevated PRMT5 expression in cancers of the colon, pancreas, ovary, kidney, lung, bladder, liver, breast, prostate, cervix, and skin. This suggests that high levels of this enzyme may promote tumorigenesis, at least in part by facilitating NF-κB-induced gene expression [22, 38]. For instance, by conducting colorectal cancer (CRC) tissue microarray (TMA), we found that PRMT5 is overexpressed in polyps, advanced stages of colorectal cancer, and in the metastatic stage [39]. Similarly, PRMT5 is also overexpressed in various stages of pancreatic cancer, especially in the metastatic stage [39]. We proved that overexpression of PRMT5 promotes CRC HT29 cell and pancreatic cancer PANC1 cell proliferation, anchorage-independent growth, and cell migration ability. Knockdown of PRMT5 by shRNA showed the opposite effect, confirming PRMT5 functions as a tumor promoter in these cancers [39].

Additionally, overexpression of PRMT5 has been shown to be associated with poor epithelial ovarian cancer prognosis [40]. In a clinical study with 150 ovarian cancer patient samples, the overexpression of PRMT5 is found to be highly correlated with the Federation of Gynecology and Obstetrics (FIGO) advanced stage, which includes poor cell differentiation, high proliferation activity, and lymph node involvement. The overall survival rate of patients with low PRMT5 expression is 90%. In contrast, only 30% of patients with high PRMT5 expression survived. The progression-free survival rate is 50% for patients with low PRMT5 expression, but in those with high PRMT5 expression the rate is only 10% [40].

Moreover, Kumar and colleagues showed that the expression level of PRMT5 is inversely correlated with oropharyngeal squamous cell carcinoma (OPSCC) patient outcome. For instance, high PRMT5 expression correlated with low overall survival and had over 1.7 times higher death risk than the patient who has low PRMT5 expression [41]. Together, these studies have identified PRMT5 as a promising therapeutic target in cancers.

To date, multiple efforts have been made to develop the small molecule inhibitors of PRMT5. For instance, EPZ015666 was reported [39, 42] to inhibit PRMT5 methyltransferase activity in panels of mantle cell lymphoma (MCL) cell lines (Maver-1, Mino, Granta-519, Jeko-1and Z-138). It also significantly inhibits tumor growth in Z-138 and Maver-1 MCL xenograft mouse model as compare with vehicle control.

Recently, by adapting the AlphaLISA technique into a sensitive high throughput screening platform, our lab identified PR5-LL-CM01 as a potent PRMT5 small molecule inhibitor. PR5-LL-CM01 showed greater potency than EPZ015666 in both PDAC and CRC model [39].

These examples highlight the great potential of using histone methylases, such as PRMT5, as novel therapeutic targets in cancer.

Likewise, other histone methylases (**Table 1**) that methylate NF-κB may also play critical roles in the development and progression of cancer and other hyper NF-κB driven diseases. Therefore, they constitute a group of highly promising future therapeutic targets for these pathological conditions.

6. Conclusion, perspective, and future directions

The implications of methylation of NF-κB are multi-fold and far reaching. Methylation provides a snapshot of the complexity underlying the regulation of this important transcription factor. Even with the studies done to date, researchers have just begun to understand the crosstalk between these different PTMs and their implications in normal cellular function and disease. Two interesting questions remain. First, how does methylation of these residues on the same subunit affect NF-κB function? Second, can we reconcile the effects of other kinds of PTMs coupled with methylation both in normal and diseases states? A deeper understanding of these aspects will shed important light on the overall strategies for the development of new therapeutic approaches to treat the affected diseases.

Cancer is one of the leading causes of morbidity and mortality worldwide. Methylation of NF-κB as described in this review highlights its significance in cancers and other inflammatory diseases. Over the past decade, several transformative discoveries in epigenetics have led to the development of novel therapies that target epigenetic enzymes. However, the inquiries into acetylation and methylation modifications of lysines and arginines have been mainly focused on histone proteins. Important research identifying methylation residues on important non-histone proteins like NF-κB may be crucial to developing therapeutic interventions that target these modifications. For instance, the PRMT5 inhibitor identified in our laboratory has paved the way for future drug development to treat cancers and other disease with hyper PRMT5-driven NF-κB activity [22, 39]. In addition to PRMT5, other histone methylases, such as NSD1, have been reported by us and others as a significant player in cancer development [20, 43–45]. Although researchers have been trying to develop a small NSD1 inhibitor for cancer treatment, no NSD1 specific inhibitor has yet been reported due to the large size of NSD1 enzyme and the lack of sufficiently sensitive assay development. Future effort on this front and other histone methylases are equally as important in developing new medicines that target PRMT5.

Additionally, as mentioned in the Introduction, the prototypical NF-κB is comprised of a heterodimer of p65 and p50 subunits. Though multiple sites of methylation have been discovered on the p65 subunit of NF-κB, the potential methylation of the p50 subunit is quite understudied. With recent advances in proteomics and prediction software, novel methylation site(s) on p50 could arise in the near future. The study on p50 methylation could provide more a complete picture in terms of NF-κB regulation, and may possibly lead to novel discoveries regarding the methylation-mediated regulation of this subunit as well.

Since NF-κB is an important transcription factor that also plays a fundamental role in normal cells, one must consider important factors such as specificity of inhibiting modification only in cancer cells but not in normal cells. Multi-targeted approaches that simultaneously cripple several signaling pathways in cancer cells would be ideal, and a better understanding of the crosstalk between these pathways will advance the drug development process. In the future, a combination of advanced animal models, Cas9/CRISPR system, and more sophisticated bioinformatics approaches will serve as invaluable tools to study the implications of methylation on NF-κB and its interactions with other critical cellular factors that are important in the disease context. This will help to expedite the development of therapeutic tools to combat these deadly diseases.

Acknowledgements

We thank Ms. Lisa King from the Department of Pharmacology and Toxicology at Indiana University School of Medicine for her professional help with revising this book chapter. This work is supported by NIH-NIGMS Grant (# 1R01GM120156-01A1 to TL), NIH-NCI Grant (# 1 R03 CA223906-01 to TL), V foundation Kay Yow Cancer Fund (Grant 4486242 to TL), and 100 VOH Grant (# 2987613 to TL).

Abbreviation

BAF	B-cell activation factor
BMDM	bone marrow-derived macrophages
CD40L	CD40 ligand
ChIP-seq	chromatin immunoprecipitation (ChIP) with DNA sequencing
CRC	colorectal cancer
CXCL10	C-X-C motif chemokine 10 (also known as IP10)
EGR1	early growth response protein
FBXL11	F-box and leucine-rich repeat protein 11
FIGO	Federation of Gynecology and Obstetrics
GLP	G9A-like protein
IHC	immunohistochemistry
IKK	IκB kinase
IL-1β	interleukin 1 β
IL-8	Interleukin 8

MCL	mantle cell lymphoma
MEFs	mouse embryonic fibroblast cells
NF-κB	nuclear factor κB
NIK	NF-κB-inducing kinase
NSD1	nuclear receptor-binding SET domain-containing protein 1
OPSCC	oropharyngeal squamous cell carcinoma
PHF20	plant homeodomain finger protein 20
PKC-ζ	Protein kinase C zeta
PRMT1	protein arginine methyltransferase 1
PRMT5	protein arginine methyltransferase 5
PTM	post-translational modifications
RHD	Rel homology domain
Set9	Set domain-containing protein 9
TAD	transactivation domain
TMA	tissue microarray
TNFα	tumor necrosis factor α

Author details

Han Wei[1], Lakshmi Prabhu[1], Antja-Voy Hartley[1], Matthew Martin[1], Emily Sun[1], Guanglong Jiang[2], Yunlong Liu[2] and Tao Lu[1,2,3*]

*Address all correspondence to: lut@iupui.edu

1 Department of Pharmacology and Toxicology, Indiana University School of Medicine, Indianapolis, IN, USA

2 Department of Medical and Molecular Genetics, Indiana University School of Medicine, Indianapolis, IN, USA

3 Department of Biochemistry and Molecular Biology, Indiana University School of Medicine, Indianapolis, IN, USA

References

[1] Kumar A, Takada Y, Boriek AM, Aggarwal BB. Nuclear factor-kappaB: Its role in health and disease. Journal of Molecular Medicine (Berlin). 2004;**82**:434-448. DOI: 10.1007/s00109-004-0555-y

[2] Hayden MS, Ghosh S. Shared principles in NF-kappaB signaling. Cell. 2008;**132**:344-362. DOI: 10.1016/j.cell.2008.01.020

[3] Oeckinghaus A, Ghosh S. The NF-kappaB family of transcription factors and its regulation. Cold Spring Harbor Perspectives in Biology. 2009;**1**:a000034. DOI: 10.1101/cshperspect.a000034

[4] Karin M. How NF-kappaB is activated: The role of the IkappaB kinase (IKK) complex. Oncogene. 1999;**18**:6867-6874. DOI: 10.1038/sj.onc.1203219

[5] Clark K, Nanda S, Cohen P. Molecular control of the NEMO family of ubiquitin-binding proteins. Nature Reviews. Molecular Cell Biology. 2013;**14**:673-685. DOI: 10.1038/nrm3644

[6] Dolcet X, Llobet D, Pallares J, Matias-Guiu X. NF-kB in development and progression of human cancer. Virchows Archiv. 2005;**446**:475-482. DOI: 10.1007/s00428-005-1264-9

[7] Sun SC. Non-canonical NF-kappaB signaling pathway. Cell Research. 2011;**21**:71-85. DOI: 10.1038/cr.2010.177

[8] Israel A. The IKK complex, a central regulator of NF-kappaB activation. Cold Spring Harbor Perspectives in Biology. 2010;**2**:a000158. DOI: 10.1101/cshperspect.a000158

[9] Schmid JA, Birbach A. IkappaB kinase beta (IKKbeta/IKK2/IKBKB)--a key molecule in signaling to the transcription factor NF-kappaB. Cytokine & Growth Factor Reviews. 2008;**19**:157-165. DOI: 10.1016/j.cytogfr.2008.01.006

[10] Huang B, Yang XD, Lamb A, Chen LF. Posttranslational modifications of NF-kappaB: Another layer of regulation for NF-kappaB signaling pathway. Cellular Signalling. 2010;**22**:1282-1290. DOI: 10.1016/j.cellsig.2010.03.017

[11] Perkins ND, Gilmore TD. Good cop, bad cop: The different faces of NF-kappaB. Cell Death and Differentiation. 2006;**13**:759-772. DOI: 10.1038/sj.cdd.4401838

[12] Neumann M, Naumann M. Beyond IkappaBs: Alternative regulation of NF-kappaB activity. The FASEB Journal. 2007;**21**:2642-2654. DOI: 10.1096/fj.06-7615rev

[13] Jamaluddin M, Wang S, Boldogh I, et al. TNF-alpha-induced NF-kappaB/RelA Ser(276) phosphorylation and enhanceosome formation is mediated by an ROS-dependent PKAc pathway. Cellular Signalling. 2007;**19**:1419-1433. DOI: 10.1016/j.cellsig.2007.01.020

[14] Vermeulen L, De Wilde G, Van Damme P, et al. Transcriptional activation of the NF-kappaB p65 subunit by mitogen- and stress-activated protein kinase-1 (MSK1). The EMBO Journal. 2003;**22**:1313-1324. DOI: 10.1093/emboj/cdg139

[15] Kiernan R, Bres V, Ng RW, et al. Post-activation turn-off of NF-kappa B-dependent transcription is regulated by acetylation of p65. The Journal of Biological Chemistry. 2003;**278**:2758-2766. DOI: 10.1074/jbc.M209572200

[16] Chen LF, Williams SA, Mu Y, et al. NF-kappaB RelA phosphorylation regulates RelA acetylation. Molecular and Cellular Biology. 2005;**25**:7966-7975. DOI: 10.1128/MCB.25.18.7966-7975.2005

[17] Ishinaga H, Jono H, Lim JH, et al. TGF-beta induces p65 acetylation to enhance bacteria-induced NF-kappaB activation. The EMBO Journal. 2007;**26**:1150-1162. DOI: 10.1038/sj.emboj.7601546

[18] Ea CK, Baltimore D. Regulation of NF-kappaB activity through lysine monomethylation of p65. Proceedings of the National Academy of Sciences of the United States of America. 2009;**106**:18972-18977. DOI: 10.1073/pnas.0910439106

[19] Yang XD, Huang B, Li M, et al. Negative regulation of NF-kappaB action by Set9-mediated lysine methylation of the RelA subunit. The EMBO Journal. 2009;**28**:1055-1066. DOI: 10.1038/emboj.2009.55

[20] Lu T, Jackson MW, Wang B, et al. Regulation of NF-kappaB by NSD1/FBXL11-dependent reversible lysine methylation of p65. Proceedings of the National Academy of Sciences of the United States of America. 2010;**107**:46-51. DOI: 10.1073/pnas.0912493107

[21] Lu T, Yang M, Huang DB, et al. Role of lysine methylation of NF-kappaB in differential gene regulation. Proceedings of the National Academy of Sciences of the United States of America. 2013;**110**:13510-13515. DOI: 10.1073/pnas.1311770110

[22] Wei H, Wang B, Miyagi M, et al. PRMT5 dimethylates R30 of the p65 subunit to activate NF-kappaB. Proceedings of the National Academy of Sciences of the United States of America. 2013;**110**:13516-13521. DOI: 10.1073/pnas.1311784110

[23] Levy D, Kuo AJ, Chang Y, et al. Lysine methylation of the NF-kappaB subunit RelA by SETD6 couples activity of the histone methyltransferase GLP at chromatin to tonic repression of NF-kappaB signaling. Nature Immunology. 2011;**12**:29-36. DOI: 10.1038/ni.1968

[24] Ryo A, Suizu F, Yoshida Y, et al. Regulation of NF-kappaB signaling by Pin1-dependent prolyl isomerization and ubiquitin-mediated proteolysis of p65/RelA. Molecular Cell. 2003;**12**:1413-1426. DOI: 10.1016/S1097-2765(03)00490-8

[25] Kelleher ZT, Matsumoto A, Stamler JS, Marshall HE. NOS2 regulation of NF-kappaB by S-nitrosylation of p65. The Journal of Biological Chemistry. 2007;**282**:30667-30672. DOI: 10.1074/jbc.M705929200

[26] Liu Y, Bridges R, Wortham A, Kulesz-Martin M. NF-kappaB repression by PIAS3 mediated RelA SUMOylation. PLoS One. 2012;**7**:e37636. DOI: 10.1371/journal.pone.0037636

[27] Yang XD, Tajkhorshid E, Chen LF. Functional interplay between acetylation and methylation of the RelA subunit of NF-kappaB. Molecular and Cellular Biology. 2010;**30**:2170-2180. DOI: 10.1128/MCB.01343-09

[28] Nowak DE, Tian B, Jamaluddin M, et al. RelA Ser276 phosphorylation is required for activation of a subset of NF-kappaB-dependent genes by recruiting cyclin-dependent kinase 9/cyclin T1 complexes. Molecular and Cellular Biology. 2008;**28**:3623-3638. DOI: 10.1128/MCB.01152-07

[29] Reber L, Vermeulen L, Haegeman G, Frossard N. Ser276 phosphorylation of NF-kB p65 by MSK1 controls SCF expression in inflammation. PLoS One. 2009;**4**:e4393. DOI: 10.1371/journal.pone.0004393

[30] Zhong H, Voll RE, Ghosh S. Phosphorylation of NF-kappa B p65 by PKA stimulates transcriptional activity by promoting a novel bivalent interaction with the coactivator CBP/p300. Molecular Cell. 1998;**1**:661-671. DOI: 10.1016/S1097-2765(00)80066-0

[31] Pathak SK, Basu S, Bhattacharyya A, et al. TLR4-dependent NF-kappaB activation and mitogen- and stress-activated protein kinase 1-triggered phosphorylation events are central to helicobacter pylori peptidyl prolyl cis-, trans-isomerase (HP0175)-mediated induction of IL-6 release from macrophages. Journal of Immunology. 2006;**177**:7950-7958. DOI: 10.4049/jimmunol.177.11.7950

[32] Chen LF, Greene WC. Shaping the nuclear action of NF-kappaB. Nature Reviews. Molecular Cell Biology. 2004;**5**:392-401. DOI: 10.1038/nrm1368

[33] Nadiminty N, Lou W, Lee SO, et al. Stat3 activation of NF-{kappa}B p100 processing involves CBP/p300-mediated acetylation. Proceedings of the National Academy of Sciences of the United States of America. 2006;**103**:7264-7269. DOI: 10.1073/pnas.0509808103

[34] Zhang T, Park KA, Li Y, et al. PHF20 regulates NF-kappaB signalling by disrupting recruitment of PP2A to p65. Nature Communications. 2013;**4**:2062. DOI: 10.1038/ncomms3062

[35] Reintjes A, Fuchs JE, Kremser L, et al. Asymmetric arginine dimethylation of RelA provides a repressive mark to modulate TNFalpha/NF-kappaB response. Proceedings of the National Academy of Sciences of the United States of America. 2016;**113**:4326-4331. DOI: 10.1073/pnas.1522372113

[36] Wei H, Mundade R, Lange KC, Lu T. Protein arginine methylation of non-histone proteins and its role in diseases. Cell Cycle. 2014;**13**:32-41. DOI: 10.4161/cc.27353

[37] Albert M, Helin K. Histone methyltransferases in cancer. Seminars in Cell & Developmental Biology. 2010;**21**(2):209-2020. DOI: 10.1016/j.semcdb.2009.10.007

[38] Lu T, Stark GR. NF-kappaB: Regulation by methylation. Cancer Research. 2015;**75**:3692-3695. DOI: 10.1158/0008-5472.CAN-15-1022

[39] Prabhu L, Wei H, Chen L, et al. Adapting AlphaLISA high throughput screen to discover a novel small-molecule inhibitor targeting protein arginine methyltransferase 5 in pancreatic and colorectal cancers. Oncotarget. 2017;**8**:39963-39977. DOI: 10.18632/oncotarget.18102

[40] Bao X, Zhao S, Liu T, et al. Overexpression of PRMT5 promotes tumor cell growth and is associated with poor disease prognosis in epithelial ovarian cancer. The Journal of Histochemistry and Cytochemistry. 2013;**61**:206-217. DOI: 10.1369/0022155413475452

[41] Kumar B, Yadav A, Brown NV, et al. Nuclear PRMT5, cyclin D1 and IL-6 are associated with poor outcome in oropharyngeal squamous cell carcinoma patients and is inversely associated with p16-status. Oncotarget. 2017;**8**:14847-14859. DOI: 10.18632/oncotarget.14682

[42] Chan-Penebre E, Kuplast KG, Majer CR, et al. A selective inhibitor of PRMT5 with in vivo and in vitro potency in MCL models. Nature Chemical Biology. 2015;**11**:432-437. DOI: 10.1038/nchembio.1810

[43] Shiba N, Ichikawa H, Taki T, et al. NUP98-NSD1 gene fusion and its related gene expression signature are strongly associated with a poor prognosis in pediatric acute myeloid leukemia. Genes, Chromosomes & Cancer. 2013;**52**:683-693. DOI: 10.1002/gcc.22064

[44] Ostronoff F, Othus M, Gerbing RB, et al. NUP98/NSD1 and FLT3/ITD coexpression is more prevalent in younger AML patients and leads to induction failure: A COG and SWOG report. Blood. 2014;**124**:2400-2407. DOI: 10.1182/blood-2014-04-570929

[45] Vougiouklakis T, Hamamoto R, Nakamura Y, Saloura V. The NSD family of protein methyltransferases in human cancer. Epigenomics. 2015;**7**:863-874. DOI: 10.2217/epi.15.32

Chapter 15

SOX Genes and Cancer

Li Cui, Xinyuan Zhao and Shen Hu

Additional information is available at the end of the chapter

http://dx.doi.org/10.5772/intechopen.72433

Abstract

Transcription factors play a critical role in regulating the gene expression programs that establish and maintain specific cell states in humans. Deregulation of these gene expression programs can lead to a broad range of diseases including cancer. SOX transcription factors are a conserved group of transcriptional regulators that mediates DNA binding by a highly conserved high-mobility group (HMG) domain. Numerous evidence has recently demonstrated that SOX transcription factors critically control cell fate and differentiation in major developmental processes, and that their upregulation may be important for cancer progression. In this review, we discuss recent advances in our understanding of the role of SOX genes in cancer.

Keywords: transcription factors, cancer, SOX2, SOX4, SOX9, SOX11

1. Introduction

Cancer is caused by alterations in the control and activity of genes that in turn regulate cell growth and differentiation, leading to abnormal cell proliferation [1]. It is a multi-step process leading to profound metabolic and behavioral changes in a cell. The hallmarks of cancer include sustaining proliferative signaling, evading growth suppressors, resisting cell death, enabling replicative immortality, inducing angiogenesis, activating invasion and metastasis, genome instability, inflammation, reprogramming of energy metabolism and evading immune destruction [2]. Most human malignancies are caused by somatic alterations within the cancer genome either through gain-of-function mutations in proto-oncogenes or loss-of-function mutations in tumor suppressor genes. Remarkable progress in cancer research has been made in the last 10 years. However, the detailed molecular mechanisms of cancer remain largely un-elucidated.

A transcription factor (TF) might be defined as any molecule participating, alone or as part of a complex, in the binding to a gene's enhancer response element or promoter, with the ultimate outcome being the up- or down-regulation of expression of that gene [3]. TFs are key genes involved in the regulation of gene expression. The human genome encodes over 2000 different TF-coding genes, many of which are expressed in a cell type-specific manner to coordinate gene expression programs underlying a vast array of cellular processes [4]. TFs are commonly deregulated in the pathogenesis of human cancer. For instance, *TP53* and *MYC*, which encode the TFs p53 (tumor suppressor protein 53) and c-Myc respectively, are among the most frequently changed genes across all cancers [5, 6].

Sex determining region Y (SRY)-related high-mobility group (HMG) box (SOX) family comprises more than 20 members, which have been shown to involve in regulation of many biological processes such as embryonic development, cell-fate decision, lineage commitment, determination and differentiation [7–9]. This transcription factor family is divided into 10 subgroups based on the level of amino acid conservation within the HMG box and the presence of other motifs. In this review, we discuss the current understanding on the association between SOX genes and cancer. We particularly emphasize the role of several representative SOX subgroup proteins (SOX2, SOX4, SOX9 and SOX11) in cancer initiation and development.

2. The biological functions of SOX gene family

SOX genes are part of a larger family of HMG proteins. SOX proteins bind similar DNA motifs [(A/T)(A/T)CAA(A/T)G] through their HMG domain, which is highly conserved among SOX gene family. Due to the low affinity between SOX proteins and DNA, cofactors are usually required to stabilize their interactions with DNA [9]. Based on the degree of conservation of their HMG-box and the presence of defined HMG-independent structural domains, SOX proteins are organized into 10 subfamilies: SOXA-SOXJ. For example, the SOXA group consists only of SRY; SOXB group comprises of two subgroups (SOXB1 and SOXB2); SOXB1 includes SOX1, SOX2, and SOX3, whereas SOXB2 proteins include SOX14 and SOX21; SOXC group includes SOX4, SOX11, and SOX12; SOXD group includes SOX5, SOX6, and SOX13; SOXE group includes SOX8, SOX9, and SOX10; and SOXF group includes SOX7, SOX17, and SOX18; SOXG (SOX15) and SOXH (SOX30) proteins are structurally related to SOXB1 and SOXD proteins, respectively [10–13]. Individual members within the same SOX group share similar biochemical properties and thus have overlapping biological functions. However, SOX proteins from different groups have distinct biological functions [9]. SOX gene family has been demonstrated to play important roles in various biological processes including, but not limited to development, tissue homeostasis and regeneration, reprogramming [9, 14–16].

In vertebrates, SOX genes are well known regulators of numerous developmental processes. Accumulating evidences have shown that SOX proteins are co-expressed in various developing tissues in an overlapping manner and show functional redundancy. The transcriptional activities of SOX proteins are regulated via three major pathways: (1) the expression levels of SOX proteins are regulated in specific cell types and tissues with precise timing (2) SOX proteins are regulated by posttranslational modification (3) the partners of SOX proteins are regulated to not only influence the specific recognition of the binding sites of SOX-partner complexes on the target genes, but also determine transcription activities and significantly enhance the activation/repression potential. For instance, SOXB1 and SOXB2 proteins are important for the development of the central nervous system and foregut system [17–19]. SOXD proteins are important for the development of cartilage tissues. In mouse embryos, SOX5, SOX6, SOX9 and collagen II are co-expressed in all cartilaginous sites at around 12.5 dpc. After 17.5 dpc, the chondrocytes become hypertrophic in the growth plate cartilages, the expression of above SOX genes are inhibited and disappear in the hypertrophic chondrocytes [20]. The expression patterns of SOXE genes are important for the development of reproductive system. SOX8, SOX9 and SOX10 are expressed in the overlapping temporal and spatial expression patterns during gonads development, indicating the overlapping roles of these genes in mammalian sex determination and subsequent male sexual development [21, 22]. The members of SOXF group play important roles in the development of cardio-vascular system and extraembryonic endoderm. SOX7 and SOX17 are crucial endoderm lineage-determining regulators and are involved in the later stage of extraembryonic differentiation [23–25].

SOX2 is an important marker for stem and progenitor cell populations in many adult tissues. SOX2 positive cells have been detected in progenitors of various tissues such as adult retina, trachea, tongue epithelium, dermal papilla of the hair follicle, adult testes, forestomach, glandular stomach, anus, cervix, esophagus, lens and dental epithelium [26–30]. Conditional SOX2 deletion significantly influences cell proliferation. In trachea, SOX2 expression is required to sustain tissue homeostasis by controlling the number of proliferating epithelial cells as well as the proportion of basal, ciliated and Clara cells [28]. However, whether SOX2 expression is required for homeostasis in other adult tissues needs further investigation. In addition to maintaining tissue homeostasis, SOX2 plays an important role for tissue regeneration and repair. For instance, the basal stem cells could repair the damaged tracheal epithelium in mice within 7–10 days. The number of basal stem cells was significantly lower in the trachea with SOX2-deficience. Therefore, the injured trachea was unable to undergo efficient tissue repair. SOX2 is also important for peripheral nerve regeneration. When there is injury, mature adult Schwann cells dedifferentiate to a progenitor cell-like state by re-expressing Sox2 [31].

The expression of four transcription factors, Oct4/Sox2/cMyc/Klf4, was able to convert differentiated cells to pluripotent cells [32]. SOX2 is indispensable for the success of this reprogramming process. However, the biological function of SOX2 seems to be closely correlated with its levels. SOX2 overexpression can promote differentiation and reduce the reprogramming efficiency of neural progenitor cells. In addition to SOX2, SOX1 and SOX3, which are also members of SOXB1 family, can replace SOX2 during the reprogramming process. SOX15 or SOX18 was also able to generate the pluripotent cells but less efficient than SOXB1 family [33].

Many members of SOX gene family have been demonstrated to be closely correlated with tumorigenesis [34, 35]. Below, we discuss the involvement of several SOX genes that have been most extensively studied in human malignancies so far. **Table 1** listed these SOX genes and their clinical relevance in cancers.

SOX genes	Deregulation	Potential clinical significance	Reference
SOX2	Lung, esophagus and oral cancer↑	Promote tumor progression	[36]
	Melanoma↑	Enhance the self-renewal capacity of cancer stem cells	[37]
	Glioblastoma ↑	Associated with tumor aggressiveness and worse prognosis	[38, 39]
	Gastric cancer↓	Promote tumor progression	[40]
SOX4	Oral cancer ↑	Promote tumor initiation and development	[41, 42]
	Prostate cancer↑	Associated with worse prognosis	[43, 44]
	Leukemia↑	Promote tumor progression	[45]
	Primary gallbladder carcinoma↓	Associated with worse prognosis	[46]
SOX9	Papillary thyroid cancer↑	Promote tumor progression	[47]
	Breast cancer ↑	Associated with chemoresistance	[48]
	Gastric cancer ↑	Promote tumorigenesis	[49]
	Cervical carcinoma↓	Promote tumor progression	[50]
SOX11	Breast cancer↑	Promote tumor progression	[51]
	Mantle cell lymphoma↑	Promote tumor progression	[52–54]
	Epithelial ovarian cancer↓	Associated with worse prognosis	[55]
	Gastric cancer↓	Associated with worse prognosis	

Table 1. Deregulation of typical SOX genes and their clinical relevance in cancers.

3. SOX2 and cancer

The SOX2 gene is located on chromosome 3q26.3–q27, it belongs to the SOXB1 group and encodes for 317 amino acids [56, 57]. SOX2 is one of the key transcription factors for induced pluripotent stem cells establishment, stem cell maintenance, and lineage fate determinant. Deregulation of SOX2 has been associated with various diseases such as anophthalmia-esophageal-genital (AEG) syndrome and bilateral anaphthalmia/microphthalmia, anterior pituitary hypoplasia, hypogonadotropic hypogonadism hypothalamic hamartoma, sensorineural hearing loss, and esophageal atresia [58, 59]. In addition to the above diseases, increasing evidence has revealed there is a strong relationship between SOX2 and cancer. Cancer stem cells are key drivers of tumorigenesis and may be responsible for tumor initiation, growth and spawning metastases. SOX2-postive cancer stem cells were able to drive tumor initiation and therapy resistance in various types of cancers, indicating that it is a common phenomenon that SOX2 might mastermind the tumor initiating potential of cancer cells [60].

SOX2 silencing significantly suppresses the tumorigenicity of glioblastoma tumor-initiating cells (TICs) [38]. Importantly, high levels of SOX2 have been associated with tumor aggressiveness and worse prognosis in glioblastoma, indicating targeting SOX2 might be an effective strategy for the treatment of glioblastoma [39]. SOX2 is also amplified in squamous cell carcinomas of the lung, the esophagus, and the oral cavity. SOX2 amplification and SOX2 protein overexpression might be responsible for the tumor initiation and progression in squamous cell carcinomas derived from different organ sites [36]. SOX2 was found to be critical for maintaining the sphere-forming capacity of DU145 prostate cancer stem cells (PCSCs). It promoted the self-renewal of the PCSC population by regulating downstream of EGFR signaling [61]. Similarly, SOX2 was highly expressed in melanoma stem cells. SOX2 suppression remarkably inhibited self-renewal in melanoma spheres and in putative melanoma stem cells with high aldehyde dehydrogenase activity. On the contrary, SOX2 overexpression in melanoma cells enhanced their self-renewal *in vitro*. Animal models showed that SOX2 was critical for tumor initiation and continuous tumor growth. These data suggested that SOX2 was an important factor for self-renewal and tumorigenicity of melanoma-initiating cells [37].

There are conflicting results regarding the role of SOX2 in gastric cancer. For instance, SOX2 was dispensable for self-renewal of gastric stem cells. In addition, loss of SOX2 promoted tumor formation in Apc-deficient gastric cells *in vivo* and *in vitro* by inducing Tcf/Lef-dependent transcription and upregulating intestinal metaplasia-associated genes, suggesting SOX2 acted as a tumor suppressor in gastric cancer [62]. In addition, the expression level of *SOX2* expression was frequently downregulated in gastric cancers. Ectopic expression of SOX2 inhibited cell growth through cell-cycle arrest and apoptosis in gastric cells. Moreover, the gastric cancers with SOX2 methylation had a significantly worse survival than those without this methylation [40]. However, SOX2 was found to enhance the tumorigenicity and chemoresistance of cancer stem-like cells derived from gastric cancer, suggesting SOX2 plays an oncogenic role in gastric cancer [63]. SOX2 inhibition reduced cell proliferation and migration, promoted apoptosis and induced changes in cell cycle *in vitro* as well as suppressed the tumorigenic potential of gastric cancer cells *in vivo* [64]. The contradictory findings regarding the role of SOX2 in gastric cancer further support the fact that the outcome of SOX2 activation is closely correlated with tumor origin and cellular context. Future experiments with lineage tracing and gain- and loss-of-function mouse models are required to clarify the role of SOX2 in gastric cancer. SOX2 is frequently regarded as an oncogene in lung SCCs, but previous studies indicated that higher SOX2 levels predicted favorable outcome in lung SCCs [65, 66]. The underlying reasons accounting for the contradictory role of SOX2 in lung SCCs warrant further exploration.

4. SOX4 and cancer

SOX4, one of group-C SOX genes, plays an important role in the regulation of transcription during developmental processes such as embryonic cardiac development, nervous system development, osteoblastic differentiation, and thymocyte development [67]. SOX4 gene is located on 6p22.3 and encodes a protein of 474 amino acids with three distinguishable domains: an HMG box, a glycine-rich region, and a serine-rich region. SOX4 is considered as one of the members of epithelial-mesenchymal transition (EMT)-transcriptional inducers. EMT is a key developmental program that is often activated during organismal development and the progression of epithelial tumors to metastatic cancers and may promote therapeutic resistance, indicating that SOX4 might be a potential therapeutic target for cancer treatment.

Recently, multiple studies have reported altered expression of SOX4 in human cancers. Our group demonstrated that SOX4 was significantly upregulated when oral lichen planus (OLP) progressed to oral squamous cell carcinoma (OSCC). In addition, downregulation of SOX4 suppressed the proliferation, migration and invasion of oral cancer cells. These findings suggest that SOX4 might play a critical role in the progression of OLP to OSCC [41]. Similarly, the expression level of SOX4 was remarkably overexpressed in OSCC tissues compared to adjacent normal mucosa. Also SOX4 was important for maintaining the oncogenic phenotypes of oral cancer cells by promoting cell survival and increasing chemoradioresistance [68]. High SOX4 expression levels were positively correlated with adverse clinicopathological parameters of OSCC, indicating that SOX4 might be significantly associated with poor prognosis of OSCC [42]. In addition to OSCC, SOX4 plays an oncogenic role in other malignancies. SOX4 was overexpressed in prostate cancer (PCa) and higher SOX4 levels predicted unfavorable prognosis [43]. Upregulation of SOX4 in PCa was mechanistically induced by PTEN loss due to the activation of PI3K-AKT–mTOR signaling [44]. SOX4 was able to directly regulate the expression of the epigenetic modifier Ezh2 in breast cancer, indicating SOX4 might be indispensable for tumor progression [69]. SOX4 might combine with oncogenic Ras together to promote tumorigenesis *in vivo* [70]. SOX4 was a direct target of C/EBPα and SOX4 suppression reduced the self-renewal of leukemic cells and restored their differentiation, indicating that SOX4 overexpression resulting from inactivation of C/EBPα promoted leukemia development [45].

However, it should be noted that SOX4 might also function as a tumor suppressor in tumorigenesis. For instance, SOX4 was indispensable for p53 activation in response to DNA damage. In addition, SOX4 could stabilize p53 protein by inhibiting Mdm2-mediated p53 ubiquitination and degradation, suggesting that SOX4 might suppress the progression DNA damage response-associated cancer [71]. In primary gallbladder carcinoma (PGC), SOX4 upregulation was significantly associated with favorable clinical parameters. In addition, SOX4 overexpression predicted better survival [46]. The expression level of SOX4 was significantly reduced in metastatic melanoma compared with that in dysplastic nevi and primary melanoma. In addition, SOX4 suppression promoted the migration and invasion of melanoma cells in an NF-κB p50-dependent manner [72]. Taken together, these findings indicate that the concrete role of SOX4 is closely associated with tumor microenvironment and might be tissue specific.

5. SOX9 and cancer

The SOXE group comprises three members named SOX8, SOX9 and SOX10. SoxE proteins are important for the development of nervous system and neural crest progenitors. SOX9 was first described as a candidate gene for campomelic dysplasia (CD), a genetic condition that affects the development of the skeleton and reproductive system [73]. SOX9 has been demonstrated to greatly contribute to the organogenesis and development of many tissue types, such as the stomach, pancreas, tooth and craniofacial tissues. In addition, SOX9 is also a master regulator of cartilage development. It is indispensable for roles in the chondrogenic lineage progression of mesenchymal stem cells [74].

Recent studies have reported that SOX9 is aberrantly expressed in several types of cancers. Higher expression levels of SOX9 are correlated with a poor prognosis in patients with Chordoma. In

http://dx.doi.org/10.5772/intechopen.72433

addition, SOX9 downregulation suppressed the oncogenic behaviors of Chordoma cell *in vitro*, suggesting that SOX9 might function as an oncogene in Chordoma [75]. The expression of SOX9 was upregulated in papillary thyroid cancer (PTC) tissues and cell lines. Downregulation of SOX9 inhibited the proliferation, colony formation, migration, invasion, as well as EMT phenotype of PTC cells. ERα–RUNX2 complex activated the SOX9 expression and promoted endocrine resistance and metastases [76]. In breast cancer, up-regulation of SOX9 expression was closely correlated with tamoxifen (TAM) resistance [77]. The SOX9 levels were significantly higher in osteosarcoma tissues compared with the adjacent normal tissues. However, CLDN8 expression was significantly lower in osteosarcoma tissues. Knockdown of SOX9 inhibited the proliferation and migration but promoted the apoptosis of human osteosarcoma cell lines by downregulating CLDN8 [47]. FOXK2 was overexpressed in colorectal cancer tissues and associated with poor prognosis. In fact, FOXK2 was shown to be transcriptionally activated by SOX9, suggesting that SOX9-FOXK2 axis plays a critical role in the development of colorectal cancer [48]. SOX9 upregulation was associated with *Helicobacter pylori* infection, elevated carcinoembryonic antigen–related cell adhesion molecule 1 (CEACAM1) and gastrokine 1 (GKN1) inactivation. SOX9 knockdown suppressed the tumorigenic capacity of gastric cancer cells by inhibiting the downstream β-catenin signaling pathway [49]. Interestingly, SOX2 was expressed in highly proliferative but minimally invasive lung cancer cells; in contrast, cells with highly invasiveness capacity exhibited increased SOX9 expression but reduced SOX2 expression. The switch between SOX2 and SOX9 expression is epigenetically controlled and is important for determining cancer cell plasticity and metastatic progression [78]. Ectopic expression of SOX9 enhanced growth, invasion, and angiogenesis, whereas silencing of endogenous SOX9 markedly impaired tumor growth in prostate cancer. High SOX9 levels drove tumorigenesis by reactivating the Wnt/β – catenin signaling in a subset of prostate cancer, indicating WNT inhibition might beneficial for the effective treatment of prostate cancer [79]. SOX9 was critical for maintaining proliferation, self-renewal, and tumorigenicity in liver cancer stem cells (CSCs), and SOX9 overexpression was positively correlated with worse survival in HCC patients [80]. Although most studies showed that SOX9 played an oncogenic role in cancer development. Excopic expression of SOX9 was found to suppress cell growth, clonal capacity and colonosphere formation by inhibiting Wnt/ß-catenin signaling pathway and c-myc expression in colorectal cancer, suggesting that SOX9 might be a tumor suppressor in colorectal cancer [81]. SOX9 expression was progressively decreased in cervical carcinoma *in situ* and especially in invasive cervical carcinoma, compared with normal cervix tissue. Lastly, SOX9 overexpression in cervical carcinoma cells inhibited cell growth *in vitro* and tumor formation *in vivo*, and *vice versa* [50].

6. SOX11 and cancer

Similar to SOX4, SOX11 is also a transcriptional activator that falls in the subgroup C. The Sox11 gene is mapped at chromosome 2p25.3 and the human SOX11 protein has 441 amino acids and 46.7 kDa molecular weight. It contains two functional domains: a HMG box DNA-binding domain and a transactivation domain [82]. SOX11 plays an important role in embryogenesis and tissue remodeling. Sox11 expression in most tissues is transient and thus little SOX11 expression has been found in terminally differentiated adult tissues. The role of SOX11 in the tumor microenvironment is cancer type-dependent.

Our recent studies have demonstrated that SOX11 plays a tumor promotion role in the development of head and neck cancer (HNC) [83]. We have employed a liquid chromatography–tandem mass spectrometry (LC–MS/MS) based approach to identify novel targets that may interact with SOX11 in HNC cells. The proteins that strongly bind to SOX11 in HNC cells may be important for maintaining the activity, stability and function of SOX11 or be regulated by SOX11. Gene ontology and Kyoto Encyclopedia of Genes and Genomes (KEGG) pathway analysis indicated that many potential SOX11-binding partners were associated with protein synthesis, cell metabolism and cell–cell adhesion. We speculated that upregulation of SOX11 might firstly activate the aggressive phenotypes of HNC cells by modulating the oncoprotein synthesis and altering cellular metabolism. Then it might further promote invasion and metastasis by affecting cell–cell adhesion system and formation and release of extracellular exosomes. One of the identified proteins, heat shock protein 90 alpha (HSP90α), was selected for further investigation. A biochemical interaction is validated between SOX11 and HSP90α through the co-immunoprecipitation with Western blot analysis. In addition, we have found that downregulation of HSP90α inhibits the malignant phenotypes of HNC cells and HSP90α upregulation is significantly associated with worse clinical outcome of HNC, suggesting HSP90α might serve as a potential prognostic biomarker and therapeutic target for HNC [84].

Aberrant expression of SOX11 has been reported in other types of cancer. SOX11 levels were negatively correlated with the tumorigenic capacity of glioma-initiating cells [85]. Similarly, epithelial ovarian cancer patients with lower SOX11 suffered poorer recurrence-free survival [55]. SOX11 mRNA was downregulated in both gastric cancer (GC) cell lines and primary GC tissues. SOX11 gene promoter hyper-methylation was significantly associated with worse clinical parameters and poorer prognosis, suggesting that SOX11 might function as a tumor suppressor in gastric cancer [86]. The methylation frequency of serum SOX11 promoter in hepatocellular carcinoma (HCC) patients was significantly higher than that in chronic hepatitis B (CHB) patients. In addition, significant difference of serum SOX11 promoter methylation in HCC patients with vascular invasion and those without vascular invasion was found. Moreover, serum SOX11 promoter methylation was found to be more sensitive than serum alpha-fetoprotein for discriminating HCC from CHB [87]. Previous studies also reported SOX11 functions an oncogene during tumorigenesis. SOX11 upregulation can promote oncogenic behaviors of ductal carcinoma in situ (DCIS) cells both *in vitro* and *in vivo,* indicating that SOX11 contributes to the progression of ductal carcinoma in situ to invasive breast cancer [88]. Similarly, SOX11 is an important regulator of multiple basal-like breast cancers (BLBCs) phenotypes, including growth, migration, invasion, and expression of signature BLBC genes. In addition, high SOX11 expression was also found to be a poor prognostic indicator of survival in women with breast cancer [51].

SOX11 is expressed in virtually all aggressive mantle cell lymphoma (MCL) and at lower levels in a subgroup of Burkitt and acute lymphoblastic lymphomas, but not in other lymphoid neoplasms. The *in vivo* tumorigenic potential of SOX11 in a MCL xenograft model has been demonstrated, indicating that SOX11 functions as an oncogene in MCL [52]. In addition, SOX11 can block the terminal B-cell differentiation through direct positive regulation of PAX5 and promote angiogenesis in MCL through regulating platelet-derived growth factor

A [52, 53]. Patients with SOX11-negative MCL exhibited more frequent non-nodal presentation and better survival compared with patients with SOX11-positive MCL [54]. However, there is contradictory result bout the association between SOX11 and survival in MCL. The overall survival was shorter in patients with SOX11-negative MCL compared to the patients with SOX11-positive MCL [89]. The relationship between SOX11 expression and survival of patients with MCL remains uncertain.

7. Conclusion

In conclusion, recent studies have started to uncover important functions of the SOX genes as regulators of cancer initiation and progression. Our understanding of the role of SOX genes is, however, still at its infancy. Contradicting results regarding the role of SOX genes have been reported in different types of cancer. This suggests that the molecular functions of SOX genes in tumorigenesis need to be examined carefully in tissue-specific setting.

Abbreviation list

SOX	sex determining region Y box
HMG	high mobility group
MCL	mantle cell lymphoma
HNC	head and neck cancer
EMT	epithelial-mesenchymal transition
TF	transcription factor
HSP90α	heat shock protein 90 alpha
KEGG	Kyoto Encyclopedia of Genes and Genomes
LC–MS/MS	liquid chromatography–tandem mass spectrometry

Author details

Li Cui[1], Xinyuan Zhao[2] and Shen Hu[1]*

*Address all correspondence to: shenhu@ucla.edu

1 School of Dentistry and Jonsson Comprehensive Cancer Center, University of California, Los Angeles, CA, USA

2 Stomatological Hospital, Southern Medical University, Guangzhou, Guangdong, China

References

[1] Weir B, Zhao X, Meyerson M. Somatic alterations in the human cancer genome. Cancer Cell. 2004;**6**:433-438. DOI: 10.1016/j.ccr.2004.11.004

[2] Hanahan D, Weinberg RA. Hallmarks of cancer: The next generation. Cell. 2011;**144**:646-674. DOI: 10.1016/j.cell.2011.02.013

[3] Nebert DW. Transcription factors and cancer: An overview. Toxicology. 2002;**181-182**: 131-141. DOI: 10.1016/S0300-483X(02)00269-X

[4] Lee TI, Young RA. Transcriptional regulation and its misregulation in disease. Cell. 2013; **152**:1237-1251

[5] Lee EY, Muller WJ. Oncogenes and tumor suppressor genes. Cold Spring Harbor Perspectives in Biology. 2010;**2**:a003236. DOI:10.1101/cshperspect.a003236

[6] Bretones G, Delgado MD, León J. Myc and cell cycle control. Biochim Biophys Acta. 2015;**1849**:506-516. DOI: 10.1016/j.bbagrm.2014.03.013

[7] She ZY, Yang WX. SOX family transcription factors involved in diverse cellular events during development. European Journal of Cell Biology. 2015;**94**:547-563. DOI:10.1016/j.ejcb.2015.08.002

[8] Kamachi Y, Kondoh H. Sox proteins: Regulators of cell fate specification and differentiation. Development. 2013;**140**:4129-4144. DOI:10.1242/dev.091793

[9] Sarkar A, Hochedlinger K. The sox family of transcription factors: Versatile regulators of stem and progenitor cell fate. Cell Stem Cell. 2013;**12**:15-30. DOI:10.1016/j.stem.2012.12.007

[10] Bowles J, Schepers G, Koopman P. Phylogeny of the SOX family of developmental transcription factors based on sequence and structural indicators. Developmental Biology. 2000;**227**:239-255. DOI:10.1006/dbio.2000.9883

[11] Chew LJ, Gallo V. The Yin and Yang of Sox proteins: Activation and repression in development and disease. Journal of Neuroscience Research. 2009;**87**:3277-3287. DOI: 10.1002/jnr.22128

[12] Castillo SD, Sanchez-Cespedes M. The SOX family of genes in cancer development: Biological relevance and opportunities for therapy. Expert Opinion on Therapeutic Targets. 2012;**16**:903-919. DOI: 10.1517/14728222.2012.709239

[13] Schepers GE, Teasdale RD, Koopman P. Twenty pairs of sox: Extent, homology, and nomenclature of the mouse and human sox transcription factor gene families. Developmental Cell. 2002;**3**:167-170. DOI:10.1016/S1534-5807(02)00223-X

[14] Kiefer JC. Back to basics: Sox genes. Developmental Dynamics. 2007;**236**:2356-2366. DOI: 10.1002/dvdy.21218

[15] Pevny LH, Lovell-Badge R. Sox genes find their feet. Current Opinion in Genetics and Development. 1997;**7**:338-344. DOI: 10.1016/S0959-437X(97)80147-5

[16] Abdelalim EM, Emara MM, Kolatkar PR. The SOX transcription factors as key players in pluripotent stem cells. Stem Cells Development. 2014;**23**:2687-2699. DOI:10.1089/scd.2014.0297

[17] Pevny LH, Nicolis SK. Sox2 roles in neural stem cells. International Journal of Biochemistry and Cell Biology. 2010;**42**:421-424. DOI: 10.1016/j.biocel.2009.08.018

[18] Pevny L, Placzek M. SOX genes and neural progenitor identity. Current Opinion in Neurobiology. 2005;**15**:7-13. DOI:10.1016/j.conb.2005.01.016

[19] Wang TW, Stromberg GP, Whitney JT, Brower NW, Klymkowsky MW, Parent JM. Sox3 expression identifies neural progenitors in persistent neonatal and adult mouse forebra ingerminative zones. The Journal of Comparative Neurology. 2006;**497**:88-100. DOI: 10.1002/cne.20984

[20] Lefebvre V, Li P, de Crombrugghe B. A new long form of Sox5 (L-Sox5), Sox6 and Sox9 are coexpressed in chondrogenesis and cooperatively activate the type II collagen gene. The EMBO Journal. 1998;**17**:5718-5733. DOI: 10.1093/emboj/17.19.5718

[21] She ZY, Yang WX. Sry and SoxE genes: How they participate in mammalian sex determination and gonadal development? Seminars in Cell & Developmental Biology. 2017;**63**:13-22. DOI: 10.1016/j.semcdb.2016.07.032

[22] Barrionuevo F, Scherer G. SOX E genes: SOX9 and SOX8 in mammalian testis development. The International Journal of Biochemistry & Cell Biology. 2010;**42**:433 436. DOI: 10.1016/j.biocel.2009.07.015

[23] Niakan KK, Ji H, Maehr R, Vokes SA, Rodolfa KT, Sherwood RI, Yamaki M, Dimos JT, Chen AE, Melton DA, McMahon AP, Eggan K. Sox17 promotes differentiation in mouse embryonic stem cells by directly regulating extraembryonic gene expression and indirectly antagonizing self-renewal. Genes & Development. 2010;**24**:312-326. DOI: 10.1101/gad.1833510

[24] Engert S, Liao WP, Burtscher I, Lickert H. Sox17-2A-iCre: A knock-in mouse line expressing Cre recombinase in endoderm and vascular endothelial cells. Genesis. 2009;**47**:603-10. DOI: 10.1002/dvg.20540

[25] Francois M, Koopman P, Beltrame M. SoxF genes: Key players in the development of the cardio-vascular system. The International Journal of Biochemistry & Cell Biology. 2010;**42**:445-458. DOI: 10.1016/j.biocel.2009.08.017

[26] Arnold K, Sarkar A, Yram MA, Polo JM, Bronson R, Sengupta S, Seandel M, Geijsen N, Hochedlinger K. Sox2 (+) adult stem and progenitor cells are important for tissue regeneration and survival of mice. Cell Stem Cell. 2011;**9**:317-29. DOI: 10.1016/j.stem.2011.09.001

[27] Taranova OV, Magness ST, Fagan BM, Wu Y, Surzenko N, Hutton SR, Pevny LH. SOX2 is a dose-dependent regulator of retinal neural progenitor competence. Genes & Development. 2006 May 1;**20**:1187-202. DOI:10.1101/gad.1407906

[28] Que J, Luo X, Schwartz RJ, Hogan BL. Multiple roles for Sox2 in the developing and adult mouse trachea. Development. 2009;**136**:1899-1907. DOI: 10.1242/dev.034629

[29] Okubo T, Clark C, Hogan BL. Cell lineage mapping of taste bud cells and keratinocytes in the mouse tongue and soft palate. Stem Cells. 2009;**27**:442-450. DOI: 10.1634/stemcells.2008-0611

[30] Biernaskie J, Paris M, Morozova O, Fagan BM, Marra M, Pevny L, Miller FD. SKPs derive from hair follicle precursors and exhibit properties of adult dermal stem cells. Cell Stem Cell. 2009;**5**:610-23. DOI: 10.1016/j.stem.2009.10.019

[31] Parrinello S, Napoli I, Ribeiro S, Wingfield Digby P, Fedorova M, Parkinson DB, Doddrell RD, Nakayama M, Adams RH, Lloyd AC. EphB signalling directs peripheral nerve regeneration through Sox2-dependent Schwann cell sorting. Cell. 2010;**143**:145-55. DOI: 10.1016/j.cell.2010.08.039

[32] Qi H, Pei D. The magic of four: Induction of pluripotent stem cells from somatic cells by Oct4, Sox2, Myc and Klf4. Cell Research. 2007;**17**:578-580. DOI:10.1038/cr.2007.59

[33] Nakagawa M, Koyanagi M, Tanabe K, Takahashi K, Ichisaka T, Aoi T, Okita K, Mochiduki Y, Takizawa N, Yamanaka S. Generation of induced pluripotent stem cells without Myc from mouse and human fibroblasts. Nature Biotechnology. 2008;**26**:101-106. DOI: 10.1038/nbt1374

[34] Weina K, Utikal J. SOX2 and cancer: Current research and its implications in the clinic. Clinical and Translational Medicine. 2014;**3**:19. DOI: 10.1186/2001-1326-3-19

[35] Dong C, Wilhelm D, Koopman P. Sox genes and cancer. Cytogenetic and Genome Research. 2004;**105**:442-447. DOI:10.1159/000078217

[36] Maier S, Wilbertz T, Braun M, Scheble V, Reischl M, Mikut R, Menon R, Nikolov P, Petersen K, Beschorner C, Moch H, Kakies C, Protzel C, Bauer J, Soltermann A, Fend F, Staebler A, Lengerke C, Perner S. SOX2 amplification is a common event in squamous cell carcinomas of different organ sites. Human Pathology. 2011;**42**:1078-1088. DOI: 10.1016/j.humpath.2010.11.010

[37] Santini R, Pietrobono S, Pandolfi S, Montagnani V, D'Amico M, Penachioni JY, Vinci MC, Borgognoni L, Stecca B. SOX2 regulates self-renewal and tumorigenicity of human melanoma-initiating cells. Oncogene. 2014;**33**:4697-4708. DOI: 10.1038/onc.2014.71

[38] Gangemi RM, Griffero F, Marubbi D, Perera M, Capra MC, Malatesta P, Ravetti GL, Zona GL, Daga A, Corte G. SOX2 silencing in glioblastoma tumor-initiating cells causes stop of proliferation and loss of tumorigenicity. Stem Cells. 2009;**27**:40-48. DOI: 10.1634/stemcells.2008-0493

[39] Garros-Regulez L, Garcia I, Carrasco-Garcia E, Lantero A, Aldaz P, Moreno-Cugnon L, Arrizabalaga O, Undabeitia J, Torres-Bayona S, Villanua J, Ruiz I, Egaña L, Sampron N, Matheu A. Targeting SOX2 as a therapeutic strategy in glioblastoma. Frontiers in Oncology. 2016;**6**:222. DOI: 10.3389/fonc.2016.00222

[40] Otsubo T, Akiyama Y, Yanagihara K, Yuasa Y. SOX2 is frequently downregulated in gastric cancers and inhibits cell growth through cell-cycle arrest and apoptosis. British Journal of Cancer. 2008;**98**:824-831. DOI: 10.1038/sj.bjc.6604193

[41] Liu Y, Cui L, Huang J, Ji EH, Chen W, Messadi D, Hu S. SOX4 promotes progression in OLP-associated squamous cell carcinoma. Journal of Cancer. 2016;**7**:1534-1540. DOI: 10.7150/jca.15689

[42] Watanabe M, Ohnishi Y, Wato M, Tanaka A, Kakudo K. SOX4 expression is closely associated with differentiation and lymph node metastasis in oral squamous cell carcinoma. Medical Molecular Morphology. 2014;**47**(3):150-155. DOI: 10.1007/s00795-013-0057-5

[43] Wang L, Zhang J, Yang X, Chang YW, Qi M, Zhou Z, Zhang J, Han B. SOX4 is associated with poor prognosis in prostate cancer and promotes epithelial-mesenchymal transition *in vitro*. Prostate Cancer and Prostatic Diseases. 2013;**16**:301-307. DOI: 10.1038/pcan.2013.25

[44] Bilir B, Osunkoya AO, Wiles WG 4th, Sannigrahi S, Lefebvre V, Metzger D, Spyropoulos DD, Martin WD, Moreno CS. SOX4 is essential for prostate tumorigenesis initiated by PTEN ablation. Cancer Research. 2016;**76**:1112-21. DOI: 10.1158/0008-5472.CAN-15-1868

[45] Zhang H, Alberich-Jorda M, Amabile G, Yang H, Staber PB, Di Ruscio A, Welner RS, Ebralidze A, Zhang J, Levantini E, Lefebvre V, Valk PJ, Delwel R, Hoogenkamp M, Nerlov C, Cammenga J, Saez B, Scadden DT, Bonifer C, Ye M, Tenen DG. Sox4 is a key oncogenic target in C/EBPα mutant acute myeloid leukemia. Cancer Cell. 2013;**24**:575-588. DOI: 10.1016/j.ccr.2013.09.018

[46] Wang C, Zhao H, Lu J, Yin J, Zang L, Song N, Dong R, Wu T, Du. X. Significance of SOX4 expression in primary gallbladder carcinoma. Diagnostic Pathology. 2012;**7**:41. DOI: 10.1186/1746-1596-7-41

[47] Qi J, Yang Y, Hao P, Xu J. Transcription factor SOX9 promotes osteosarcoma cell growth by repressing Claudin-8 expression. The Tohoku Journal of Experimental Medicine. 2017;**241**:55-63. DOI: 10.1620/tjem.241.55

[48] Qian Y, Xia S, Feng Z. Sox9 mediated transcriptional activation of FOXK2 is critical for colorectal cancer cells proliferation. Biochemical and Biophysical Research Communications. 2017;**483**:475-481. DOI: 10.1016/j.bbrc.2016.12.119

[49] Santos JC, Carrasco-Garcia E, Garcia-Puga M, Aldaz P, Montes M, Fernandez-Reyes M, de Oliveira CC, Lawrie CH, Araúzo-Bravo MJ, Ribeiro ML, Matheu A. SOX9 elevation acts with canonical WNT signaling to drive gastric cancer progression. Cancer Research. 2016;**76**:6735-6746. DOI: 10.1158/0008-5472.CAN-16-1120

[50] Wang HY, Lian P, Zheng PS. SOX9, a potential tumor suppressor in cervical cancer, transactivates p21WAF1/CIP1 and suppresses cervical tumor growth. Oncotarget. 2015; **6**:20711-20722. DOI:10.18632/oncotarget.4133

[51] Shepherd JH, Uray IP, Mazumdar A, Tsimelzon A, Savage M, Hilsenbeck SG, Brown PH. The SOX11 transcription factor is a critical regulator of basal-like breast cancer growth, invasion, and basal-like gene expression. Oncotarget. 2016;**7**:13106-13121. DOI: 10.18632/oncotarget.7437

[52] Vegliante MC, Palomero J, Pérez-Galán P, Roué G, Castellano G, Navarro A, Clot G, Moros A, Suárez-Cisneros H, Beà S, Hernández L, Enjuanes A, Jares P, Villamor N,

Colomer D, Martín-Subero JI, Campo E, Amador V. SOX11 regulates PAX5 expression and blocks terminal B-cell differentiation in aggressive mantle cell lymphoma. Blood. 2013;**121**:2175-2185. DOI: 10.1182/blood-2012-06-438937

[53] Palomero J, Vegliante MC, Rodríguez ML, Eguileor A, Castellano G, Planas-Rigol E, Jares P, Ribera-Cortada I, Cid MC, Campo E, Amador V. SOX11 promotes tumor angiogenesis through transcriptional regulation of PDGFA in mantle cell lymphoma. Blood. 2014;**124**:2235-2247. DOI: 10.1182/blood-2014-04-569566

[54] Fernàndez V, Salamero O, Espinet B, Solé F, Royo C, Navarro A, Camacho F, Beà S, Hartmann E, Amador V, Hernández L, Agostinelli C, Sargent RL, Rozman M, Aymerich M, Colomer D, Villamor N, Swerdlow SH, Pileri SA, Bosch F, Piris MA, Montserrat E, Ott G, Rosenwald A, López-Guillermo A, Jares P, Serrano S, Campo E. Genomic and gene expression profiling defines indolent forms of mantle cell lymphoma. Cancer Research. 2010;**70**:1408-1418. DOI: 10.1158/0008-5472.CAN-09-3419

[55] Brennan DJ, Ek S, Doyle E, Drew T, Foley M, Flannelly G, O'Connor DP, Gallagher WM, Kilpinen S, Kallioniemi OP, Jirstrom K, O'Herlihy C, Borrebaeck CA. The transcription factor Sox11 is a prognostic factor for improved recurrence-free survival in epithelial ovarian cancer. European Journal of Cancer. 2009;**45**:1510-1517. DOI: 10.1016/j.ejca.2009.01.028

[56] Stevanovic M, Zuffardi O, Collignon J, Lovell-Badge R, Goodfellow P. The cDNA sequence and chromosomal location of the human SOX2 gene. Mammalian Genome. 1994;**3**:640-642

[57] Collignon J, Sockanathan S, Hacker A, Cohen-Tannoudji M, Norris D, Rastan S, Stevanovic M, Goodfellow PN, Lovell-Badge R. A comparison of the properties of Sox-3 with Sry and two related genes, Sox-1 and Sox-2. Development. 1996;**3**:509-520

[58] Williamson KA, Hever AM, Rainger J, Rogers RC, Magee A, Fiedler Z, Keng WT, Sharkey FH, McGill N, Hill CJ, Schneider A, Messina M, Turnpenny PD, Fantes JA, van Heyningen V, FitzPatrick DR. Mutations in SOX2 cause anophthalmia-esophageal-genital (AEG) syndrome. Human Molecular Genetics. 2006;**15**:1413-1422. DOI: 10.1093/hmg/ddl064

[59] Kelberman D, Rizzoti K, Avilion A, Bitner-Glindzicz M, Cianfarani S, Collins J, Chong WK, Kirk JM, Achermann JC, Ross R, Carmignac D, Lovell-Badge R, Robinson IC, Dattani MT. Mutations within Sox2/SOX2 are associated with abnormalities in the hypothalamo-pituitary-gonadal axis in mice and humans. The Journal of Clinical Investigation. 2006;**116**:2442-2455. DOI:10.1172/JCI28658

[60] Boumahdi S, Driessens G, Lapouge G, Rorive S, Nassar D, Le Mercier M, Delatte B, Caauwe A, Lenglez S, Nkusi E, Brohée S, Salmon I, Dubois C, del Marmol V, Fuks F, Beck B, Blanpain C. SOX2 controls tumour initiation and cancer stem-cell functions in squamous-cell carcinoma. Nature. 2014;**511**:246-250. DOI: 10.1038/nature13305

[61] Rybak AP, Tang D. SOX2 plays a critical role in EGFR-mediated self-renewal of human prostate cancer stem-like cells. Cell Signal. 2013;**25**:2734-2742. DOI: 10.1016/j.cellsig.2013.08.041

[62] Sarkar A, Huebner AJ, Sulahian R, Anselmo A, Xu X, Flattery K, Desai N, Sebastian C, Yram MA, Arnold K, Rivera M, Mostoslavsky R, Bronson R, Bass AJ, Sadreyev R, Shivdasani RA, Hochedlinger K. Sox2 suppresses gastric tumorigenesis in mice. Cell Reports. 2016;**16**:1929-1941. DOI:10.1016/j.celrep.2016.07.034

[63] Tian T, Zhang Y, Wang S, Zhou J, Xu S. Sox2 enhances the tumorigenicity and chemoresistance of cancer stem-like cells derived from gastric cancer. Journal of Biomedical Research. 2012;**26**:336-345. DOI: 10.7555/JBR.26.20120045

[64] Hütz K, Mejías-Luque R, Farsakova K, Ogris M, Krebs S, Anton M, Vieth M, Schüller U, Schneider MR, Blum H, Wagner E, Jung A, Gerhard M. The stem cell factor SOX2 regulates the tumorigenic potential in human gastric cancer cells. Carcinogenesis. 2014; **35**:942-950. DOI: 10.1093/carcin/bgt410

[65] Hussenet T, Dali S, Exinger J, Monga B, Jost B, Dembelé D, Martinet N, Thibault C, Huelsken J, Brambilla E, du Manoir S. SOX2 is an oncogene activated by recurrent 3q26.3 amplifications in human lung squamous cell carcinomas. PLoS One. 2010;**5**:e8960. DOI: 10.1371/journal.pone.0008960

[66] Zheng S, Pan Y, Wang R, Li Y, Cheng C, Shen X, Li B, Zheng D, Sun Y, Chen H. SOX2 expression is associated with FGFR fusion genes and predicts favorable outcome in lung squamous cell carcinomas. OncoTargets and Therapy. 2015;**8**:3009-3016. DOI: 10.2147/OTT.S91293

[67] Huang YW, Liu JC, Deatherage DE, Luo J, Mutch DG, Goodfellow PJ, Miller DS, Huang TH. Epigenetic repression of microRNA-129-2 leads to overexpression of SOX4 oncogene in endometrial cancer. Cancer Research. 2009;**69**:9038-9046. DOI: 10.1158/0008-5472.CAN-09-1499

[68] Tae Mi Yoon, Sun-Ae Kim, Wan Seok Cho, Dong Hoon Lee, Joon Kyoo Lee, Young-Lan Park, Kyung-Hwa Lee, Jae Hyuk Lee, Sun-Seog Kweon, Ik-Joo Chung, Sang Chul Lim, Young-Eun Joo. SOX4 expression is associated with treatment failure and chemoradioresistance in oral squamous cell carcinoma. BMC Cancer. 2015;**15**:888. DOI: 10.1186/s12885-015-1875-8

[69] Tiwari N, Tiwari VK, Waldmeier L, Balwierz PJ, Arnold P, Pachkov M, Meyer-Schaller N, Schübeler D, van Nimwegen E, Christofori G. Sox4 is a master regulator of epithelial-mesenchymal transition by controlling Ezh2 expression and epigenetic reprogramming. Cancer Cell. 2013;**23**:768-783. DOI: 10.1016/j.ccr.2013.04.020

[70] Zhang J, Liang Q, Lei Y, Yao M, Li L, Gao X, Feng J, Zhang Y, Gao H, Liu DX, Lu J, Huang B. SOX4 induces epithelial mesenchymal transition and contributes to breast cancer progression. Cancer Res. 2012;**72**:4597-4608. DOI: 10.1158/0008-5472.CAN-12-1045

[71] Pan X, Zhao J, Zhang WN, Li HY, Mu R, Zhou T, Zhang HY, Gong WL, Yu M, Man JH, Zhang PJ, Li AL, Zhang XM. Induction of SOX4 by DNA damage is critical for p53 stabilization and function. Proceedings of the National Academy of Sciences of the United States of America. 2009;**106**:3788-3793. DOI: 10.1073/pnas.0810147106

[72] Jafarnejad SM, Wani AA, Martinka M, Li G. Prognostic significance of Sox4 expression in human cutaneous melanoma and its role in cell migration and invasion. The American Journal of Pathology. 2010;**177**:2741-2752. DOI: 10.2353/ajpath.2010.100377

[73] Lee YH, Saint-Jeannet JP. Sox9 function in craniofacial development and disease. Genesis. 201;**49**:200-208. DOI: 10.1002/dvg.20717

[74] Nishimura R, Hata K, Takahata Y, Murakami T, Nakamura E, Yagi H. Regulation of cartilage development and diseases by transcription factors. Journal of Bone Metabolism. 2017;**24**:147-153. DOI: 10.11005/jbm.2017.24.3.147

[75] Chen H, Garbutt CC, Spentzos D, Choy E, Hornicek FJ, Duan Z. Expression and therapeutic potential of SOX9 in Chordoma. Clinical Cancer Research. 2017;**23**:5176-5186. DOI: 10.1158/1078-0432

[76] Huang J, Guo L. Knockdown of SOX9 inhibits the proliferation, invasion, and EMT in thyroid cancer cells. Oncology Research. 2017;**25**:167-176. DOI: 10.3727/096504016X14732772150307

[77] Jeselsohn R, Cornwell M, Pun M, Buchwalter G, Nguyen M, Bango C, Huang Y, Kuang Y, Paweletz C, Fu X, Nardone A, De Angelis C, Detre S, Dodson A, Mohammed H, Carroll JS, Bowden M, Rao P, Long HW, Li F, Dowsett M, Schiff R, Brown M. Embryonic transcription factor SOX9 drives breast cancer endocrine resistance. Proceedings of the National Academy of Sciences of the United States of America. 2017;**114**:4482-4491. DOI: 10.1073/pnas.1620993114

[78] Lin SC, Chou YT, Jiang SS, Chang JL, Chung CH, Kao YR, Chang IS, Wu CW. Epigenetic switch between SOX2 and SOX9 regulates cancer cell plasticity. Cancer Research. 2016;**76**:7036-7048. DOI: 10.1158/0008-5472.CAN-15-3178

[79] Ma F, Ye H, He HH, Gerrin SJ, Chen S, Tanenbaum BA, Cai C, Sowalsky AG, He L, Wang H, Balk SP, Yuan X. SOX9 drives WNT pathway activation in prostate cancer. The Journal of Clinical Investigation. 2016;**126**:1745-1758. DOI: 10.1172/JCI78815

[80] Kawai T, Yasuchika K, Ishii T, Miyauchi Y, Kojima H, Yamaoka R, Katayama H, Yoshitoshi EY, Ogiso S, Kita S, Yasuda K, Fukumitsu K, Komori J, Hatano E, Kawaguchi Y, Uemoto S. SOX9 is a novel cancer stem cell marker surrogated by osteopontin in human hepatocellular carcinoma. Scientific Reports. 2016;**6**:30489. DOI: 10.1038/srep30489

[81] Prévostel C, Rammah-Bouazza C, Trauchessec H, Canterel-Thouennon L, Busson M, Ychou M, Blache P. SOX9 is an atypical intestinal tumor suppressor controlling the oncogenic Wnt/ß-catenin signaling. Oncotarget. 2016;**7**:82228-82243. DOI: 10.18632/oncotarget.10573

[82] Jay P, Gozé C, Marsollier C, Taviaux S, Hardelin JP, Koopman P, Berta P. The human SOX11 gene: Cloning, chromosomal assignment and tissue expression. Genomics. 1995;**29**:541-545. DOI: 10.1006/geno.1995.9970

[83] Ji EH. SOX11 Promotes Head and Neck Cancer Progression Via the Regulation of SDCCAG8. PhD Dissertation. Los Angeles: University of California; 2017

[84] Elzakra N, Cui L, Liu T, Li H, Huang J, Hu S. Mass spectrometric analysis of SOX11-binding proteins in head and neck cancer cells demonstrates the interaction of SOX11 and HSP90α. Journal of Proteome Research. 2017. DOI: 10.1021/acs.jproteome.7b00247

[85] Hide T, Takezaki T, Nakatani Y, Nakamura H, Kuratsu J, Kondo T. Sox11 prevents tumorigenesis of glioma-initiating cells by inducing neuronal differentiation. Cancer Research. 2009;**69**:7953-7959. DOI: 10.1158/0008-5472.CAN-09-2006

[86] Xu X, Chang X, Li Z, Wang J, Deng P, Zhu X, Liu J, Zhang C, Chen S, Dai D. Aberrant SOX11 promoter methylation is associated with poor prognosis in gastric cancer. Cellular Oncology (Dordrecht). 2015;**38**:183-194. DOI: 10.1007/s13402-015-0219-7

[87] Teng Y, Fan YC, Mu NN, Zhao J, Sun FK, Wang K. Serum SOX11 promoter methylation is a novel biomarker for the diagnosis of Hepatitis B virus-related hepatocellular carcinoma. Neoplasma. 2016;**63**:419-426. DOI: 10.4149/311_151029N552

[88] Oliemuller E, Kogata N, Bland P, Kriplani D, Daley F, Haider S, Shah V, Sawyer EJ, Howard BA. SOX11 promotes invasive growth and ductal carcinoma in situ progression. The Journal of Pathology. 2017;**243**:193-207. DOI: 10.1002/path.4939

[89] Nygren L, Baumgartner Wennerholm S, Klimkowska M, Christensson B, Kimby E, Sander B. Prognostic role of SOX11 in a population-based cohort of mantle cell lymphoma. Blood. 2012;**119**:4215-4223. DOI: 10.1182/blood-2011-12-400580